Laparoscopic Surgery

Springer
New York
Berlin
Heidelberg
Barcelona
Budapest
Hong Kong
London
Milan
Paris
Singapore
Tokyo

Ronald C. Merrell, MD, FACS

Lampman Professor and Chairman, Department of Surgery,
Yale University School of Medicine, New Haven, Connecticut
Editor

Robert M. Olson III, MD

Fellow, Department of Surgery, Yale University School of
Medicine, New Haven, Connecticut
Associate Editor

Laparoscopic Surgery
A Colloquium

With 112 Illustrations

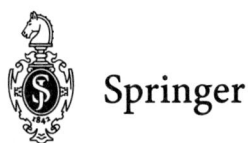

Springer

Ronald C. Merrell, MD, FACS
Lampman Professor and Chairman
Department of Surgery
Yale University School of Medicine
New Haven, CT 06510, USA

Library of Congress Cataloging-in-Publication Data
Laparoscopic surgery : a colloquium / [edited by] Ronald C. Merrell.
        p. cm.
    Includes bibliographical references and index.
    ISBN 0-387-98396-1 (hardcover : alk. paper)
    1. Laparoscopic surgery. 2. Abdomen—Endoscopic surgery.
  I. Merrell, Ronald C., 1953– .
    [DNLM: 1. Surgical Procedures, Laparoscopic congresses.   WO 505
  L2992   1998]
  RD540.L2775   1998
  617'.05—DC21   98-15837

Printed on acid-free paper.

Production coordinated by Chernow Editorial Services, Inc., and managed by Tim Taylor;
manufacturing supervised by Jacqui Ashri.
Typeset by Best-set Typesetter Ltd., Hong Kong.
Printed and bound by Maple-Vail Book Manufacturing Group, York, PA.
Printed in the United States of America.

9 8 7 6 5 4 3 2 1

ISBN 0-387-98396-1 Springer-Verlag New York Berlin Heidelberg   SPIN 10660755

*This book is dedicated to C. Elton Cahow, MD
Carmalt Professor of Surgery at Yale*

*We acknowledge his leadership;
we seek to emulate his clinical skill;
we celebrate his life.*

Preface

In May 1997 the Faculty of Surgery from the University of Athens and elsewhere gathered with colleagues in Athens for the third time in 6 years to continue our discussions on the progress, problems, realization, and future of laproscopic surgery. The topics were rather inclusive with regard to the issues that defined the field, and the assembled investigators, educators, and clinicians brought a rich experience and clear vision of the field in the coming years. The decision had been made months before to collect our thoughts and experience as a colloquium of the state of laproscopic surgery in the tenth year following the report of Mouret on laparoscopic cholecystectomy, not as the proceedings of the specific meeting. At the end of a decade of mercurial advance, heated debate, professional turmoil, and very little science, it was clear that general surgery would never be the same. Laproscopic surgery is now fully established and requires accommodation in the curriculum, practice, and research of surgery for the foreseeable future. This book is called a colloquium on laparoscopy because it collects the thoughts of many workers in the form of consensus presentations. It is offered to any surgeon who is ready to survey this field with clear eyes, absent of emotion or hyperbole, in our evolution of a better standard of care for surgical patients. I offer my profound gratitude to Professor Basil Golematis for his friendship and collegiality in planning the meetings between Yale and the University of Athens. I thank the contributing authors for their efforts and the scholarship that supports these pages. All of us express our gratitude for the life and work of our friend Professor Elton Cahow, Carmalt Professor of Surgery at Yale, for his leadership, vision, and energy in making laparoscopic surgery a matter of excellence and common effort in our work as surgeons. Professor Cahow initiated this conference, and to him we dedicate the colloquium.

Ronald C. Merrell, MD, FACS

Acknowledgment

The support of the United States Surgical Corporation is gratefully acknowledged. Its funds permitted the interactions and personal contacts that led to this work.

Ronald C. Merrell

Contents

Part III   Other Abdominal Procedures

Part IV   Education and Training

Part V   Laparoscopic Surgery in the Future

Contributors

Dana K. Andersen, MD
Department of Surgery, Yale University School of Medicine, New Haven, CT 06520, USA

Robert Bell, MD
Department of Surgery, Yale University School of Medicine, New Haven, CT 06520, USA

Harold Brem, MD
Department of Surgery, Mount Sinai Medical Center, New York, NY 10029-6574, USA

Spyros G. Condos, MD
Department of Surgery, Yale University School of Medicine, New Haven, CT 06520, USA

Theodore Diamantis, MD
Department of Surgery, University of Athens, Athens, Greece

John L. Flowers, MD
Department of Surgery, University of Maryland Medical Center, Baltimore, MD 21201, USA

Michael Georgiou, MD
Iatrikon Kentron Hospital, Athens, Greece

Ioannis G. Kaklamanos, MD, PhD
Department of Surgery, Yale University School of Medicine, New Haven, CT 06520, USA

Barbara K. Kinder, MD
Department of Surgery, Yale University School of Medicine, New Haven, CT 06520, USA

Konstantinos Konstantinidis, MD
Iatrikon Kentron Hospital, Athens, Greece

M.M. Konstadoulakis, MD
Hippokrateion Hospital, University of Athens, Athens, Greece

G.D. Kymionis, MD
Hippokrateion Hospital, University of Athens, Athens, Greece

Vasillis Laopodis, MD
Red Cross Hospital, Athens, Greece

Rifat Latifi, MD
Department of Surgery, Yale University School of Medicine, New Haven,
CT 06520, USA

E.A. Leandros, MD
Hippokrateion Hospital, University of Athens, Athens, Greece

Ronald C. Merrell, MD, FACS
Department of Surgery, Yale University School of Medicine, New Haven,
CT 06520, USA

Margret Oddsdottir, MD
Department of Surgery, University of Iceland Medical School, IS-101
Reykjavik, Iceland

Robert M. Olson III, MD
Department of Surgery, Yale University School of Medicine, New Haven,
CT 06520, USA

Joseph B. Petelin, MD
Department of Surgery, University of Kansas School of Medicine, Kansas
City, KS 66160-7300, USA

Andreas A. Polydorou, MD
Hippokrateion Hosital, University of Athens, Athens, Greece

Ronnie Ann Rosenthal, MD
Department of Surgery, Yale University School of Medicine, New Haven,
CT 06520, USA

James C. ("Butch") Rosser Jr., MD
Department of Surgery, Yale University School of Medicine, New Haven,
CT 06520, USA

George Sambalis, MD
Iatrikon Kentron Hospital, Athens, Greece

Richard M. Satava, MD
Department of Surgery, Yale University School of Medicine, New Haven,
CT 06520, USA

Frank G. Scholl, MD
Department of Surgery, Yale University School of Medicine, New Haven, CT 06520, USA

Periclis J. Tzardis, MD
Red Cross Hospital, Athens, Greece

Michael Vorias, MD
Iatrikon Kentron Hospital, Athens, Greece

Part I
Biliary Surgery

1
Avoidance of Complications in Laparoscopic Cholecystectomy

Margret Oddsdottir

Cholecystectomy for cholelithiasis is a commonly performed procedure. More than 500,000 cholecystectomies are done every year in the United States alone.[1] Laparoscopic cholecystectomy is presently the surgical procedure of choice for most patients with symptomatic cholelithiasis. For a trained surgeon with good equipment and assistance, laparoscopic cholecystectomy can be a quick and easy procedure; however, it can also be a nightmare where just about every step can be difficult and go wrong. The list of complications reported during laparoscopic cholecystectomy is long, but most of the complications reported are minor and, when compared with open cholecystectomy, the total number is much lower.[1-6] The incidence of extrahepatic bile duct injuries, however, which is the worst complication of a cholecystectomy, increased significantly with the introduction of laparoscopic cholecystectomy.[2,7-11] This increase in the incidence of bile duct injuries raised the concerns of surgeons as well as of health authorities. Several surgeons and institutions have subsequently published guidelines for the training for and the performance of laparoscopic cholecystectomy.[1,7,12-14] The data supports the view that bile duct injuries mostly occur early in a surgeon's experience and that they are associated with the learning curve for laparoscopic cholecystectomy.[1,15] The incidence of bile duct injury seems to be decreasing, and there are suggestions that the pattern of injury may be changing.[8,15,16] By identifying these problems and by analyzing how, why, and when they occur, several authors have come up with a list of preventive measures to avoid complications during laparoscopic cholecystectomy.[1,6,7,9,12,14,16-19]

What Can We Do to Avoid Complications?

In general, laparoscopic cholecystectomy should be performed by a surgeon trained in laparoscopy. In the near future this will probably not be an issue because most residents today will finish their surgical residency well trained in laparoscopic cholecystectomy. Difficult cases should be avoided to begin with, and it is important to remember that it is not a defeat or a complication to convert to an open procedure. It may be hard to identify difficult cases preoperatively; however, laparoscopic cholecystectomy in patients with cholecystitis, in the elderly, and in the morbidly obese tend to be rather difficult.[2,20] It is also important not to start off with inadequate equipment and poorly trained staff. A surgeon working with a trained laparoscopic team is both almost twice as fast as the one working with a randomly assigned operating room (OR) team, and it has a significantly lower conversion rate.[21]

In this chapter we will deal with complications that are specific for laparoscopic cholecystectomy, but leave out general laparoscopic perioperative complications.

Bile Duct Injuries

It became clear soon after the introduction of laparoscopic cholecystectomy that the incidence of bile duct injuries had increased two- to ten-fold (0.1–0.2% to 0.3–1.0%).[2,7,8,16] There are several centers that show decreasing numbers of injury and conclude that the high numbers early on are associated with the surgeons' learning curve. There are also data indicating that the bile duct injuries are not decreasing, and that late injury is on the rise.[11,16]

In 1991, Dr. Hunter outlined five steps that would provide optimal exposure of the critical anatomy during laparoscopic cholecystectomy, thereby minimizing the risk of common bile duct (CBD) injury (Table 1.1).[9] First, a 30-degree forward-oblique viewing telescope offers different angles of the surgical field and gives the surgeon more information to guide the safe dissection of Calot's triangle than a 0-degree forward-viewing telescope. The use of a 30-degree forward-oblique viewing telescope virtually eliminates the duodenum as an obstacle to cystic duct exposure. Second, firm cephalic retraction on the fundus of the gallbladder will reduce redundancy in the gallbladder infundibulum. Adequate retraction of the gallbladder and liver has been achieved when the gallbladder infundibulum can be seen tapering into the region of the cystic duct. Third, lateral traction on the infundibulum of the gallbladder to place the cystic duct perpendicular to

TABLE 1.1. Laparoscopic avoidance of bile duct injuries.

1. 30-degree scope
2. Reduce redundant infundibulum
3. Retract infundibulum laterally
4. Thorough dissection of Calot's triangle visualize the cystic duct and gallbladder junction
5. Routine intraoperative cholangiogram

Source: Hunter, Am J Surg 1991;162:71.

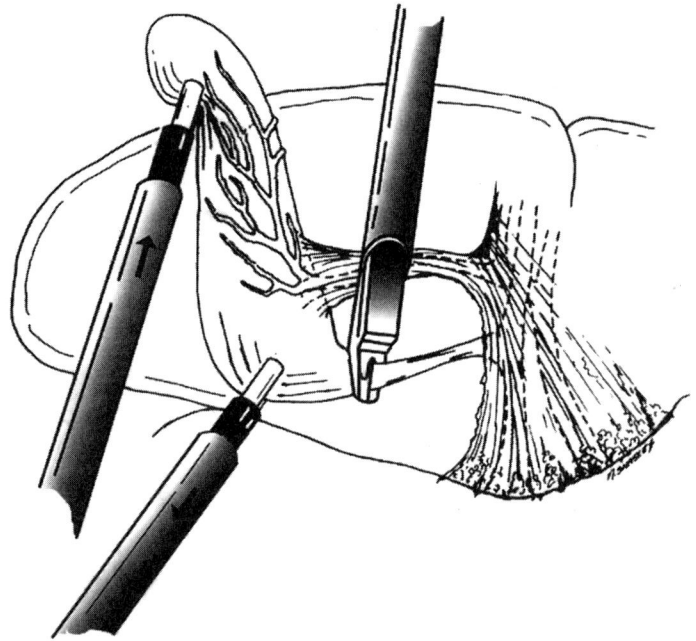

FIGURE 1.1. Lateral traction of the infundibulum of the gallbladder will place the cystic duct perpendicular to the CBD, and open the triangle of Calot for laparoscopic view [From Hunter JG (1991), Avoidance of bile duct injury during laparoscopic cholecystectomy. Reprinted from *American Journal of Surgery*. Volume 162, Hunter, JG, Avoidance of Bile Duct Injury during Laparoscopic Cholecystectomy, pp. 71–76, 1991, with permission from Excerpta Medica, Inc.].

the CBD (Fig. 1.1). If one is using a 0-degree forward-viewing telescope, then the triangle of Calot will lie in the plane of the telescope and cannot be adequately visualized without tilting the plane. This can be accomplished by pulling the infundibulum posterolaterally. Fourth, once the peritoneum overlying the gallbladder infundibulum is divided, it is stripped with a fine dissecting grasper to reveal the presumed origin of the cystic duct. The cystic duct is dissected out from the gallbladder down to the cystic duct. The cystic duct must be seen widening into the gallbladder infundibulum in all cases. No attempt should be made to dissect the cystic duct down to the common duct. A 1.5-cm length of cystic duct is adequate for cholangiography and ligature.

Finally, a routine cholangiography using digital fluoroscopy with a portable C-arm can give valuable anatomical information. It helps to identify dissection errors as well as anatomical aberrations and prevent CBD injury when correctly done and interpreted.[9,13,17,19,22] Only when fluoroscopic cholangiography is routinely performed, will the surgeon become skilled in accessing the duct, interpreting the cholangiogram and be able to work proficiently and quickly with his team. When done routinely, intraoperative cholangiography (IOC) adds only 5 to 10 minutes to the procedure time.

Dr. Hunter reported that cholangiograms performed routinely in his first 100 laparoscopic cholecystectomies prevented serious CBD injuries in three patients, identified low-inserting accessory right hepatic ducts in other three patients, and identified unsuspected filling defects in three patients.[9] In combined data from seven institutions, the impact of IOC on occurrence, recognition and correction of biliary tract complications was examined.[12] Significantly more injuries were detected intraoperatively in the group having an IOC. Conversion to a laparotomy, which is often for repair of the injury, occurred more commonly in the group having a correctly interpreted IOC. The conversion resulted in detection of injuries sooner, which lead to significantly fewer operative procedures to correct the injury. A transecting injury to a bile duct was prevented in at least seven patients when no visualization of the proximal biliary tree was documented by IOC. Incorrect interpretation of the IOC occurred in at least eight patients, with no identification of the proximal biliary tree in six. If the surgeon is unsure of an IOC finding, then a radiologist's opinion should be obtained prior to proceeding. Because most surgeons are now doing a fluoroscopic cholangiogram, the radiologists are not directly involved in interpreting intraoperative cholangiograms. To improve the interpretation of intraoperative cholangiograms, a few medical centers now have a link between the OR and the radiology department. The radiologists and the surgeon thus can watch and discuss the cholangiograms as they are being done in the OR.

Biliary anomalies occur in approximately 24% of patients, and hazardous anatomical variations that could predispose to ductal injury if unrecognized occur in at least 3.5% of patients.[12] A low confluence of the hepatic ducts is the most common of these hazards. An IOC will aid in the identification of these anomalies. Injuries occurring after a correctly interpreted IOC are rare and usually minor.[8,12,17] A cystic duct leak, which will be discussed later, can usually be handled nonoperatively.

Detection of CBD stones was the foremost purpose of using IOC in elective open cholecystectomy, whereas delineation of the extrahepatic biliary anatomy and prevention of injuries have attained greater importance in laparoscopic cholecystectomy. Selective IOC was therefore attractive in the era of open cholecystectomy. As pointed out by Cuschieri et al., however, the arguments for selective use of IOC during laparoscopic cholecystectomy are flawed.[22] Anomalies relating to the anatomy of cystic duct drainage are not visible by simple laparoscopic inspection of the structures of the triangle of Calot, and unsuspected calculi can occur in visually normal ducts. They suggest that there are no persistently reliable intraoperative criteria upon which a selective IOC policy can be based and that a selective policy means recourse to intraoperative cholangiography when the surgeon is in trouble.[22] Another practical argument for the routine use of IOC is to gain practice in performing them, both for the surgeon and the resident performing them and for all the OR staff. When doing the IOC selectively, the surgeon may simply not have the skills to access the cystic duct when needed.

Laparoscopic ultrasonography is gaining popularity; however, it does require considerable training in interpretation. When used for assessment of ductal anatomy and calculi in 209 patients in a prospective multicenter trial, it required less time than IOC, but it was less reliable at defining anatomy and complete duct visualiztion.[23] Ultrasound was more sensitive for stones than was the IOC; however, as more surgeons gain experience with laparoscopic ultrasonography, and intraoperative ultrasonic equipment improves and becomes widely available in the OR, ultrasound may become a winner. The use of monopolar electrocautery during laparoscopic cholecystectomy has been a controversial issue.[1,3,16,24] Monopolar electrocautery can result in thermal injury to the bile ducts if used liberally inside Calot's triangle or if used blindly to control bleeding. When used carefully, however, monopolar electrocautery will decrease bleeding, improve visibility, and, therefore, decrease likelihood of bile duct injury. Low cautery settings should be used in the portal area. When using cautery, instruments should always be directed away from important structures and never be used to divide the cystic duct as this may result in thermal necrosis of the cystic duct stump and the adjacent bile duct. The use of a laser has not proven to be safer or more effective than monopolar electrocautery during laparoscopic cholecystectomy. It appears that electrosurgical dissection may be faster than laser dissection and is generally less costly.[24]

Bile Leaks

Bile in the hilum after ligation of the cystic duct must be carefully inspected. Are the clips on the cystic duct tight and properly placed? Is there an accessory duct or do we have a bile duct injury? If the presence of bile is not fully explained, then the IOC should be reread and/or repeated. If it is still not clear, then the procedure should be converted to an open procedure. An accessory duct or a laceration of a small bile duct in the liver parenchyma can usually be dealt with without conversion. Postoperative drainage is only appropriate if a major bile duct injury is suspected; however, if the expertise is not available, then the patient should therefore be referred to a tertiary care facility.

Cystic duct leaks usually present in the early postoperative period. They comprise about 20% of bile duct injuries and usually require some form of intervention for treatment.[8,16] Cystic duct leaks may result from inaccurate clip placement, perforations proximal to the clips, or stump necrosis possibly from a thermal injury. According to Woods et al. they present with pain (76%) and nausea and/or vomiting (35%).[18] Most of these leaks can be outlined and treated with an endoscopic retrograde cholangiography (ERC) and sphincterotomy or biliary stent placement. A few require reoperation. If a reoperation becomes necessary, then a suture ligation of the cystic duct or a T-tube placement is required as well as closed suction drainage. Preventive measures to avoid cystic duct leaks include the use of endoscopic ligature if the cystic duct is wide and thick, closed suction drainage of the subhepatic space and avoidance of cautery to divide the cystic duct. Although cystic duct leaks are not a major ductal injury, it may pose a real potential problem, not only in the immediate postoperative period, but also over the long term, with the threat of late biliary stricture caused by periductal inflammation and fibrosis.[10,18,25]

Bleeding

Bleeding does not have to be massive to obscure the view and absorb the light during laparoscopic cholecystectomy. A good suction-irrigation device and a high flow insufflator technically make a big difference when dealing with bleeding. One must identify the bleeding site clearly before applying electrocautery or clips. Blind application of electrocautery or clips in the portal area is a common cause of ductal injury during laparoscopic cholecystectomy.[1,16] Only bleeding from the liver bed away from the Hilar structures allows for liberal use of electrocautery and clips for control. If irrigation and suction do not clearly identify the bleeding site, and the view is obscured by the bleeding, then one must convert to an open procedure. Bleeding is reported as the reason for conversion from laparoscopic to open cholecystectomy in 7.7–20% of the converted procedures.[2,5,15]

Enterotomy

These are rare, and they unfortunately often go unrecognized because they occur outside the field and are frequently thermal injuries. Colon injuries can occur when adhesions from the omentum and the proximal transverse colon to the gallbladder are being taken down with electrocautery. The duodenal injuries are also usually thermal and occur either when adherent tissue is dissected off the gallbladder or when hook-cautery is used and is pulled in the direction of the duodenum. If recognized during the procedure, then a stitch along with perioperative antibiotics may be all that is needed.

Are the Patterns of Injury Changing?

It has been 10 years since the first laparoscopic cholecystectomy was performed in France.[26] The learning curve for laparoscopic cholecystectomy for most practicing surgeons has passed, but has the incidence and the pattern of injury changed? Both the incidence and the pattern of bile duct injuries at UCSF, from 1989 to 1995, are shown in Figure 1.2. There was a steady increase in the number of laparoscopic cholecystectomies performed

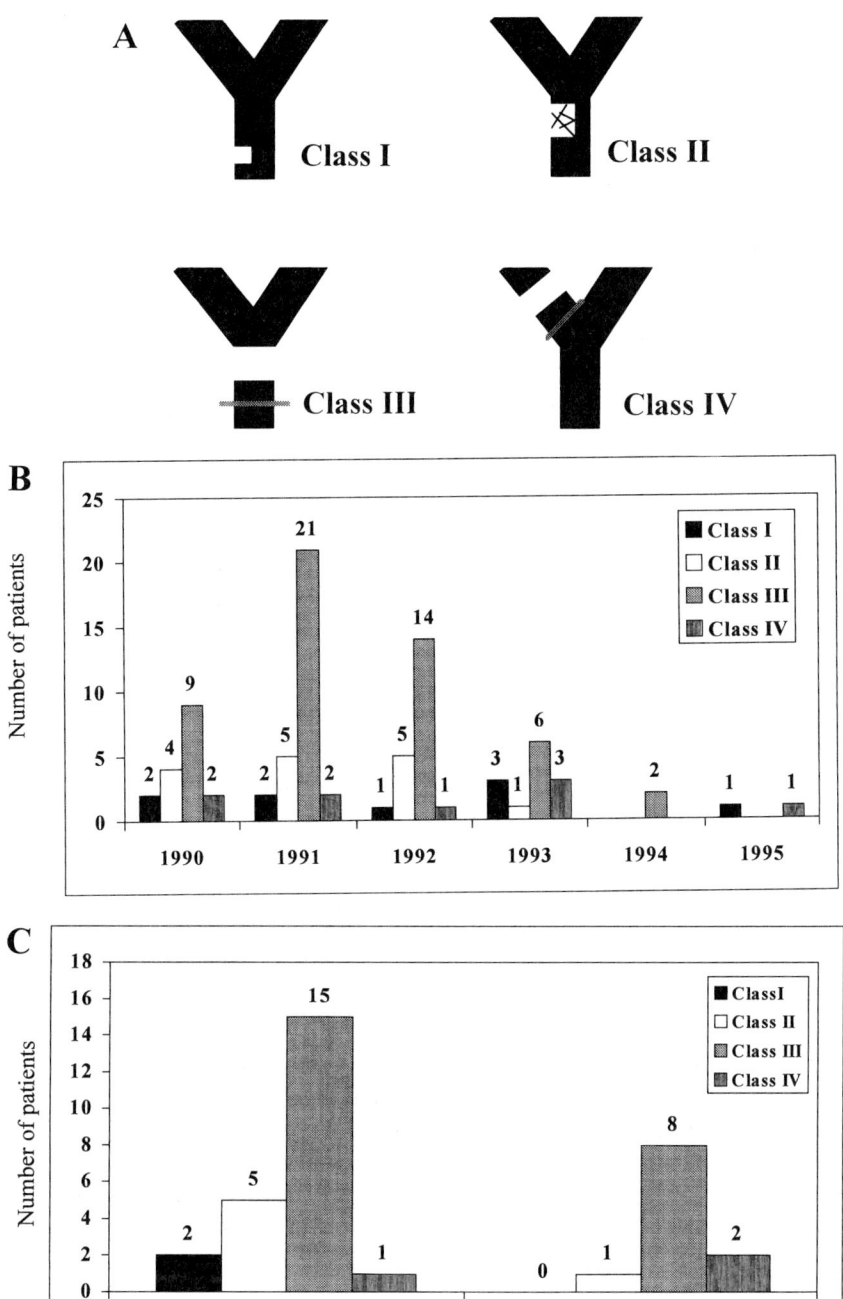

FIGURE 1.2. (A) The "Stewart-Way Classification" of laparoscopic bile duct injuries. (B) The incidence and type of laparoscopic bile duct injuries treated at UCSF 1989–1995 (A and B), personal communication, with permission from Dr. Lygia Stewart and Dr. Lawrence W. Way). (C) The incidence and type of laparoscopic bile duct injuries treated at Emory University Hospital (personal communication, with permission from Dr. John G. Hunter).

from 1991 to 1995; however, there is a rapid decline in the incidence of bile duct injuries at the same time. If we look at the pattern of bile duct injury for these years, we see that in addition to decreasing overall numbers, the incidence of the more serious injuries seem to have decreased the most. Similar analysis from Emory University Hospital shows a significant decline in the number of bile duct injuries, but the pattern there has not changed (personal communication). These figures indicate that the incidence of bile duct injuries may be decreasing; however, these are institutional reports. We will only get the exact picture when large statewide or nationwide registry is analyzed.[11,16] Another issue of great concern is late strictures. Unpublished data from Duke indicates that although the incidence of acute bile duct injury has decreased as much as 75%, the number of chronic bile duct problems have increased (personal communication). Half of these late-occurring problems are injuries that were not recognized at the time of the operation, but present later, with a stricture. The other half is anastomotic strictures from previously repaired bile duct injuries. It will take several years until we can assess the incidence, the severity, and the reasons for these late-occurring bile duct strictures.[8,26–28]

Conclusion

Laparoscopic cholecystectomy is the new gold standard for removal of the gallbladder. It seems that the increased number of bile duct injuries reported initially have decreased, but it is still too early to state whether late strictures are on the rise. Only careful dissection using standard technique and instruments, recognition of anatomical aberration, and the use of intraoperative cholangiography will help to avoid complications.

Acknowledgment. With respect and gratitude, I would like to pay tribute to the late Dr. Elton Cahow, my mentor, with whom I did my first cholecystectomy, during my residency at Yale (1987–1992). Dr. Cahow was a fine surgeon and excellent teacher. Special thanks are also due to my mentor, Dr. John G. Hunter, who, like the late Dr. Cahow, is an excellent surgeon and teacher. The subject of bile duct injury has been of great importance to both of them, and many of the issues in this chapter come directly from their teaching.

References

1. Horvath KD. Strategies for the prevention of laparoscopic common bile duct injuries. Surg Endosc 1993;7:439–444.
2. Bonatsos G, Leandros E, Dourakis N, et al. Laparoscopic cholecystectomy; intraoperative findings and postoperative complications. Surg Endosc 1995; 9:889–893.

3. Airan M, Appel M, Berci G, et al. Retrospective and prospective multi-institutional laparoscopic cholecystectomy study organized by the Society of American Gastrointestinal Endoscopic Surgeons. Surg Endosc 1992;6:169–176.
4. Jones DB, Dunnegan DL, Soper NJ. The influence of intraoperative gallbladder perforation on long-term outcome after laparoscopic cholecystectomy. Surg Endosc 1995;9:977–980.
5. Cagir B, Rangraj M, Maffuci L, et al. A retrospective analysis of laparoscopic and open cholecystectomies. J Laparoendosc Surg 1994;4:89–100.
6. Saunders CJ, Leary BF, Wolfe BM. Is outpatient laparoscopic cholecystectomy wise? Surg Endosc 1995;9(10):1263–1268.
7. Bernard HR, Hartman TW. Complications after laparoscopic cholecystectomy. Am J Surg 1993;165:533–535.
8. Woods MS, Traverso W, Kozarek RA, et al. Characteristics of biliary tract complications during laparoscopic cholecystecomy: a multi-institutional study. Am J Surg 1994;167:27–34.
9. Hunter JG. Avoidance of bile duct injury during laparoscopic cholecystectomy. Am J Surg 1991;162:71–76.
10. Ferguson CM, Rattner DW, Warshaw AL. Bile duct injury in laparoscopic cholecystectomy. Surg Laparosc Endosc 1992;2:1–7.
11. Adamsen S, Hansen OH, Funch-Jensen P, et al. Bile duct injury during laparoscopic cholecystectomy: a prospective nationwide series. J Am Coll Surg 1997;184:571–578.
12. Woods MS, Traverso LW, Kozarek RA, et al. Biliary tract complications of laparoscopic cholecystectomy are detected more frequently with routine intraoperative cholangioography. Surg Endosc 1995;9:1076–1080.
13. Hawasli A. Does routine cystic duct cholangiogram during laparoscopic cholecystectomy prevent common bile duct injury? Surg Laparoscopy Endosc 1993;3:290–295.
14. Guidelines for the clinical application of laparoscopic biliary tract surgery. Revision of SAGES Publication #6 (1994) SAGES, 2716 Ocean Park Avenue, Suite 3000, Santa Monica, CA 90025.
15. Southern Surgeon's Club. A prospective analysis of 1581 laparoscopic cholecystectomies. N Engl J Med 1991;324:1073–1078.
16. Strasberg SM, Hertl M, Soper NJ. An analysis of the problem of biliary injury during laparoscopic cholecystectomy. J Am Coll Surg 1995;180:101–125.
17. Bruhn EW, Miller FJ, Hunter JG. Routine fluoroscopic cholangiography during laparoscopic cholecystectomy: an argument. Surg Endosc 1991;5:111–115.
18. Woods MS, Shellito JL, Santoscly GS, et al. Cystic duct leaks in laparoscopic cholecystectomy. Am J Surg 1994;168:560–565.
19. McIntyre RC, Bensard DD, Stiegmann GV, et al. Exposure for laparoscopic cholecystectomy dissection adversely alters biliary ductal anatomy. Surg Endosc 1996;10:41–43.
20. Angrisani L, Lorenzo M, De Palma G. Laparoscopic cholecystectomy in obese patients compared with nonobese patients. Surg Laparosc Endosc 1995;5:197–201.
21. Kenyon TA, Lenker MP, Bax TW, et al. Cost and benefit of the trained laparoscopic team. A comparative study of a designated nursing team vs a nontrained team. Surg Endosc 1997;11:812–814.

22. Cuschieri A, Shimi S, Banting S, et al. Intraoperative cholangiography during laparoscopic cholecystectomy. Surg Endosc 1994;8:302–305.
23. Stiegmann GV, Soper NJ, Filipi CJ, et al. Laparoscopic ultrasonography as compared with static or dynamic cholangiography at lapaorscopic cholecystectomy. A prospective multicenter trial. Surg Endosc 1995;9:1269–1273.
24. Hunter JG. Laser or Electrocautery for laparoscopic cholecystectomy? Am J Surg 1991;161:345–349.
25. Kozarek RA. Endoscopic treatment of biliary injuries. Gastroenterol Clin North Am 1993;3:261–270.
26. Dubois F, Icard P, Berthelot G, et al. Coelioscopic cholecystectomy: preliminary report of 36 cases. Ann Surg 1990;221:60–62.
27. Stewart L, Way LW. Bile duct injuries during laparoscopic cholecystectomy. Factors that influence the result of treatment. Arch Surg 1995;130:1123–1128.
28. Blumgart LH, Kelley CJ, Benjamin IS. Benign bile duct stricture following cholecystectomy: critical factors in management. Br J Surg 1984;71:836–843.

2
Common Bile Duct Stones: Endoscopic Extraction or Laparoscopic Management

Andreas A. Polydorou

Starting in the early 1990s, laparoscopic cholecystectomy (LC) has become the treatment of choice for patients with symptomatic gallbladder stones, and more than 85% of all patients are now treated this way. Among these patients a proportion of 7–20% suffer from choledocholithiasis.[1] The preoperative clinical and laboratory evaluation of possibly coexisting common bile duct (CBD) pathology is therefore important for making the appropriate management decision. The management of CBD stones has changed considerably. Therapeutic endoscopy has become firmly established as the most effective minimally invasive approach to CBD stones, and it is now preferable to surgery in the majority of patients. Laparoscopic CBD exploration was the logical extension of laparoscopic cholecystectomy, as experience and laparoscopic technology has grown. The advent of laparoscopic techniques for CBD stone treatment has introduced the alternative of a single-stage treatment for these patients, and it has given rise to debate regarding the optimal management of choledocholithiasis. Laparoscopic surgery has improved the management of gallbladder stones in many aspects, and, after the extension of laparoscopic techniques to common duct pathology, many questions have arisen regarding the proper CBD stone treatment. It is not clear now whether the management of these patients should be conducted in two stages [preoperative endoscopic retrograde cholangiography (ERC) and endoscopic sphincterotomy (EST) followed by LC], or as a one-stage surgical procedure with ductal stone extraction being performed at the time of LC. This chapter will focus on some of the controversies in the management of ductal stones in patients undergoing laparoscopic cholecystectomy, and an attempt will be made to give some guidelines to the optimal therapy of patients with gallbladder and common duct stones in the era of laparoscopic surgery.

Diagnosis of Bile Duct Stone

The management of CBD stones is influenced to a large degree by the time of diagnosis in relation to the LC. It is therefore essential to be aware whether or not CBD stones are present in patients undergoing LC before their operation begins. Ultrasonography is routinely performed in every patient with gallbladder stones. The overall sensitivity in detecting CBD stones ranges from 19% to 55%, with a higher degree of accuracy in jaundiced patients.[2] One important piece of information, which can be derived from ultrasonography, is the CBD diameter. The incidence of CBD stones rises with increased CBD diameter; therefore, dilated CBD on ultrasonography will alert the surgeon to perform more detailed investigation to diagnose or exclude choledocholithiasis. One more widely accepted policy for selective preoperative application of more extensive investigation of the biliary tree is based on clinical history (acute cholangitis, pancreatitis, jaundice), ultrasonography, and elevated levels of serum bilirubin and liver enzymes. This method will isolate almost 25% of patients, of whom 33% may have bile duct stones. Normal ultrasonographic findings and liver function tests are associated with a very low incidence of CBD stones (0–3%).[3]

Intravenous cholangiography is associated with a high rate of diagnostic error (40%) along with the risk of adverse reactions, despite the use of new, less-allergenic contrast agents. The use of this method increased in the era of laparoscopic surgery in an attempt to diagnose CBD stones or ductal variations preoperatively. This technique proved less accurate compared with ERCP or intraoperative cholangiography, and it is not routinely used in patients undergoing LC when CBD stones are suspected.[4] Since the mid 1990s the new technique of magnetic resonance cholangiography (MRC) has developed with promising initial results. It has the advantage of being a totally noninvasive method, but needs more improvement to be competitive with ERC or intraoperative cholangiography.

Endoscopic retrograde cholangiography (ERC) provides excellent pictures of the biliary tree in more than 95% of patients, depending mainly on the experience of the endoscopist. Its diagnostic accuracy is high enough to be the gold standard for evaluation of the other methods of CBD stone diagnosis. The major disadvantages of the technique are certain complications (2–5%) and mortality (<0.5%) rates with which it is associated. This test is not well accepted by patients due to discomfort and distress during the examination. The routine use of ERC prior to LC is not recommended in view of the associated morbidity and mortality rate, and, mainly, because of the normal findings in about 80–90% of the patients with successful cholangiography. ERC should be restricted to patients in whom CBD stones are suspected on the basis of history, laboratory examinations, and ultrasonographic findings.[5] The advantage of the method is the possibility of treatment application in patients with stones in the CBD after the initial diagnostic cholangiography. The combined endoscopic and laparoscopic treatments of these patients seems to be a valuable therapeutic approach that is minimally invasive and promises a short hospital stay, as well as an alternative to open surgery in centers where laparoscopic CBD exploration is not available.

Intraoperative cholangiography (IOC) has played a major role in both the diagnosis of CBD stones and in reducing the number of unnecessary bile duct explorations and retained stones. The procedure is not commonly associated with major complications, and it can be safely completed within 5–15 minutes in most cases. The number of false positive and false negative results is less than 5%, depending mainly on the diagnostic criteria that have been used rather than the technique.[6] The preexisting laparoscopic era debate about routine versus selective use of the technique is still going on. Several authors have shown the safety of using selective laparoscopic IOC. Others have argued against the policy because routine cholangiography can diagnose unsuspected CBD stones and ductal anomalies along with possible ductal injuries. Unsuspected stones are found in about 6% of patients with CBD stones (range: 1–12%).[7] The majority of these stones are small in diameter and will most likely pass spontaneously into the duodenum without creating problems for the patient. The initial impression that intraoperative cholangiography can reduce the incidence of ductal injuries seems inaccurate, although some benefits from the use of the technique have been obtained. The ductal injury rate is dependent mainly on the experience of the surgeon rather than on the use of IOC. The initial high incidence of ductal injury during the learning curve of laparoscopic cholecystectomy has fallen down rapidly into the range of that previously reported for open cholecystectomy. The majority of surgeons are using this method selectively and rely on postoperative ERCP and EST in cases of missed CBD stones after LC.[8]

Ultrasonography is used for intraoperative CBD stone detection after the development of special high frequency (7.5 MHz) probes. Some authors have reported good results, which are comparable to intraoperative cholangiogram in detecting stones of the biliary tree, but the presence of small CBD stones still remains difficult to diagnose. This technique is difficult to perform compared with intraoperative cholangiography; it is not expected to replace it simply because IOC gives more information about the entire biliary tree and ultrasonography cannot be applied to the entire liver surface due to technical limitations.[9]

The majority of surgeons are presently using both ERC preoperatively and IOC selectively for CBD stone detection. The patients are selected on the basis of positive history, abnormal liver function tests, and abnormal findings on ultrasonography. They rely on postoperative ERCP and EST in cases of missed or unsuspected CBD stones after LC if and when they produce symptoms in the patients.

Therapeutic Approach to Common Duct Stones

We presently have many options available to treat patients with CBD stones who are about to undergo LC. First, we have the endoscopic removal of the stones, which is now a well-established method and is used by the majority of surgeons. Second, there is laparoscopic removal of the stones either via the transcystic route or with choledochotomy in a single-stage procedure combined with LC. This approach is gaining wide acceptance today, and the majority of laparoscopic surgeons are trying to obtain training in advanced laparoscopic CBD exploration. Traditional open cholecystectomy and CBD exploration is another choice for all surgeons in case of inability to perform the previously mentioned minimally invasive techniques. The final option is to observe patients with small CBD stones and treat them if and when they develop symptoms due to stones. This option is controversial because with only a few sporadic reports in the literature there is not enough data to support it. It is based on the observation of some authors that small asymptomatic CBD stones will pass spontaneously into the duodenum without creating any problem to the patient and that they therefore do not require any form of treatment.[7]

Selection of Treatment for CBD Stones

In those centers where there are many methods available for CBD stone removal, the surgeon has to choose the most appropriate method for each patient in order to achieve the best results and, at the same time, lessen the patient's discomfort from the procedure. The criteria that must be taken into account for treatment selection are shown in Table 2.1. The time of CBD stone diagnosis is important and determines to some degree the choice of the treatment. Stones diagnosed before the LC are best treated by endoscopic or laparoscopic techniques if they are available. If these techniques are not feasible options, then the open approach is indicated. When the stones are found after IOC during LC, laparoscopic removal must be attempted. If this fails, the surgeon has two options: the first is to finish the LC and rely on postoperative ERCP and EST, and the second is to convert

TABLE 2.1. Parameters influencing the selection of treatment of CBD stones.

1. Time of CBD stone diagnosis in relation to laparoscopic cholecystectomy
2. Patient's parameters
   a. Age
   b. Comorbid diseases
   c. CBD diameter
   d. Size, number and location of stones
   e. Anatomic variations
   f. Previous UGI surgery
3. Surgeon's parameters
4. Availability of instruments

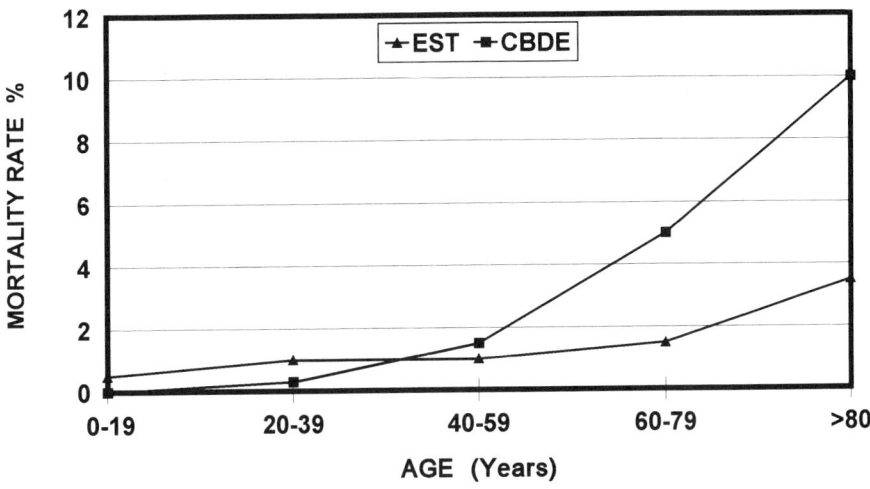

EST is superior to CBDE in patients >60 years
CBDE is preferred to EST in patients <40 years
Both methods have the same results in patients 40-60 years

FIGURE 2.1. Mortality rate following surgical and endoscopic treatment of common bile duct stones. The older aged group (>60 years) is most benefited by the endoscopic method, although the younger group of patients (<40 years) is best treated by choledochotomy.[7]

the operation to open and remove the stones. If the stones are found after the LC then the endoscopic removal is the procedure of choice.[7]

Many patient-related parameters are important in choosing the best method for CBD stone treatment. One of the most important is the age of the patients because that determines the morbidity associated with endoscopic and surgical treatment of CBD stones (Fig. 2.1). In young patients, under 40 years, the surgical CBDE is superior to the endoscopic techniques in terms of mortality and complications. Both methods are equally safe in patients between 40 and 60 years old, although a great difference is observed in patients over 60 years of age, in whom the endoscopic treatment seems to be quite safe compared with surgical alternatives, which have a mortality rate of 8–10%. This observation stands to reason because both morbidity and mortality associated with the endoscopic techniques are mainly procedure related. On the other hand, most of the complications following surgical treatment are related to the general condition of the patient, which reflects the presence of many comorbid diseases in the older age group.[7,10]

The diameter of the CBD is another important factor that influences the selection of the method used to remove the ductal stones. Endoscopic sphincterotomy or laparoscopic transcystic CBDE rather than choledo-

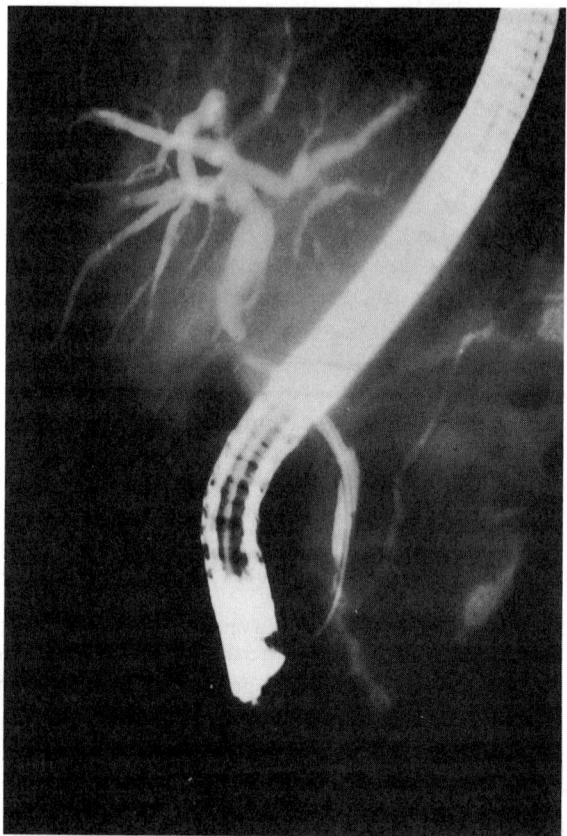

Figure 2.2. Postoperative stricture of the bile duct due to surgical exploration and T-tube placement. This cholangiogram was taken 3 months after the removal of the T-tube. It would be better to avoid surgical exploration in this small diameter bile duct and prefer the endoscopic therapy or transcystic removal of the stones.

chotomy best treat patients with CBD diameter less than 6mm. By following this policy we can avoid complications like the one shown in Figure 2.2, which is a stricture in a CBD with small diameter after choledochotomy and T-tube removal. It has been reported that the complication rate from EST increases in patients with small CBD diameters. Sherman et al. reported a complication rate of 10.4% after EST in patients with CBD diameters less than 10mm compared with 2.6% in those with diameters of 10mm or more.[11] Other studies have not identified any difference in complication rates, and this has been our experience at Hippocration Hospital after more than 4,000 ESTs during the last 8 years. An experienced endoscopist can remove small stones (<10mm) without EST through an intact papilla and after pharmacological or mechanical dilation of the sphincter of Oddi. This approach may become more widely applicable with other adjuvant techniques, such as solvent dissolution and endoscopic lithotripsy.[12]

Other features, such as the size, number, and location of the stones, as well as many anatomic variations of the CBD, have to be taken into account in selecting the method of treatment. Choledochotomy, rather than any other method, best treats large stones, such as those in Figure 2.3. On the other hand, one must be very cautious when treating patients with small asymptomatic CBD stones in the small duct. It is not clear whether all these patients require treatment. A number of the small stones will remain asymptomatic or will pass spontaneously into the duodenum without creating problems to the patients. This is clearly shown in Figure 2.4.[13] If we decide to treat these patients for their stones, we will eventually end up having submitted our patients to a number of possible unnecessary procedures along with the associated mortality, morbidity, and cost of treatment.

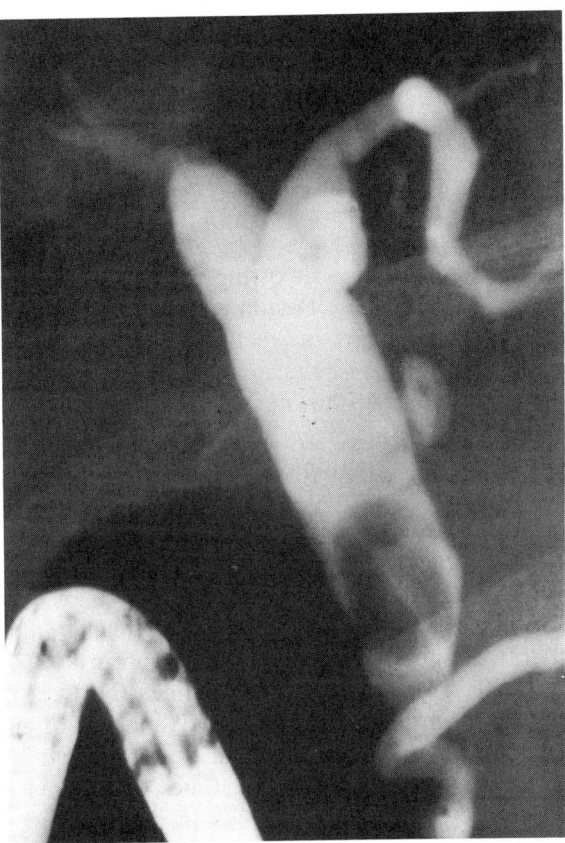

FIGURE 2.3. Large CBD stones difficult to be removed endoscopically. This patient is best treated by choledochotomy.

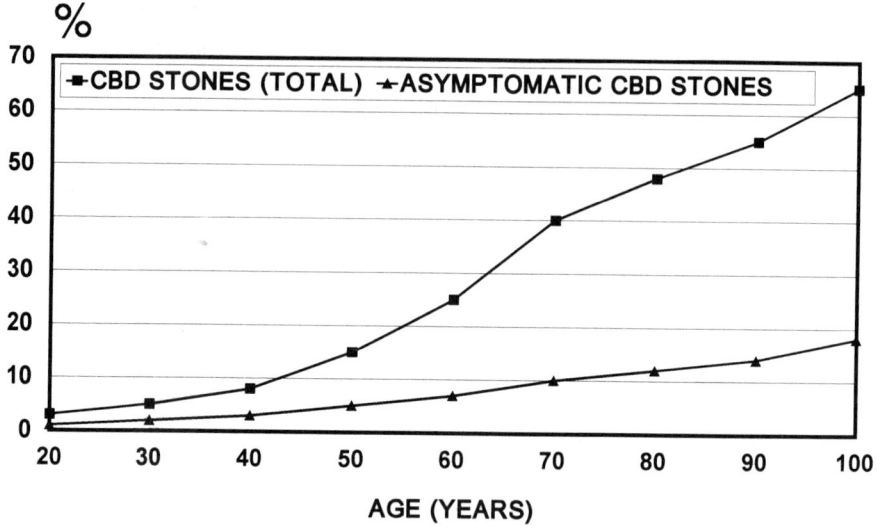

FIGURE 2.4. Incidence of CBD stones in patients with gallbladder stones in relation to the age of patients. In every age group there is a proportion of patients with asymptomatic stones, some of which will remain asymptomatic or will pass into the duodenum without any significant problem to the patients.[13]

At the present time there is no existing data available to guide us in selecting which patients with CBD stones require observation alone and which must undergo some form of treatment. In patients with low cystic duct–bile duct junction the transcystic approach is impossible due to technical reasons; therefore, one of the other techniques should be employed, depending on the time of stone diagnosis (Fig. 2.5). The endoscopic route or choledochotomy best treats multiple stones. Previous upper gastrointestinal operations, which have altered the anatomy, make the endoscopic approach difficult or even impossible.

The experience and the competence of the surgeon performing the laparoscopic CBDE, as well as the presence of an experienced endoscopist, will influence the choice of the optimal treatment of CBD stones. Another factor is the availability of the appropriate instrumentation in each institution, which very often determines the treatment decision. It is easier to make an appointment for ERCP and EST in many hospitals that have excellent endoscopic units rather than to spend 2 or 3 hours in the operating theater to remove the CBD stones. Thus, the ERCP appointment seems appealing because it shortens theater time and reduces the possibility of future operations. This is the case in our hospital, and this is the main reason that more than 90% of CBD stones are removed endoscopically.

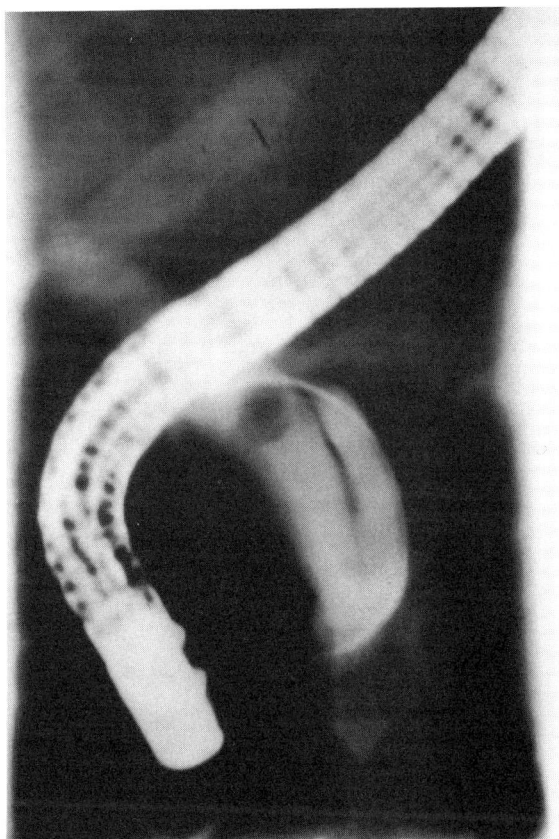

FIGURE 2.5. Low cystic duct—bile duct junction with a stone above it. Transcystic CBDE is technically impossible and choledochotomy is best avoided due to the small diameter of the duct. The endoscopic treatment seems the most appropriate for this patient.

Endoscopic Treatment of CBD Stones

The endoscopic extraction of CBD stones is successful in about 90% of cases as long as the endoscopist gains access to the papilla. By incorporating the use of lithotripsy techniques this success rate can rise to 95–98%; it is practically 100% in very experienced endoscopic units. It must be emphasized that the success rate in routine community service is lower and we often see successful CBD clearance rates of 80% in the literature, which is very low, and is often followed by high complication rates. These results guide us to a wrong conclusion concerning the efficacy and safety of the endoscopic procedures. Endoscopic sphincterotomy is not always necessary for stone removal, although more than one procedure is required for complete duct clearance in some cases. However, the endoscopic methods can be repeated without a significant burden to the patient. This is obviously not the case with the surgical methods, which can not be repeated as easily.[10,12]

The complication rate after endoscopic sphincterotomy for CBD stones is less than 10% (usually 5–7%), and the mortality rate less than 1%. These values are representative of all patients undergoing EST for different indications. The age of the patients does not have any effect on the complication rate. Vaira et al. reported a procedural mortality rate of 0.3% in 303 patients less than 65 years old, and 9.4% in 697 patients over 65 years of age. The complication rate in these two groups was 4% and 6.5%, respectively.[10] The indication for EST is important in determining the complication and mortality rates. In our hospital the total procedure-related morbidity rate after EST was 7.2% (305 out of 4,243). In patients with CBD stones it was 5.6% (138 out of 2,463), and in patients who underwent EST prior to LC, 4.4% (16 out of 360). If we want to have reliable results when comparing the endoscopic and surgical groups, then we must use the values from the last group of patients who had the EST performed prior to LC, and not the total number of patients with ductal stones.

The disadvantage of performing ERCP prior to LC in patients with suspected CBD stones is the large number of negative tests, which ranges between 20% and 50% (23% in our hospital), although the patients were selectively referred for ERCP. Routing use of ERCP prior to LC is not indicated, as many studies have recommended.[5,7,12]

ERCP is usually performed prior to LC so that the surgeon may choose an alternative treatment for CBD stones in case of failure. It is better to do the LC the next day so new stones do not have time to pass into the bile duct from the gallbladder. It can be performed during the same anesthetic administration for LC, but there are problems related to the presence of large numbers of personnel and instruments in theater, as well as to bowel distention, which makes the LC difficult. If we decide to send the patient for ERCP after the LC, then we must be sure that the endoscopist is experienced enough to guarantee ductal clearance. Otherwise the patient will need another operation, which is a result that must be avoided. In this case it is recommended that the surgeon place a catheter or a guide wire through the cystic duct and bile duct into the duodenum to facilitate the canulation of the bile duct with a special sphincterotome, and to eliminate any possibility of failure. ERCP after LC is most often done to detect or exclude bile duct injuries, leaks, or other missed pathology.[14]

Laparoscopic CBD Extraction

Extraction of CBE stones can be accomplished laparoscopically using either the transcystic duct approach or the direct choledochotomy approach. Most surgeons prefer the transcystic approach for small stones, especially because it avoids the difficult and tedious task of laparoscopic suturing required in the choledochotomy technique. The disadvantage of this technique is that the anatomy of the cystic duct and bile duct junction usually limits access to the proximal hepatic ducts (Fig. 2.5), and only stones that lie distal to the junction are amenable to removal by this technique. Stones larger than 1 cm can not be removed via the cystic duct. One of the most important parts of the procedure is the dilation of the cystic duct. Balloon dilated catheters are safer and more successful than sequential bougie catheters. Dilation must be performed slowly and under direct visualization, and care must be taken in order to avoid avulsion of the cystic duct, which is usually the most common cause of failure. A short cystic duct lying perpendicular to the bile duct is ideal and permits access to the proximal bile duct; however, this is only feasible in 10–15% of the cases. Stones can be removed with a dormia basket under fluoroscopy control or under direct visualization using the choledochoscope. Small stones or fragments after lithotripsy can be flushed out through the papilla, with or without dilation or pharmacological relaxation of the sphincter of Oddi. All these procedures may be prolonged and may cause unseen perforation of the posterior wall of the bile duct, which necessitates the performance of a completion cholangiography.[15,16]

When the transcystic approach fails or is contraindicated, then the surgeon must resort to laparoscopic choledochotomy. This approach is much more demanding as it requires the technical expertise on the part of the surgeon to be able to perform intracorporeal suturing. This method does not have restrictions concerning the site and size of the stones; therefore, it is superior to the transcystic approach in this regard. The major disadvantage is that it cannot be applied in CBDs with a diameter less than 6 or 7 mm due to the high possibility of postoperative complications, as seen in Figure 2.2, which shows a postoperative stricture after CBDE and T-tube removal. A choledochoscope is most often used and the stones are retrieved with a dormia basket or balloon catheter. Lithotripsy techniques can be applied and the T-tube is used in the majority of patients.

There has been increasing experience with the laparoscopic techniques for CBD stone extraction. The proper patient selection and the appropriate training have made these techniques the preferred treatment of CBD stones in many centers. Many centers report high success rates (about 90%) and a variable complication rate ranging from 4% to almost 20%, although a complication rate of about 10% is acceptable and comparable to the endoscopic methods (Table 2.2). The advantage of the laparoscopic approach over combined endoscopic and laparoscopic treatment is that the former can be accomplished in one session with minimal discomfort to the patient. The hospital stay of the patient is short, usually 3–5 days, and the patients who undergo transcystic stone removal have the shortest hospital stay.[7,14–16]

Discussion

The rapid changes in the management of CBD stones following the establishment of endoscopic techniques and the introduction of laparoscopic techniques resulted in the development of a confused status about the most

TABLE 2.2. Complication and success rates of laparoscopic CBDE (Transcystic or Choledochotomy).

Author	*n* pts	Complication	Success
Petelin JB, 1993	77	8 (10.4%)	74 (96%)
Caroll BJ, 1994	88	17 (19.3%)	82 (93%)
Phillips EH, 1994	115	20 (17.4%)	105 (91%)
DePaula AL, 1994	114	7 (6.2%)	108 (95%)
Lezorche E, 1995	120	8 (6.8%)	77 (64%)
Kelley WE, 1995	24	—	18 (75%)
Swanstrom LL, 1996	18	2 (4%)	15 (83%)
E.A.E.S. study, 1996	82	10 (10%)	68 (83%)

CBDE: Common Bile Duct Exploration.

effective and safe treatment of the CBD lithiasis in the era of laparoscopic surgery. In order to avoid the traditional open operation and have all the benefits of minimally invasive surgery ERCP and EST became the procedures of choice for the extraction of ductal stones prior to or after the LC soon after the application of the laparoscopic cholecystectomy. The number of ERCPs and ESTs increased rapidly and most laparoscopic centers started a close collaboration with endoscopic centers to treat patients with gallbladder and CBD stones.[12] This collaboration of the endoscopic and surgical approach had been attempted in the prelaparoscopic era and the results were compared with open surgery. Some authors suggested that preoperative ERCP and EST might increase the overall morbidity and perhaps the mortality rates, and that they should be avoided on a routine basis although it is beneficial for selected patients who present with cholangitis, pancreatitis, belong to a high surgical risk group, or are more than 70 years of age.[17] On the contrary, others have shown significant decrease in the morbidity and mortality rates in groups of patients treated with EST and cholecystectomy.[18] It is true that the patients included in these studies were inadequately matched, and the studies were criticized for this. These results, however, cannot be applied to the laparosocpic era because laparoscopic techniques have proved superior to open surgery in many aspects. In this field of uncertainty and controversy regarding the optimal management of CBD stones today, each center has developed its own expertise with a certain strategy of management. The variety of decision making is clearly shown in results of different major centers. Perissat et al. have treated 83.6% (107 out of 128) of patients with CBD stones endoscopically, whereas the laparoscopic approach was used in only 7% (9 out of 128), with the rest (9.4% or 12 out of 128) treated surgically.[7] On the other hand, Petelin reported successful laparoscopic ductal clearance in EST in 19% (18/95) and open surgery in 5% (5/95).[15] Results from other centers simply confirm the lack of adequate data to rely on and follow a certain strategy for treating the patients safely and with minimal discomfort. Our preference in Hippocration Hospital is similar to that reported by Perissat et al. with the use of ERCP and EST in selected patients preoperatively followed by LC. We found 360 (77%) patients with ductal stones among 468 referred to ERCP and possible EST. In 334 (93%), the stones were successfully extracted endoscopically with no mortality, and the morbidity was 4.4% (16 out of 360). Patients with failed endoscopic treatment were referred for laparoscopic or open surgical therapy. The disadvantage of our strategy is the large number of unnecessary ERCPs (108 or 23%) due to negative finding. Our attempt to reduce this number of unnecessary procedures using more strict criteria for preoperative ERCP resulted in an increase of patients presenting with CBD stones after the LC requiring postoperative ERCP and EST.[19]

In an effort to present guidelines for the optimal therapeutic strategies of patients with GB and CBD stones, the European Association of Endoscopic Surgery (E.A.E.S.) adapted and is performing a multicenter randomized trial comparing the endoscopic and laparoscopic treatment of CBD stones. The preliminary results have been published and showed that both methods have similar success rates around 80% (Table 2.3). The complication and the mortality rates were similar in both groups. The only statistically significant difference was seen in the conversion rate, which was higher in the laparoscopic series. The very low success rate of the endoscopic therapy in this trial must be noted and given further explanation. It is obvious that surgeons who are doing the laparoscopic CBDE are

TABLE 2.3. Clinical outcome of patients in E.A.E.S. study.

	ES + LC	LC + CBDE
Total number	105	101
n with other pathology	2	2
n with CBD stones	78/105 (74%)	82/101 (91%)
Successful stone clearance	62/78 (80%)	68/82 (83%)
Failed procedures	16/78 (20%)	14/82 (17%)
Cholecystectomy only	87	17
Conversion	8/105 (7.6%)*	16/101 (16%)*
Total morbidity	13/105 (12.3%)	10/101 (10%)
Reoperation	1/105	0
Postoperative deaths	2/105	1/101
Hospital stay (Median, days)	9.5	6.5#

E.A.E.S. ductal stone study. Surg Endosc 1996;10:1130–1135.
*$p < 0.01$; #$p < 0.05$.
EST + LC: Endoscopic Sphincterotomy + Laparoscopic Cholecystectomy
LC + LCBDE: Laparoscopic Cholecystectomy + Common Bile Duct Exploration.

the most experienced in the centers that collaborate in this trial. This is not necessarily the case with the endoscopists who do not show the expected successful ductal clearance rate of more than 90%. We are in danger of obtaining unreliable results at the end of this trial due to the different experiences of the surgeons and the endoscopists involved. In reference to the hospital stay, the group of patients submitted to laparoscopic therapy alone remained less days than those who underwent the two-stage treatment. This difference proved statistically significant. Once again, further explanation is necessary to clarify the longer hospital stay in the group of patients with the combined endoscopic and laparoscopic treatment. This was probably due to the high failure rate of EST or the long waiting time between the procedures. The exclusion of ASA III and IV patients who would most likely benefit from the combined method because they present higher complication rates following surgical CBDE rather than endoscopic duct clearance, is another reason which influences the results. When comparing the two laparoscopic methods of CBD clearance, the group with the transcystic approach is therefore the ideal treatment for ductal stones when it is applicable.[20]

Definite conclusions should await the completion of the present E.A.E.S. study, but the preliminary data indicate that single-stage laparoscopic management of patients who are fit for surgery is at least as good, if not better, and probably more cost effective than preoperative EST followed by LC, as long as the surgical laparoscopic expertise is available. The role of the endoscopic treatment should change to selective use in those patients in whom laparoscopic CBD stone extraction has failed. While these results need to be reproduced by other centers in order to be generally adopted, we must keep in mind the possible mistakes in the design of the study and the questionable experience of the endoscopists involved in the study that may influence the results in favor of the single-stage laparoscopic approach.

Medical literature has seen the publication of many algorithmic tables, all of which propose the best option in the therapeutic management of CBD stones in patients who are about to undergo LC. Most charts actually represent the personal experience and preferences of the authors.[5,7,2,14,15,19] One of the best charts available is shown in detail in Figures 2.6, 2.7, and 2.8. An important factor, which determines the choice of the treatment, is the presence of an experienced surgeon who is able to perform laparoscopic CBD exploration. At those centers where laparoscopic CBDE is available and in patients with positive IOC, we proceed with laparosocpic CBDE. If it is unsuccessful, then the patient is either opened or is referred to the endoscopist for postoperative EST. On the other hand, peroperative ERCP is ordered in other units where laparoscopic BDE is not available, but where the endoscopic unit is competent enough to guarantee the endoscopic stone extraction or extraction of suspected CBD stones. If it is positive, then EST and stone extraction are performed, followed by LC the next day. It is important that the LC must be done immediately after the

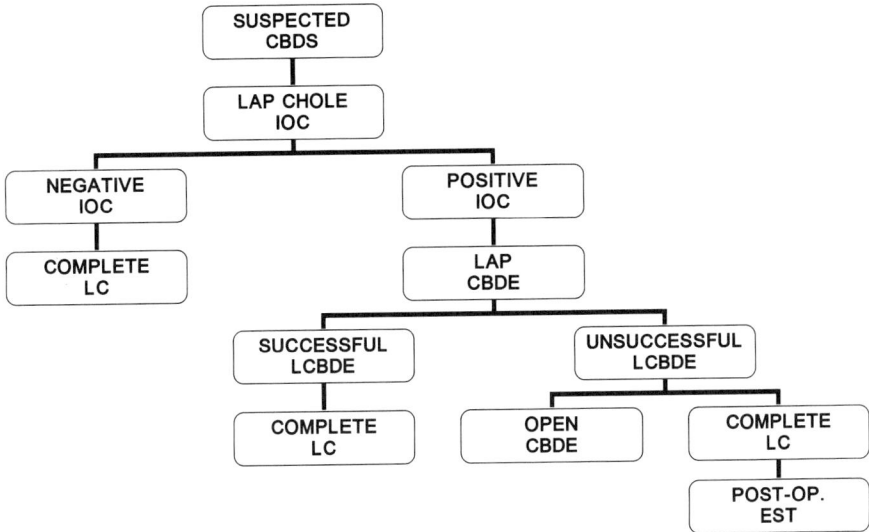

FIGURE 2.6. Proposed strategy for treatment of PTS with suspected CBD stones when laparoscopic CBDE is available.[14]

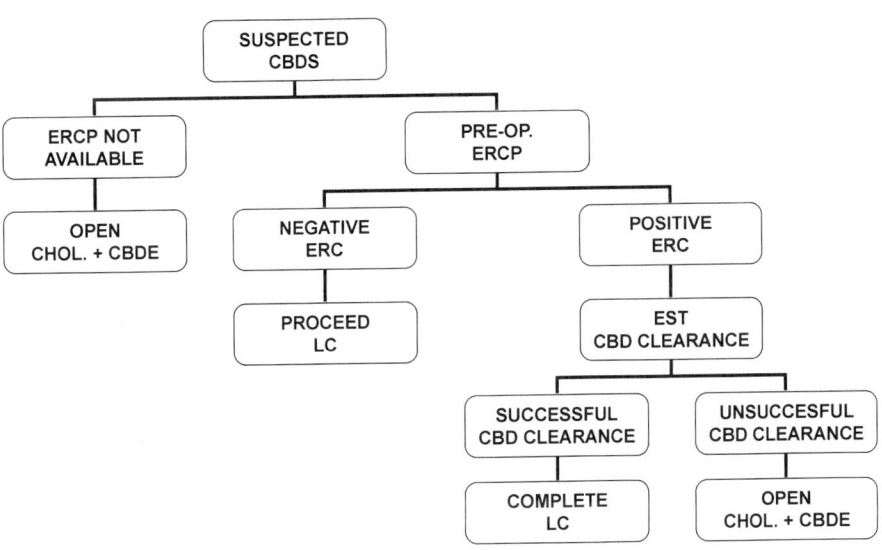

FIGURE 2.7. Proposed strategy for treatment of PTS with suspected CBD stones when laparoscopic CBDE is not available.[14]

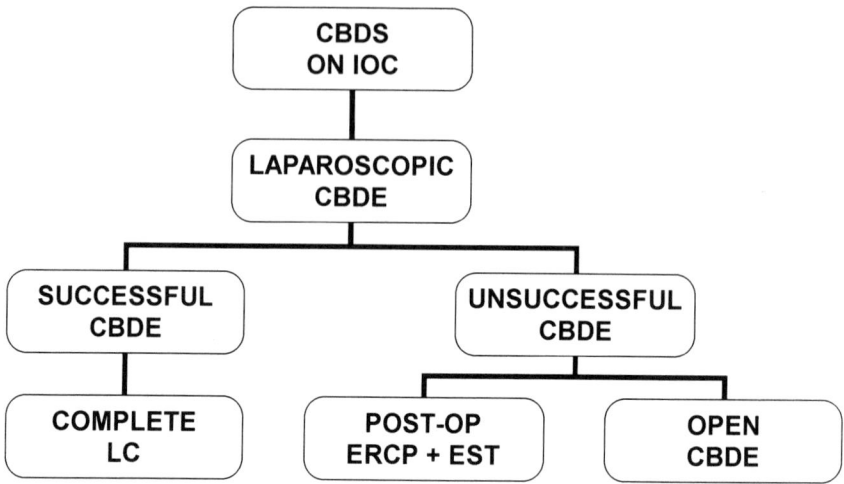

FIGURE 2.8. Proposed strategy for treatment of PTS with unsuspected CBD stones discovered at IOC.[14]

EST for two reasons. First, there is an increased incidence of acute cholecystitis after ERCP and EST which will make the LC difficult and may raise the complication rate of the procedure. Second, stones may pass through the cystic duct into the CBD after the EST and create problems for the patients, requiring further treatment. In case of failed endoscopy the patient must be submitted to open surgery. When unsuspected stones are discovered in IOC, laparoscopic extraction must be attempted. If it is unsuccessful, then we convert the operation to open or we rely on postoperative endoscopic treatment.

With the given facts available today, it is very difficult for someone to propose endoscopic or laparosocpic therapy alone for CBD stones. This means that each unit must develop and follow a therapy plan that assures the best possible results according to their experience and available instrumentation. There is a growing tendency toward decreased use of preoperative ERCP and EST, and surgeons will again start playing the main role in the management of CBD stones. When laparoscopic treatment is applied, the transcystic approach is preferred to choledochotomy. Despite all these observations and until the time when laparoscopic CBDE becomes part of all surgeons' abilities, therapeutic endoscopy will continue to play the main role in the treatment of CBD stones.

References

1. Hermann RE. The spectrum of biliary stone disease. Am J Surg 1989;158:171–173.

2. Soctt MA, Farrands PA, Guyer PB, et al. Ultrasound of the common bile duct in patients undergoing cholecystectomy. JCU J Clin Ultrasound 1991;19:73–76.

3. Hauer-Jensen M, Karesen R, Nygaard K, et al. Predictive ability of choledocholithiasis indicators: a prospective evaluation. Ann Surg 1985;202:64–68.

4. Goodman MW, Ansel HJ, Vennes JA, et al. Is intravenous cholangiography still useful? Gastroenterology 1980;79:642–645.

5. Neuhaus H, Feussner H, Ungeheuer A, et al. Prospective evaluation of the use of endoscopic retrograde cholangiography prior to laparoscopic cholecystectomy. Endoscopy 1992;24:745–749.

6. Mofti AB, Ahmed I, Tandon RC, et al. Routine or selective preoperative cholangiography. Br J Surg 1986;73:548–550.

7. Perissat J, Huibregste K, Keane FBV, et al. Management of bile duct stones in the era of laparoscopic cholecystectomy. Br J Surg 1994;81:799–810.

8. White TT, Hart MJ. Cholangiography and small duct injury. Am J Surg 1985;149:640–643.

9. Jakimowitcz JJ, Ruten H, Jurgens PJ, et al. Comparison of operative ultrasonography and radiography in screening of the common bile duct for calculi. World J Surg 1987;11:628–634.

10. Vaira D, D'Anna L, Ainley C, et al. Endoscopic sphincterotomy in 1,000 consecutive patients. Lancet 1989;2:431–434.

11. Sherman S, Ruffolo TA, Hawes RH, et al. Complications of endoscopic sphincterotomy. A prospective series with emphasis on the increased risk associated with sphincter of Oddi dysfunction and non dilated bile ducts. Gastroenterology 1991;101:1068–1075.

12. Cotton PB. Treatment of choledocholithiasis: endoscopic retrograde cholangiopancreatography and laparoscopic cholecystectomy. Am J Surg 1993;165:474–478.

13. Hermann RE. A plea for a safer technique of cholecystectomy. Surgery 1976;79:609–611.

14. Fink AS. Current dilemmas in management of common duct stones. Surg Endosc 1993;7:285–291.

15. Petelin JB. Laparoscopic approach to common duct pathology. Am J Surg 1993;165:487–491.

16. Martin IG, Curley P, McMahon MJ. Minimally invasive treatment for common bile duct stones. Br J Surg 1993;80:103–106.

17. Neoptolemos JP, Carr-Locke DL, Fossard DP. Prospective randomised study of preoperative endoscopic sphincterotomy versus surgery alone for common bile duct stones. BMJ 1987;294:470–474.

18. Heinerman PM, Boeckl O, Pimpi W. Selective ERCP and preoperative stone removal in bile duct surgery. Ann Surg 1989;209:267–272.

19. Bonatsos G, Leandros E, Polydorou A, et al. ERCP in association with laparoscopic cholecystectomy: a strategy to minimize the number of unnecessary ERCP's. Surg Endosc 1996;10:37–40.

20. Cuschieri A, Croce E, Faggioni A, et al. EAES ductal stone co-operative group. EAES ductal stone study. Surg Endosc 1996;11:30–35.

3
Techniques and Results of Laparoscopic Common Bile Duct Exploration

JOSEPH B. PETELIN

Approximately 10% of patients undergoing laparoscopic cholecystectomy harbor common bile duct stones. Although technically much more difficult than laparoscopic cholecystectomy, laparoscopic treatment of common bile duct stones is successful in clearing the ductal system in more than 90% of these patients. It offers the same minimally invasive benefits to the patient without the necessity of laparotomy or secondary procedures such as endoscopic retrograde choledocholithotomy or sphincterotomy.

Numerous techniques for laparoscopic common bile duct exploration (LCDE) have been developed. Each of them accesses the stones by one of two routes: through the cystic duct or through a choledochotomy. Both approaches are associated with equivalent success rates in removing stones, but the transcystic approach has the added benefit of being truly minimally invasive, as compared with choledochotomy.[1-22]

Indications for LCDE

An abnormal intraoperative cholangiogram is the most common indication for LCDE. Unexplained elevated liver function tests, a dilated ductal system, sonographic evidence of bile duct stones, scintigraphic, endoscopic, or radiographic evidence of common bile duct obstruction, or history of biliary pancreatitis may also lead to LCDE.

Contraindications to LCDE

Absence of any of the preceding indications, inability of the surgeon to perform the maneuvers required for common bile duct exploration, instability of the patient, and local conditions in the porta hepatis that would make exploration hazardous are the primary contraindications to LCDE. In addition, as will be explained shortly, there are relative contraindications to specific approaches to ductal exploration. There are also certain situations where a given technique of choledocholithotomy is preferred over another.

Equipment Needed for LCDE

Standard instrumentation used for laparoscopic cholecystectomy includes forceps, scissors, dissecting instruments, cholangiographic accessories, and a fluoroscope. In addition to this set, specialized tools are usually needed to perform common bile duct exploration.

Some or all of the following equipment may be required for ductal exploration:

1. Glucagon, 1–2 mg (given IV by the anesthetist)
2. Balloon-tipped catheters (4 French preferred over 3 French and 5 French)
3. Segura type baskets (4-wire, flat, straight in-line configuration)
4. 0.035 inch diameter long guide wire
5. Mechanical "over-the-wire" dilators (7 to 12 French)
6. High pressure "over-the-wire" pneumatic dilator
7. IV tubing (for saline instillation through the choledochoscope)
8. Atraumatic grasping forceps (for choledochoscope manipulation)
9. Flexible choledochoscope with light source (smaller (3 mm) diameter, with (1.1 mm) working channel preferred)
10. Second camera
11. Second monitor (or second viewing area on the primary laparoscopic monitor)
12. Video switcher (for simultaneous same monitor display of choledochoscopic and laparoscopic images)
13. Waterpik
14. Electrohydraulic lithotripter
15. Absorbable suture (polyglycolic acid suture, 4-0 or 5-0 size)
16. T-tube (transductal) or C-tube (transcystic)
17. Stent (straight, 7 French or 10 French)
18. Sphincterotome (for antegrade sphincterotomy)

For most efficient performance, this equipment should be available on a separate cart near the OR and specific items arranged on a separate sterile cart or Mayo stand near the surgeon (Fig. 3.1).

Techniques of LCDE

Cholangiography and Preparation of the Porta Hepatis

Intraoperative imaging of the ductal system is an integral part of managing choledocholithiasis. The surgeon should be facile with his or her favorite

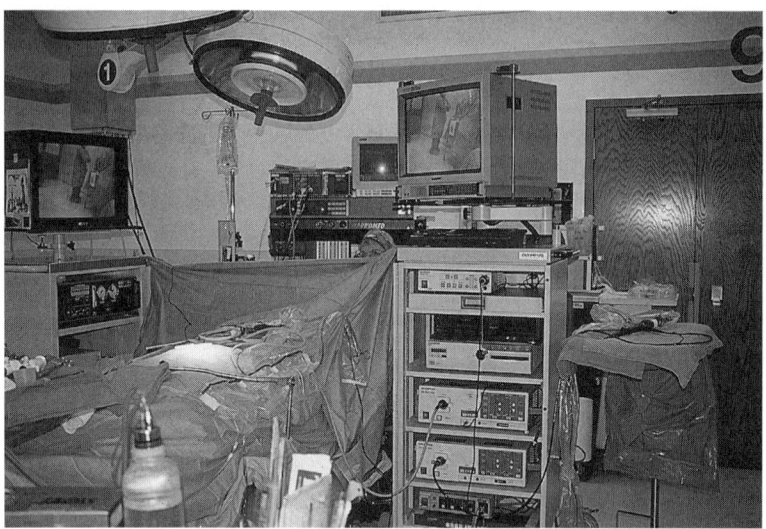

FIGURE 3.1. CBD Mayo stand adjacent to surgeon location.

method: percutaneous cholangiography, portal cholangiography, or intra-operative ultrasonography. Fluoroscopic imaging has become the gold standard for intraoperative radiological evaluation because it is faster than other methods, it is more detailed, and it allows surgeon interaction with the images in real time (i.e. the surgeon can scan the ductal system by moving the C-arm while injecting contrast material) (Fig. 3.2).

When abnormal cholangiograms are obtained, dissection of the porta hepatis is usually carried out more thoroughly in preparation for laparoscopic duct exploration than it is for routine laparoscopic cholecystectomy. In general, the dissection of the triangle of Calot should be approached from lateral to the neck of the gallbladder and carried toward the cystic duct–common duct junction as the anatomy is further defined. This is required because access to the cystic duct–common duct junction or to the anterior surface of the common duct itself is usually necessary for ductal exploration. Intraoperative cholangiography provides a "map" that proves useful in this sometimes tedious dissection.

Transcystic or Transductal Approach

When ductal exploration is indicated, the surgeon must select the route of access: transcystic or choledochotomy. The anatomical definition of the triangle of Calot, including the cystic duct–common duct junction, the actual course of the cystic duct, and the diameter of each of the ducts affect

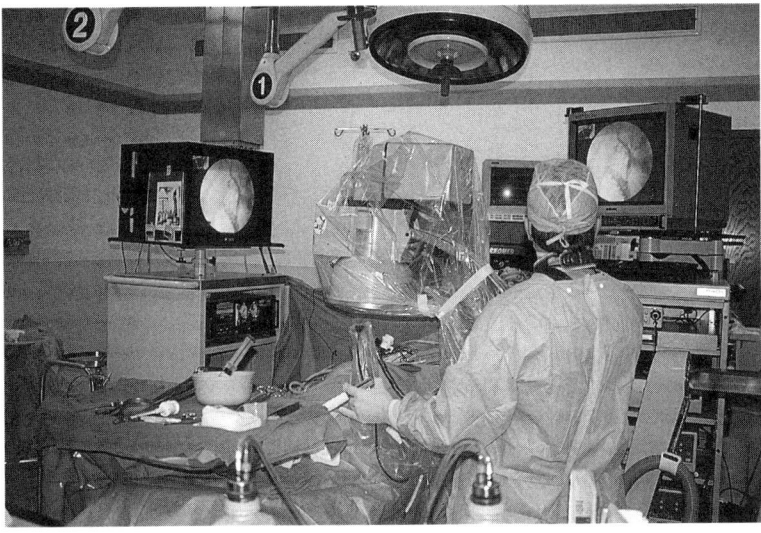

FIGURE 3.2. Fluoroscopic cholangiography.

this decision. If a transcystic approach appears feasible, then it is usually tried before choledochotomy because it is less invasive.

In most cases, transcystic ductal exploration is possible and highly successful. In others, choledochotomy is necessary or even the preferred route. Table 3.1 summarizes characteristics that are helpful in making the determination.

Negative influences listed in Table 3.1 have a more profound impact on the access route determination than do positive or neutral ones.[19] The particular techniques discussed later may be used with either access route, although there is usually less morbidity with the transcystic approach.

If a choledochotomy is to be used, then it is usually made longitudinally on the anterior surface of the duct, or by extending the cystic duct opening onto the common duct. It is limited to 1 cm in length or the diameter of the largest stone. Stay sutures are not needed to keep the choledochotomy open during exploration.

Methods of Stone Clearance

Irrigation Techniques

When very small stone (2 mm diameter), sludge, or sphincter spasm is suspected to be responsible for lack of flow of contrast into the duodenum, glucagon, 1–2 mg, may be administered intravenously by the anesthetist in order to relieve sphincter pressure. This is combined with transcystic

TABLE 3.1. Factors influencing duct exploration approach.

Factor	Transcystic	Choledochotomy
One stone	+	+
Multiple stones	+	+
Stones ≤6mm diameter	+	+
Stones >6mm diameter	−	+
Intra-depatic stones	−	+
Diameter of cystic duct <4mm	−	+
Diameter of cystic duct >4mm	+	+
Diameter of common duct <6mm	+	−
Diameter of common duct >6mm	+	+
Cystic duct entrance-lateral	+	+
Cystic duct entrance-posterior	−	+
Cystic duct entrance-distal	−	+
Inflammation-mild	+	+
Inflammation-marked	+	−
Suturing ability-poor	+	−
Suturing ability-good	+	+

positive or neutral = +; negative effect = −.

flushing of the duct with saline or contrast material in an attempt to force the debris into the duodenum. The progress, or lack thereof, is monitored fluoroscopically. Surgeons should not expect this method to be successful in clearing stones 4mm and larger from the duct (Fig. 3.3).

Balloon Techniques

Fogarty-type low pressure balloon-tipped catheters are sometimes useful in clearing the ductal system of stones or debris. A 4-French-sized catheter fits into the 14-gauge sleeve used for percutaneous cholangiography. The insertion site for the sleeve is usually located 3cm medial to the midclavicular port. The catheter is guided into the common duct through the cystic duct with forceps introduced through the medial epigastric port. For treatment of distal stones, it is advanced all the way into the duodenum, at which point the 10cm mark on the catheter will have just entered the cystic duct. At this point, the balloon is inflated and the catheter is withdrawn slightly. The location of the papilla is confirmed when the duodenum is seen to move as the catheter is moved. The balloon is deflated, withdrawn an additional centimeter, and reinflated. The catheter is then withdrawn until the balloon exits the cystic duct orifice. This maneuver is usually repeated until no debris or stones exit from the cystic duct orifice.

This method appears to be most useful in delivering small debris or stones and in cases where it is combined with glucagon administration. In the latter, it may actually facilitate migration of small stones (<2mm) into the duodenum. This balloon technique may also be used through a

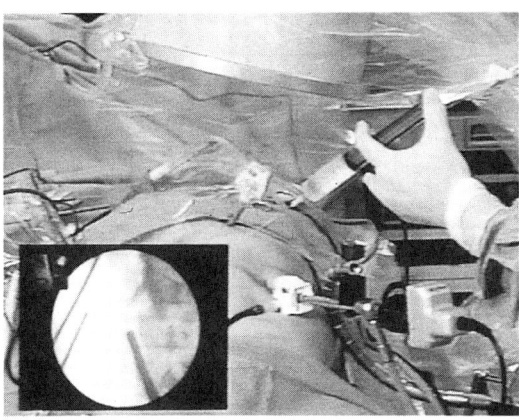

FIGURE 3.3. Irrigation techniques to clear the common bile duct.

choledochotomy if the surgeon has chosen that access route. In that case, even larger stones may be delivered through the choledochotomy with retraction on the balloon.

Balloon techniques may be combined with choledochoscopic techniques in order to retrieve hepatic duct stones and stones that defy capture with a basket. In these cases, the catheter is passed into the ductal system adjacent to the scope because the working channel of the scope is too small to admit it. The balloon is inflated distal to the stone, and the catheter is withdrawn enough to impact the stone against the scope. The entire ensemble is then removed through the duct. Combined use of these techniques requires either a large diameter cystic duct or a choledochotomy approach.

In the unlikely event that stones are displaced into the common hepatic duct during balloon manipulations, they can be flushed into the distal system again by altering the position of the table, or they can be retrieved by passing the balloon catheter proximally. This has been a rare event in my experience, and in no case were other measures necessary to retrieve common hepatic duct stones.

Basket Techniques

Basket stone retrieval methods are most often used in cases where unsuspected stones are encountered (i.e., when the duct exploration equipment is not already prepared), while the nursing team is preparing the choledochoscope. It is also useful in somewhat rare cases in which the patient's common bile duct is of such small diameter that choledochoscope passage would be difficult or hazardous.

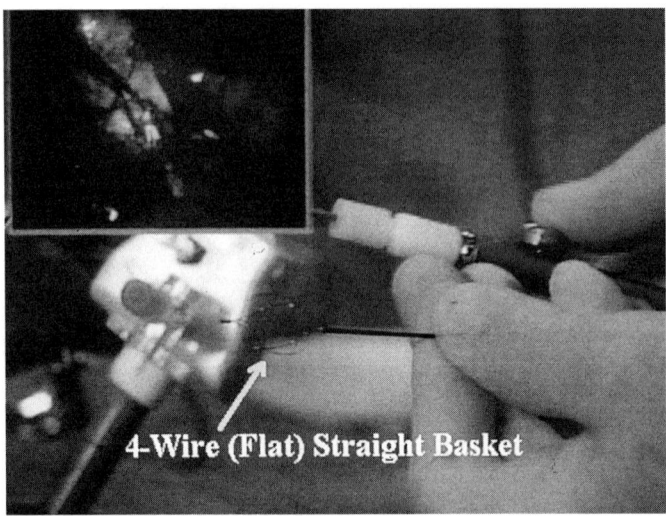

FIGURE 3.4. 4-wire straight (Segura-type) basket.

Baskets may be used to retrieve stones under fluoroscopic control, choledochoscopic control, or freely without either visual monitoring method. When used in conjunction with the choledochoscope, the basket is inserted through the working channel of the scope, and the stone is captured under direct vision. The entire ensemble is removed from the cystic duct and the stone is deposited on the omentum. The stone is then delivered through the medial epigastric or other 10 mm port (Fig. 3.4).

In the fluoroscopic method, the basket is inserted through a 14-gauge sleeve (an IV sheath) and placed 3 cm medial to the midclavicular port. It is advanced through the cystic duct into the common bile duct with forceps inserted through the medial epigastric port. The stone is then identified under fluoroscopic guidance and it is captured in the contrast-filled common bile duct. If too much contrast has drained from the ductal system after completion of the cholangiograms, then it may need to be instilled again with the cholangiocatheter. This may become cumbersome and time consuming, and it is one of the disadvantages of this method. Another disadvantage of this method is the increased radiation exposure for the patient and the team during stone capture. In addition, it is often difficult or impossible to manipulate the forceps controlling the basket while the C-arm is in place because the fluoroscope impedes movement of the forceps introduced through the medial epigastric port (Fig. 3.5).

Baskets may also be used without fluoroscopic guidance. Here, the basket is again introduced through the 14-gauge sleeve and guided into the common duct through the cystic duct. As soon as the tip of the basket passes

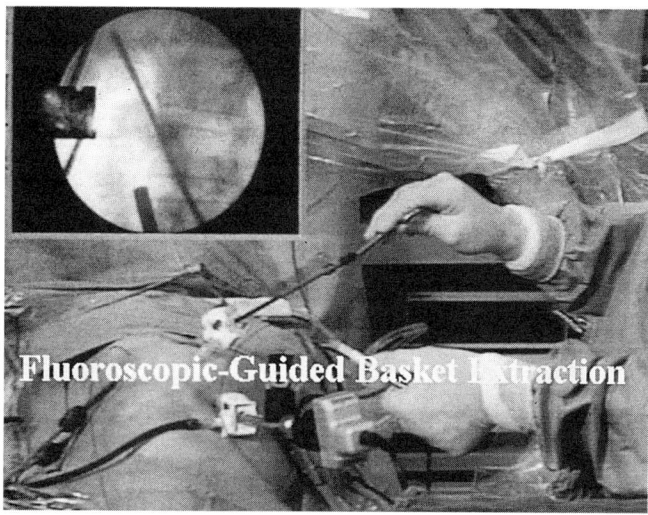

FIGURE 3.5. Fluoroscopically guided basket extraction of CBD stones.

from the cystic duct into the common bile duct, it is opened and advanced to the distal portion of the duct with forceps introduced through the medial epigastric port. There are two advantages to opening the basket when it first enters the common bile duct: (1) accidental perforation of the duct by the basket tip is minimized, and (2) accidental capture of the papilla is minimized. In both instances, it is the rounded 1 cm diameter contour of the deployed basket that causes the desired effect. In the first, it prevents excessive pressure from being applied by the basket tip. In the second, it provides increased resistance when the papilla is reached, thereby preventing easy passage into the duodenum. After the basket has reached the distal duct, it is withdrawn proximally as the basket is closed. Incomplete closure of the basket handle usually signals stone capture. The basket may have to be passed back and forth in the duct several times before the stone is captured (Fig. 3.6).

Choledochoscopic Techniques

The introduction of smaller diameter (<3 mm) flexible choledochoscopes has facilitated transcystic choledochoscopy. Nevertheless, in many cases the cystic duct must be dilated in order to allow passage of the scope. Dilatation is usually possible if the cystic duct diameter is greater than 2.5 mm.

Dilatation may be carried out with either mechanical over-the-wire graduated dilators or pneumatic over-the-wire dilators. The former are

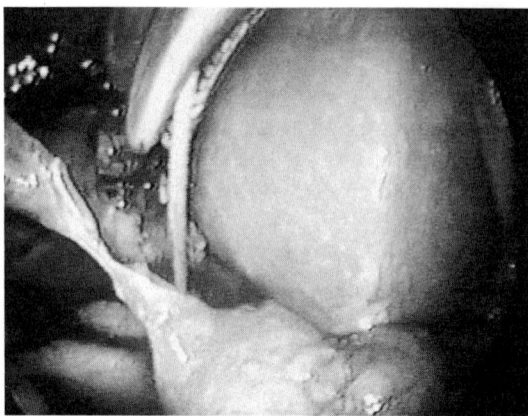

FIGURE 3.6. Basket manipulation with forceps inserted through the medial epigastric port.

found in most urology departments and are inexpensive. Each successfully larger dilator is advanced over a guide wire that is inserted through the midclavicular port and into the cystic duct and common duct. Each dilator is guided by forceps inserted through the medial epigastric port. Because these dilators exert a shearing-type force, great care must be exercised to avoid disruption of the cystic duct–common duct junction. In general, if the duct will not initially accept a 9-French-size dilator easily, then adequate dilation to the requisite 12 French is unlikely.

A more expensive way to dilate the cystic duct employs a high-pressure balloon, which is advanced over a guide wire through the midclavicular port and positioned in the cystic duct. Inflation of the balloon distends the duct with radially directed force, and it might be safer than the graduated dilators. Even with this, both the pressure on the balloon and cystic duct changes must be closely observed in order to avoid injury.

In the transcystic approach to choledochoscopy, the scope is inserted through the midclavicular port and guided into the cystic duct either through a previously placed cystic duct sleeve, or with atraumatic forceps inserted through the medial epigastric port. The surgeon should control the scope both at its insertion site on the abdominal wall and with the controls on the head of the choledochoscope. This allows rotational movements of the shaft of the scope and deflection movements of the scope tip. After the common duct is entered and the stone(s) located, the most proximal stone is captured first. To do this the basket is inserted through the working channel of the scope and advanced to the stone under direct choledochoscopic vision. When the stone is captured, the entire ensemble is removed through the cystic duct, and the stone temporarily deposited on

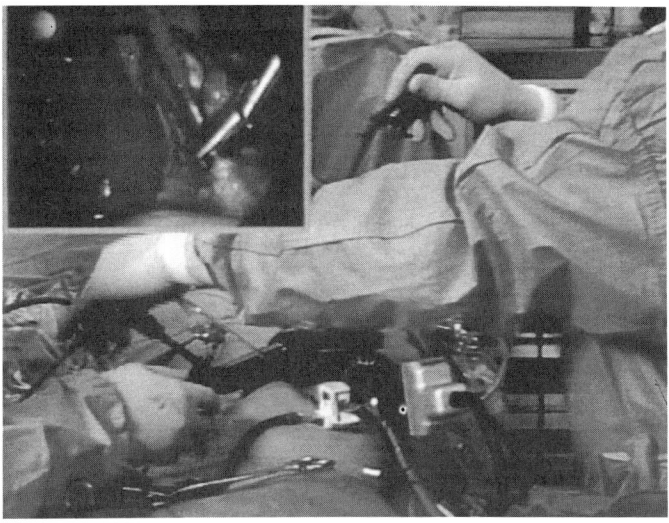

FIGURE 3.7. Transcystic duct choledochoscope insertion.

the omentum. It is removed from that site with forceps inserted through the medial epigastric port (Fig. 3.7).

When a choledochotomy approach is used, the choledochoscope may be advanced distally or proximally without difficulty. Subsequent maneuvers are essentially identical to those used in the transcystic approach.

Attaching a camera to the choledochoscope facilitates choledochoscopy. Viewing the video image then either requires a third monitor, replacement of the image on the "slave" or secondary monitor, or, preferentially, use of a video switcher to incorporate the image onto the same monitors used for the laparoscopic camera. This switcher should reside on one of the monitor towers for easy manipulation. Using such a system avoids the need for a third monitor and the clutter and chaos associated with it[1] (Fig. 3.8).

Lithotripsy

Intraoperative hydraulic or laser lithotripsy techniques have been used sporadically since the introduction of LCDE. The primary indication for intraoperative lithotripsy continues to be an impacted stone that defies less-aggressive removal techniques. Whereas the laser fragmenting devices are far too expensive to encourage widespread implementation, electrohydraulic lithotripters (EHL) are much less expensive; consequently, they have been used somewhat more frequently. The latter have the disadvantage of being somewhat more likely to cause unwanted ductal damage when the energy is directed away from the stone. With careful, direct visualization

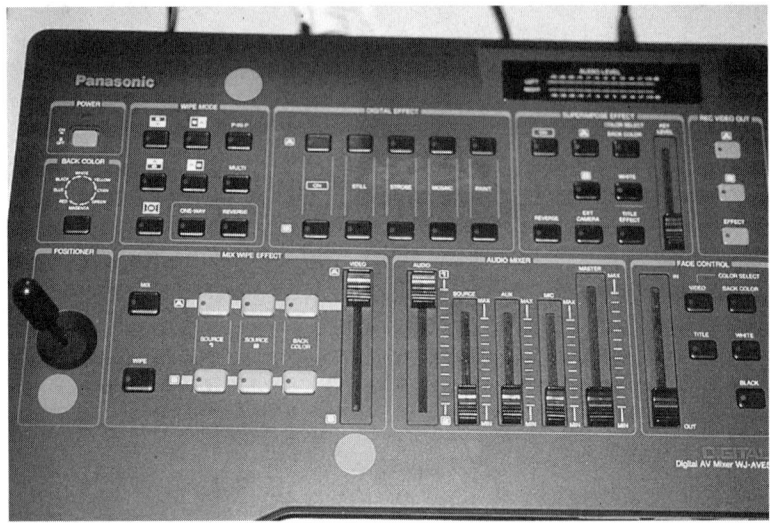

Figure 3.8. Video switcher—used for picture-in-picture effect.

and application of EHL energy to the stone surface, however, the stone may be safely fragmented without undue risk.

T-Tube Placement versus Primary Ductal Closure

The rationale for T-Tube use developed for three primary reasons: (1) decompression of the duct, in the case of residual distal obstruction, (2) ductal imaging in the postoperative period, and (3) provision of an access route for removal of residual common duct stones, should they be left after common bile duct exploration.[23]

T-Tube placement during open surgery can sometimes be difficult. This difficulty may become even more pronounced in laparoscopic surgery.[24,25] Numerous gadgets and techniques have been suggested to facilitate this maneuver, but surgeon patience and practice are the most important requirements.[26–32] Most authors prefer a longitudinal choledochotomy, a 14 French Latex T-Tube (or larger), and ductal closure with an absorbable fine suture such as 4-0 or 5-0 polyglycolic acid. Although silicone T-Tubes have been used by some authors, they are often not preferred because they do not excite the degree of tissue reaction necessary to produce a tract to the surface in the case of persistent bile leakage after removal. Silicone T-Tubes, however, have been associated with less bacterial contamination than Latex T-Tubes.[33–39]

Management of T-Tubes in the postoperative period may be associated with bacteremia, dislodgment of the tube, obstruction by the tube, or fracture of the tube.[24,25,40] Some authors recommend broad-spectrum antibiotic coverage while the T-Tube is in situ.[41] T-Tube cholangiography should be performed before removal of the tube. Removal of T-Tubes postoperatively has been suggested as early as 4 days, and as long as 6 weeks.[42] Between these two extremes lies the most appropriate management plan. Removal of T-Tubes has been associated with bile leaks, peritonitis, and reoperation.[37–39,41,43–45]

Despite the advantages of T-Tube drainage, and because of the potential complications of T-Tube placement, primary closure of the common bile duct without drainage has been advocated by some authors in open biliary tract surgery.[23,33–35,46,47] Shorter operative times, and length of stay have been observed with primary closure. No increase in bile leak or peritonitis has been noted with primary closure in the open literature. Higher patient satisfaction has been associated with primary closure.

In the author's series, primary closure of the choledochotomy laparoscopically did not result in any complications. There was no incidence of bile leak, peritonitis, or clinical evidence of retained bile duct stones. Patients reported a higher degree of comfort and satisfaction than those in whom T-Tubes had been placed.

Sphincterotomy and Drainage Procedures

Laparoscopic antegrade sphincterotomy was first described by DePaula in Brazil in 1993.[4] In this technique, a sphincterotomy is passed through the working channel of the choledochoscope and through the sphincter. The cutting action of the device is monitored by simultaneous side-viewing endoscopy of the duodenum. Whereas this technique achieves excellent results as a drainage procedure, it is logistically quite difficult to accomplish. It requires more equipment and an additional endoscopic team to be present in an already crowded operating theater. Endoscopists report that it is more difficult to perform this procedure with the patient supine. Surgeons indicate that excessive air insufflation by the endoscopist hampers laparoscopic visualization and manipulation. For all these reasons, laparoscopic antegrade sphincterotomy has not gained widespread acceptance.

In these patients with an impacted distal stone, a stone or stones located distal to a stricture, or dramatically dilated ducts with multiple stones, a choledochoenterostomy may be indicated. This may be accomplished laparoscopically, but it requires significant advanced laparoscopic suturing skills.

Results of Common Bile Duct Exploration

More than 1,000 successful laparoscopic common bile duct explorations have been reported since the introduction of laparoscopic cholecystectomy in the late 1980s. During this time techniques have evolved that enhance the likelihood of success of the procedure. Successful ductal clearance rates exceeded 90% in experienced hands.[1-19] Morbidity rates have been low in these series. Mortality has occurred in less than 1% of patients. An overview of the result of some larger series is shown in Table 3.2.

Operative Times

Laparoscopic choledocholithotomy takes longer than straightforward laparoscopic cholecystectomy. The mean operative times for some of the larger series is given here: DePaula-110 minutes, Petelin-120 minutes, Phillips-136 minutes. Not all reported series in the literature listed operative times. Assuming that mean operative time for laparoscopic cholecystectomy is less than 1 hour, it appears that LCDE adds approximately 1 hour or more to the procedure time. It is interesting that this added time is not solely due to technical manipulations; rather, it includes equipment set up time and often the need to perform additional surgery. It is also noted that these patients are often older with more chronic changes in the tissues in the porta hepatis, which makes dissection more difficult.[10,14,15]

Access Route

Most laparoscopists have generally preferred the transcystic route for ductal exploration when it is feasible. In most series it is successful in 80–90% of cases.[10,14,15] In some author's experience, (e.g., Franklin) the type and size of the ductal stones dictates the need for a transductal approach in approximately 90% of cases.[18] As discussed earlier, there are well-defined criteria that should lead a surgeon to one or the other approach.

Length of Stay

Whereas the length of stay (LOS) for laparoscopic cholecystectomy is generally less than 24 hours, the LOS for patients undergoing LCDE ranges from 1.3 to 7 days, depending on the access route, whether or not a T-Tube was placed, and whether or not a biliary enteric anastomosis was created. For transcystic LCDE, the mean length of stay is 1.5 days in reports of larger series.

Complications

Morbidity associated with LCDE occurs in approximately 8–10% of patients, and it includes those problems typically associated with general surgery and laparoscopy: nausea, diarrhea, ileus, ecchymosis, atelectasis, fever, phlebitis, urinary retention, urinary tract infection, wound infection/inflammation, biliary leak, dislodged T-Tube, subhepatic fluid collection, pulmonary embolus, and myocardial infarction. It is generally believed that

TABLE 3.2a. Results of laparoscopic common duct exploration.

Surgeon	Reference	Year	Total LCDE cases	TransCystic route	%	Choledochotomy route	%	Total successful clearance	%	Mortality	%
Petelin	14	1991	22	20	91	1	5	19	86.36	0	0
Shapiro	44	1991	16	15	94	1	6	16	100	0	0
Hunter	22	1992	20	20	100	0	0	17	85	0	0
Petelin	43	1993	77	75	97	2	3	74	96.1	1	1.3
Fielding	45	1993	21	20	95	1	5	17	80.95	0	0
Fletcher	46	1993	12	12	100	0	0	8	66.67	0	0
DePaula	47	1994	119	107	90	12	10	108	90.76	1	0.84
Phillips	48	1994	120	111	93	9	8	112	93.33	1	0.83
Dion	49	1994	59	18	31	41	69	52	88.14	0	0
Ferzli	50	1994	24	13	54	11	46	24	100	0	0
Franklin	51	1995	113	2	1.8	111	98	112	99.12	1	0.88
Philips	pc	1995	162	145	90	17	10	150	92.59	1	0.62
Petelin	pc	1996	197	173	88	24	12	189	95.94	1	0.51

Note: some authors listed more than once to show series evolution over time. pc = personal communication.

TABLE 3.2b. 1997 results.

	LCs	LCDEs	TC	TD	T-TUBE
Petelin	2,229	218	186	32	21
Franklin	2,255	141	3	138	137
Phillips et al.	1,650	179	161	16	16
Swanstrom	757	74	63	7	7
Hunter	700	69	60	4	4
Traverso*	—	48	48	0	0
Easter	850	30	28	2	2

* This series demonstrates only noncholedoschoscopic techniques used via a transcystic approach. LC = Laparoscopic Cholecystectomy; LCDE = Laparoscopic Common Duct Exploration; TC = Transcystic Duct Approach; TD = Tranductal Choledochotomy Approach.

the incidence of complications is less with a laparoscopic approach than it is with an open approach to common bile duct stones.

Mortality associated with LCDE is zero to 1% in the hands of experienced laparoscopic biliary tract surgeons. This incidence is similar to that found in open surgery and relates more to the general health status of these patients than it does to LCDE.

The Author's Experience

From September 21, 1989, through February 20, 1997, 2,255 patients presented to the author with symptomatic biliary tract disease. Laparoscopic cholecystectomy was attempted in 2,229 of them (99%). Open cholecystectomy was performed in 26 patients for the following reasons: hospital or insurance company mandate ($n = 5$), presence of common bile duct stones ($n = 4$), concomitant surgery ($n = 8$), obesity ($n = 2$), and severity of illness/general condition ($n = 7$).

Intraoperative cholangiograms were performed in 2,108 patients (95%). Abnormalities were found in 236 (13%) of these cholangiograms. This represents 11% of the entire group of 2,229 patients. Abnormal cholangiograms were managed primarily with LCDE in 211 (89%) of patients, postop ERC in 19 (8%) of patients, and conversion to open CDE in 6 (3%) of patients.

Thirty-six patients (1.5%) underwent preoperative ERCP, and 28 patients (1.3%) underwent postoperative ERCP. Laparoscopic common bile duct exploration (LCDE) was attempted in 218 cases, and it was completed successfully in 210 (96%). Mean operating times for all patients undergoing laparoscopic cholecystectomy with or without cholangiograms or LCDE was 68 minutes (17–421), and the mean length of stay was 23.6 hours

(1–622). Mean operating times for patients not undergoing LCDE was 61 minutes (17–410), and mean length of stay was 21 hours (1–622).

Ductal exploration was performed via the cystic duct in 186 (85%) of cases, and through a choledochotomy in 32 (15%) of the cases. T-Tubes were used in patients in whom there was concern for possible retained debris or stones, distal spasm, pancreatitis, or general poor tissue quality secondary to malnutrition or infection.

In cases where choledochotomy was used, placement of a T-Tube occurred in 21 (66%) and primary closure without a T-Tube occurred in 11 (34%). Mean operative times for patients undergoing transcystic duct exploration was 118 minutes (32–345). Mean length of stay for patients undergoing transcystic ductal exploration was 41 hours (1.5–540). Mean operative time for patients undergoing choledochotomy without T-Tube drainage was 187 minutes (104–355), and mean length of stay was 57 hours (19–216). Mean operative time for patients undergoing choledochotomy with T-Tube placement was 177 minutes (74–395), and mean length of stay was 88 hours (16–288).

In the group of patients in whom T-Tubes were placed, two patients had a known retained stone and one had an undetected retained stone. In one of the patients with a known retained stone, the ductal exploration was terminated because of septic complications and instability in the operating room. In both of these patients, as well as in the third patient, the retained stones were later removed by ERC +/− S.

There were no complications in the group of patients who underwent choledochotomy and primary ductal closure without T-Tube placement. There were no bile leaks, no retained stones, no sepsis, and no subsequent operations.

Summary

When laparoscopic cholecystectomy was first introduced, it was roundly criticized as a technical trick that would not allow performance of all of the tasks previously required of a biliary tract surgeon. Cholangiography and treatment of common bile duct pathology were thought to be beyond the scope of laparoscopic intervention. During the past 8 years, however, a comprehensive laparoscopic solution to the problem of common bile duct stones has been developed.

The success rate among accomplished laparoscopists should approach 90% or better. This is consistent with treatment expectations in the prelaparoscopic era; nevertheless, it is unlikely that a surgeon who has had little or no formal training in advanced laparoscopic biliary tract surgery will successfully and safely complete LCDE routinely. If a surgeon has not had enough training, or if his performance does not meet the standards listed earlier, then the surgeon should consider other options for the patient and set a plan for becoming more proficient.

Biliary tract surgeons practicing in this era should have the ability to treat all benign biliary tract pathology laparoscopically in one setting, and not require a series of patient manipulations.

References

1. Petelin J. Laparoscopic approach to common duct pathology. Surg Lap Endosc 1991;1(1):33–41.
2. Carroll BJ, Phillips EH, Daykhovsky L, et al. Laparoscopic choledochoscopy: an effective approach to the common duct. J Laparoendosc Surg 1992;2:15–21.
3. Birkett D. Technique of cholangiography and cystic duct choledochoscopy at the time of laparoscopic cholecystectomy for laser lithotripsy. Surg Endosc 1992;6:252–254.
4. DePaula A, Hashiba K, Baftitto M, et al. Laparoscopic antegrade sphincterotomy. Surg Lap Endosc 1993;3(3):157–160.
5. Kitano S, Iso Y, Moriyama M, et al. A rapid and simple technique for insertion of a T-Tube into the minimally incised common bile duct at laparoscopic surgery. Surg Endosc 1993;7:104–105.
6. Ferzli GS, Massaad A, Ozuner G, et al. Laparoscopic exploration of the common bile duct. Surg Gyn Obstet 1992;174:419–421.
7. Franklin ME, Pharand D. Laparoscopic common bile duct exploration. Proceedings—III International Congress of Laparoscopic Surgery. Brazil 1993:100–103.
8. Stoker ME, Leveillee RJ, McCann JC, et al. Laparoscopic common bile duct exploration. J Laparoendosc Surg 1991;1(5):287–293.
9. Hunter JG. Laparoscopic transcystic common bile duct exploration. Am J Surg 1992;1(63):53–58.
10. Petelin J. Laparoscopic approach to common duct pathology. Am J Surg 1993;165:487–491.
11. Shapiro SJ, Gordon LA, Daykhovsky L, et al. Laparoscopic exploration of the common bile duct: experience in 16 selected patients. J Laparoendosc Surg 1991;1(6): 333–341.
12. Fielding GA, O'Rourke NA. Laparoscopic common bile duct exploration. Aust BZ J Surg 1993;63:113–115.
13. Fletcher DR. Common bile duct calculi at laparoscopic cholecystectomy: a technique for management. Aust BZ J Surg, 1993;63:710–714.
14. DePaula AL, Hashiba K, Bafutto M. Laparoscopic management of choledocholithiasis. Surg Endosc 1994;8:1399–1403.
15. Phillips EH, Rosenthal RJ, Carroll BJ, et al. Laparoscopic trans-cystic duct common bile duct exploration. Surg Endosc 1994;8:1389–1394.
16. Dion YM, Ratelle R, Morin J, et al. Common bile duct exploration: the place of laparoscopic choledochotomy. Surg Lap Endosc 1994;(4)6:419–424.
17. Ferzli GS, Massaad A, Kiel T, et al. The utility of laparoscopic common bile duct exploration in the treatment of choledocholithiasis. Surg Endosc 1994; 8:296–298.

18. Franklin ME, Pharand D, Rosenthal D. Laparoscopic common bile duct exploration. Surg Lap Endosc 1994;(4)2:119–124.
19. Petelin JB. Laparoscopic ductal stone clearance: transcystic approach. In *Bile ducts and bile duct stones*, Berci G, Cuschieri A, eds. WB Saunders, Philadelphia, 1996, pp. 97–108.
20. Traverso LW. A cost-effective approach to the treatment of common bile duct stones with surgical versus endoscopic techniques. In *Bile ducts and bile duct stones*, Berci G, Cuschieri A, eds. WB Saunders, Philadelphia, 1996:154–160.
21. Traverso LW. The laparoscopic surgical value package and how surgeons can influence costs. Surg Clin North Am 1996;76:631–640.
22. Traverso LW, Roush TS, Koo K. Common bile duct stones outcomes and costs. Surg Endosc 1995;9:1242–1244.
23. Williams JAR, Treacy PJ, Sidey CS, et al. Primary duct closure versus T-Tube drainage following exploration of the common bile duct. Aust NZ J Surg 1994;64:823–826.
24. Berstein DE, Goldberg RI, Unger SW. Common bile duct obstruction following T-Tube placement at laparoscopic cholecystectomy. Gastrointest Endosc 1994;40(3):362–365.
25. Elewaut A, de Vos M, Huble F, et al. Unusual migration of a straight Amsterdam-type endoprosthesis for bile duct stones. Am J Gastroenterol 1989;84(6):674–676.
26. Kram HB, Garces MA, Klein SR, et al. Common bile duct anastomosis using fibrin glue. Arch Surg 1985;120:1250–1256.
27. Lange V, Rau HG, Schardey HM, et al. Laparoscopic stenting for protection of common bile duct sutures. Surg Lap Endosc 1993;3(6):466–469.
28. Kelly TR, Fink JA. A new inflatable T-Tube for completion cholangiography. Surg Gyn Obstet 1983;157(4):374–376.
29. Jacob ET, Bronsther B. A double ballooned inflatable and collapsible T-Tube for selective proximal or distal cholangiography. Surg Gyn Obstet 1988;166:85–86.
30. Fine AP. Laparoscopic, wire-guided insertion of biliary T-tubes. Surg Laparosc Endosc 1993;3(2):147–148.
31. Kitano S, Iso Y, Moriyama M, et al. A rapid and simple technique for insertion of a T-Tube into the minimally incised common bile duct at laparoscopic surgery. Surg Endosc 1993;7:104–105.
32. Lezoche E, Paganini AM, Guerrieri M. A new T-Tube applier in laparoscopic surgery. Surg Endosc 1996;10:445–448.
33. Lygidakis NJ. Choledochotomy for biliary lithiasis: T-Tube drainage or primary closure—effects on postoperative bacteremia and T-Tube bile infection. Am J Surg 1983;146:254–256.
34. Lygidakis NJ. Operative risk factors of cholecystectomy-choledochotomy in the elderly. Surg Gyn Obstet 1983;157:15–19. Payne RA, Woods WGA.
35. Lygidakis NJ. Incidence of bile infection in biliary lithiasis. Effects on postoperative bacteremia of choledochoduodenostomy, T-Tube drainage, and primary closure of the common bile duct after choledochotomy—a prospective trial. Am Surg 1984;50:236–240.
36. Koivusalo A, Makisalo H, Talja A, et al. Bacterial adherence and biofilm formation on latex and silicone T-tubes in relation to bacterial contamination of bile. Scand J Gastroenterol 1996;31(4):398–403.

37. Horgan PG, Campbell AC, Gray GR, et al. Biliary leakage and peritonitis following removal of T tubes after bile duct exploration. Br J Surg 1989; 76:1296–1297.
38. Galan CP, Alonso AC. Bile leakage after removal of T tubes from the common bile duct. Br J Surg 1990;77(9):1075.
39. Ryttov N, Rasmussen L, Pedersen SA, et al. 99m Tc-labeled HIDA scintigraphy in assessment of bile leakage after removal of T tube from the common bile duct. Br J Surg 1989;76:1319.
40. Thors H, Gudjonsson H, Oddsson E, et al. Endoscopic retrieval of a biliary T-Tube remnant. Gastrointest Endosc 1994;40(2)(1):241–242.
41. Gillatt DA, May RE, Kennedy R, et al. Complications of T-Tube drainage of the common bile duct. Ann Royal Coll Surg Engl 1985;67:369–371.
42. Noffby S, Heuman R, Anderberg B, et al. Duration of T-Tube drainage after exploration of the common bile duct. Acta Chir Scand 1988;154:113–115.
43. Cohen Z, Rosemann H, Gerber B, et al. Transient elevation of serum alkaline phosphatase after choledochotomy and T-Tube placement. J Clin Gastroenterol 1986;8(4):495–496.
44. Lygidakis NJ. Hazards following T-Tube removal after choledochotomy. Surg Gyn Obstet 1993;163:153–155.
45. Thors H, Gudjonsson H, Oddsson E, et al. Endoscopic retrieval of a biliary T-Tube remnant. Gastrointest Endosc 1994;40(2)(1):241–242.
46. Payne RA, Woods WGA. Primary Suture or T-Tube drainage after choledochotomy. Ann Royal Coll Surg Engl 1986;68:196–198.
47. Shyr-Ming sheen-Cheng, Fong-Fu Chou. Choledochotomy for biliary lithiasis: is routine T-Tube drainage necessary? A prospective controlled trial. Acta Chir Scand 1990;156:387–390.

4
Operative Strategy for Acute Cholecystitis and Other Difficult Situations

James C. Rosser Jr.

The use of advanced operative laparoscopy as a technique for performing major general surgical procedures has been one of the singular most significant advances in surgery of our lifetime. Laparoscopic cholecystectomy was the initial procedure matured, and it has now become the gold standard. Despite almost a decade of experience with this procedure, however, we continue to be plagued with a common bile duct injury rate twice that of the open procedure.

Many reasons have been suggested to be the cause for this continuing problem. The incident of common bile duct injuries is influenced by many factors, such as experience, skill, local factors, and knowledge of the anatomy, among others. Perhaps the most stable countermeasure that can be relied upon despite of the introduction of multiple operative site variables, however, is a safe, efficient, standardized operative strategy. This strategy must rely on a dissection policy that takes procedural goals into account. We will discuss this in great detail in this chapter and contribute to that necessary foundation.

Variant Anatomy

Before a field general goes into battle, one of the first things that must be done is to establish the knowledge of the terrain that will be involved at the battle site. A similar approach must be adopted whenever a laparoscopic cholecystectomy is to be performed. Knowledge and identification of anatomical variances has to be established before the operative procedure is started. These potential anatomical variants can be either vascular or ductal in origin. There are five presentations that are usually seen as far as the ductal anatomy is concerned. One includes a cystic duct that is elongated and runs parallel to the common bile duct that can at times be intimately attached to the common bile duct. This can lead to inadvertent injury. In the surgeon's efforts to ligate what he or she thinks is the cystic duct, the adhered common bile duct will also be dissected free into the operative field. This increases the possibility that a clip may be placed across both structures. The second ductal anatomical variant includes the cystic duct that either inserts into the right hepatic duct or inserts just distal to the right hepatic duct. The danger of injury is accentuated, if the cystic duct is shortened. Another presentation includes a very large right hepatic accessory duct coming from the right lobe of the liver and inserting into the common bile duct. Of course, the danger of bile duct injury may be most likely with Mirizzi's syndrome. The cystic duct is almost nonexistent with the gallbladder being associated with the common duct with various degrees of incorporation. The possibility of all these anomalies must be fully realized before the surgery. This helps in directing the dissection, especially when you have associated clinical pathology at the operative site.[1]

The next category of anatomical variants that can be very important in safely performing a laparoscopic cholecystectomy includes vascular anomalies. The knowledge of these anomalies is very important because you must avoid inadvertent serious bleeding episodes. With bleeding, the surgeon's view of the operative site becomes impaired. In addition, there is an urgent situation created with bleeding that may cause the surgeon to make a poor judgment. Both factors can increase the chance of an important structure being damaged. This danger is slightly increased in comparison with the open procedure because inadvertent bleeding cannot be stopped quickly by utilizing the Pringle maneuver. Concern over the aberrant vascular anatomy is very well founded, especially when the arterial supply of the right upper quadrant has aberrant vessels 45% of the time. The customary textbook arrangement of the common hepatic artery from the celiac trunk leading to proper left and right hepatic arteries was found only 55% of the time in the dissections of Michels.[2]

The most dangerous vascular anomaly probably includes the "high riding" right hepatic artery with a shortened cystic artery trunk. This presentation is highlighted by the presentation of the right hepatic vessel in the triangle of Calot. It is usually adherent to the fundus of the gallbladder. This exposes vessel to injury with either scissors or with inadvertent clamping. Either maneuver may lead to very brisk and startling bleeding. The most effective countermeasure against disaster is prevention. A well-considered operative strategy that acknowledges these variants from the norm can spare the surgeon and the patient from a nightmarish experience.

Local and Pathological Conditions

The anatomy at the operative site may be unclear because of the local and pathological conditions that exist at the time of surgery. Local conditions that can obscure structures in the triangle of Calot include obesity. Fibrosis from chronic cholecystitis can also make the anatomy more difficult to evaluate. We discussed earlier how acute hemorrhage at the operative site can make identification of important structures very difficult. This may be secondary to active bleeding or by staining of tissues from bleeding that subsequently was controlled. In the days of an open cholecystectomy, a local factor that has been associated with increased risk of bile duct injuries is failure to obtain exposure secondary to an inadequate length of the incision. In the laparoscopic arena, adhesions may cause the liver to be immobile and prevent the achievement of proper exposure.

There are other pathological conditions that have been identified to predispose to bile duct injury. These include hepatic neoplasm, infections, pancreatic neoplasm and pancreatitis, duodenal ulcer, hepatic cirrhosis, and polycystic disease of the liver.[3] These conditions either serve to obscure the visualization of the operative site or increase the degree of difficulty for safe dissection of the operative site. In the face of hepatic cirrhosis and sclearoatrophic gallbladder, the mobility of the liver is greatly reduced; therefore, exposure is severely limited. The most frequent pathological conditions that contribute to injury to the common bile duct, however, have to include those of the infectious nature. Perforated cholecystitis and gangrenous cholecystitis, which are the most frequently acute cholecystitis, serve to be a frequent obstacle to the successful performance of a laparoscopic cholecystectomy.[1]

Inadequate Equipment

It is traditional for a surgeon never to mention equipment as a potential cause of a complication or an inability to perform a procedure. This may be so in the open environment, but in the laparoscopic environment, the availability of equipment may be the difference between success and failure. Selection and maintenance of appropriate equipment cannot be underestimated as far as their importance in avoiding bile duct injuries.

The first equipment consideration begins with visualization equipment. If you do not have resolution and clarity of an image, you will not be able to pick up the anatomic nuances necessary to perform a laparoscopic cholecystectomy safely. We suggest, therefore that a three-chip high resolution (CCD) camera be used if more difficult cholecystectomies are going to be performed. Single-chip cameras offer very good clarity, but their resolution capability is far surpassed by three-chip technology.

A light source is the second part of the visualization equation that must be satisfied. It must be remembered that all light sources are not created equally. A xenon light source has the most intense luminance and is absolutely mandatory if you are to successfully complete a difficult cholecystectomy. Always remember to check the bulb life of the light source. If it is more than 150 usage hours, then the luminance could be greatly affected. In addition, the integrity of the light cord must always be inspected because a damaged light cord can decrease the amount of luminance delivered to the operative site. If you are operating in an acutely infected clinical situation, then visualization can become a problem when there is quite a bit of blood and infectious debris in the operative field. This material absorbs light and decreases brightness of the image shown on the monitor.

Hand instruments are very important if more difficult laparoscopic cholecystectomies are to be performed. I equate it to the way golfers use different golf clubs. Because most of the obstacles to successful completion of laparoscopic cholecystectomy are infectious in nature, it would stand to reason that the hand instruments necessary for this procedure under these circumstances are very specialized. There is frequently a need for the instruments to have long jaws that can open very wide because of induration and increased thickness of tissue. In addition, because of chronic infection, induration, and fibrosis, the grasping surface of the instrument should be aggressive. I believe that you should have at least two types of elongated jaw-grasping instruments. There should be an aggressive instrument and a highly aggressive instrument. The aggressive instrument should have a grasping surface with serrated edges. This provides an excellent gripping surface for infectious tissue that does not have a very large fibrotic component. When you have a large amount of fibrosis and chronic scar tissue, a toothed, highly aggressive grasper may be the only instrument that can adequately handle the tissue.

The ability to grasp the gallbladder is desirable but not mandatory, if a surgeon is to be able to obtain proper exposure needed to perform a laparoscopic cholecystectomy safely. If you are attempting this procedure in the face of adverse conditions and you are not able to grasp the organ, then we advise using an "influence retraction" countermeasure. The blunt end of an instrument is used to apply countertraction to the organ. This is not as efficient as direct manipulation. The organ may slip out of position frequently. It does, however, at times allow a difficult case to be successfully completed.

In addition to hand instruments, it is imperative that your irrigation and aspirator apparatus be appropriate for these procedures. I would highly recommend that you have an irrigation apparatus that has a large volume of irrigation capacity. The usual irrigation apparatus carries about 1 L capacity. If possible, an instrument with a 3 L capacity is used; if that is not possible, then you should have apparatus that has double 1 L fluid capacity hooked in series. We also suggest an aspirator that has multiple shaft diameter selections. Because of the possibility of blood with clots in the operative area, a 10 mm pool and open barrel aspirator should be available in order to efficiently evacuate debris.

You should also be able to have a tapered nozzle type of irrigation apparatus that can create a stream of fluid at a high velocity to the operative site. This greatly facilitates the use of aquadissection in order to dissect the triangle of Calot and help remove the gallbladder from the gallbladder bed. There also are other assists items, such as an ovarian aspiration needle. This can come in quite handy because the gallbladder frequently has to be decompressed before it can be grasped. This is seen in gallbladders that have had the cystic duct chronically obstructed. Early aspiration of a tense gallbladder is very important in obtaining proper exposure. It also decreases the possibility of contamination. When the gallbladder is removed from the gallbladder bed there can be a large amount of oozing that can be very difficult to control. This is because the bed is very hypervascular from the associated infectious process. Bleeding can be difficult to control because the standard Bovie electrocautery is not very effective in the face of edema. In this situation, the argon beam coagulator is much more effective in achieving hemostasis. This is a very effective instrument. Argon gas is blown in under pressure to the bleeding site to clear that site of blood. This helps greatly in being able to pinpoint the bleeding site. At this pint, electrical current is carried through the argon gas to coagulate the site where hemostasis has not been achieved. The other advantage to using this instrument is that it has very superficial coagulation penetration, therefore limiting the possibility of inadvertent injury.

Skill

Of all the factors that go into the making of a surgeon, there is none that elicits more of an emotional response than the question of skill. All surgeons have to enter the operating theater with a "controlled arrogance." The surgeon must believe that they have the innate capability to operate themselves out of trouble and successfully perform a procedure with superior results. This confidence is similar to that which we see in the personality make up of fighter pilots. This component, which illicits such an emotional response up to this point, however, has not been able to be defined objectively. When the thought of objective skill evaluation is mentioned to surgeons, this generates very aggressive arguments. Some say that the art form of surgery cannot be defined by objective boundaries. Objective evaluation of skill is an important goal in every industry except medicine. Many fear unprecedented credentialing ramifications. The use of objective parameters, however, allows the effectiveness of the training process to be monitored. It also helps to determine areas of weakness that need attention. Without objective evaluation, an individual cannot continue to refine and perfect the ability to perform a procedure well. Rosser et al. conducted the evaluation of the skill capability of experienced surgeons in the laparoscopic environment. More than 70% of the large series of surgeons from around the world could not perform an intracorporeal knot within 10 minutes.[4] This very basic skill is the most difficult task to accomplish in the laparoscopic environment, and it was found that most surgeons could not do this. If a surgeon does not have the capability to efficiently and delicately perform a dissection that allows for the identification of important structures, then the possibility for a mishap increases significantly. The surgeon depends on anatomical keys in order to make proper clinical judgment so the operation can be conducted in a safe fashion. Without the skill to perform the proper dissection to disclose these keys, inadvertent injuries to major vascular and biliary structures are highly increased. The objective evaluation and maturation of laparoscopic skills and suturing, therefore, are an absolute necessity in order to be able to perform a laparoscopic cholecystectomy safely.

All of the factors that have been discussed can converge to present obstacles to a surgeon making proper judgment. Good judgment is at the core of any successful operation. The surgeon is responsible for taking into account all of the local conditions and other factors and make decisions that will maintain the safety of the patient. The maturation of the decision-making capability of a surgeon has been mainly chiseled from experience by way of exposure to a large number of cases. This apprenticeship system has been in existence for more than 100 years, and it has served us well. We have to recognize, however, the emergence of new technology and hope to utilize that technology to allow us to develop a more effective and efficient way of developing the most important of all traits necessary to be an excellent surgical physician.

Operative Strategy

Although there are many clinical circumstances that may lead to common bile duct injuries, there are two scenarios that seem to be quite frequent.

Scenario 1

A surgeon operates on a patient that has had a long-standing history of chronic cholecystitis. This is not an acute infectious circumstance; rather, it is a chronic recurring situation that has left the hepatoduodenal ligament with quite a bit of scarring. The common bile duct is normal or less than normal in size. The first assistant in the standard Reddick-Olsen trocar placement and room setup then grabs what is thought to be the Hartman's pouch. The surgeon fails to realize that the Hartman's pouch and common bile duct are not separate. The Hartman's pouch/common bile duct angle is closed because the Hartman's pouch is adhered to the common bile duct from previous infection. Rather than starting the dissection laterally where it is safe, the surgeon, erroneously decides that the normal-to-small-sized common bile duct is the cystic duct. The dissection is begun very medial. This leads to dissection around what is thought to be the cystic duct. The surgeon sees what appears to be a tubular structure leading to the gallbladder. This tubular structure is clipped with the surgeon thinking that this is the cystic duct. The clip is usually not quite large enough to traverse the structure and others have to be added. The patient is closed and the injury is usually not detected at the time of surgery. The same scenario can present itself in an acute situation that has a chronic component.

Scenario 2

The operative team is faced with a clinical situation that has no infectious conditions. In their dissection they subsequently fail to recognize a vascular hazard. This is frequently seen in what we have previously called a "high riding" right hepatic artery that is displaced high onto the gallbladder fundus. A technical error is made and this vessel is subsequently injured. Quite a bit of bleeding then ensues, followed by a massive application of clips. The blood is cleared and the common duct is either divided or the clips have injured the duct to a point where a corrective procedure has to be done.

Despite the many clinical variables that present themselves in a case where a common bile duct injury is committed, a standardized operative strategy that is formulated with the anticipation of clinical variables can be your most reliable safeguard against injury. Proper operative strategy begins with the provision of a stable platform to conduct the procedure properly. The surgeon is traditionally in the standing position with the Reddick-Olson technique for the laparoscopic cholecystectomy (Fig. 4.1).

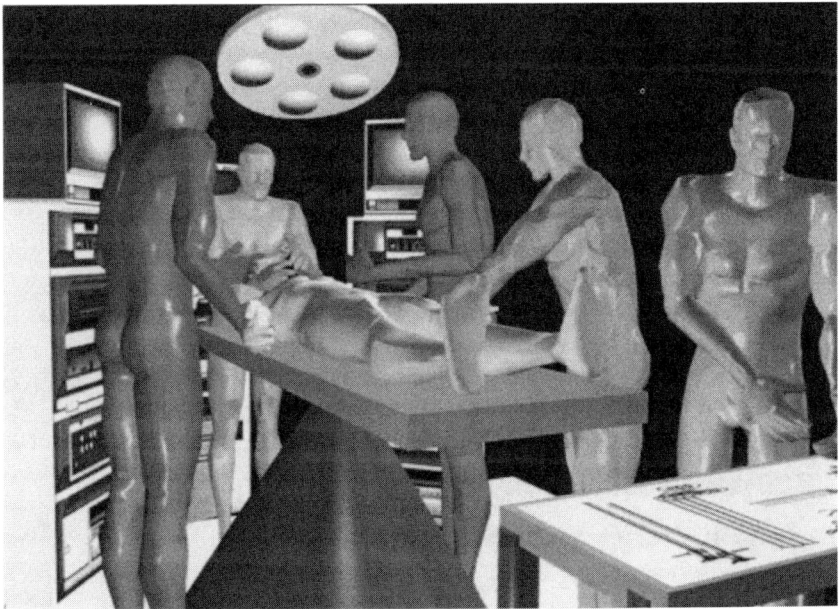

FIGURE 4.1. Schematic diagram of the personnel during the traditional Reddick-Olson technique for the laparoscopic cholecystectomy. Note that the surgeon is in the standing position.

This has some disadvantages because of current equipment designs. The surgeon has to hyperextend the neck and hyperflex the wrists. This causes the surgeon to assume the "praying mantis"-like silouhette that is ergonomically undesirable. This situation is not only for the laparoscopic cholecystectomy, but all minimally invasive procedures. By sitting down for these cases, your hands are brought into better alignment with current instrumentation. A very comfortable, ergonomically stable platform is therefore established to perform the surgery (Fig. 4.2).

If the sitting position is to be employed, then there also must be a modification to the trocar placement. In our technique, we choose to have a diamond-shaped trocar placement pattern. The umbilicus is still a primary trocar site. The laparoscope is placed at this position. The lateral port is placed along the anterior axillary line two finger breaths from the costal margin. This represents the standard technique. The modification of port placement involves the midclavicular port and xyphoid port. Instead of being to the right of the midline the xyphoid port is moved to the left. The midclavicular port is brought to the lateral edge of the left rectus muscle half way between the umbilical and xyphoid port (Fig. 4.3). The positioning is completed by placing the table 30 degrees of reverse Trendelenberg and

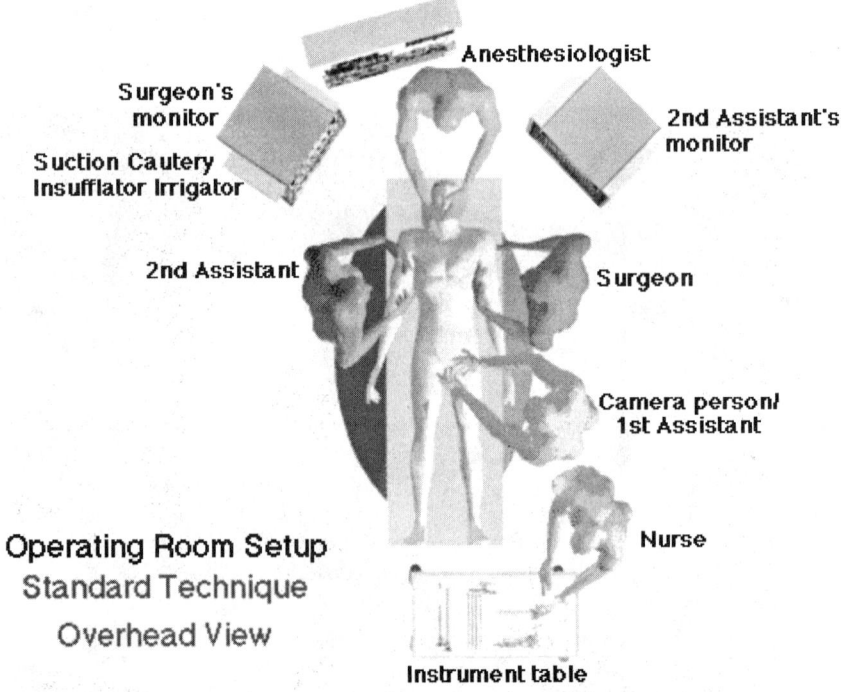

FIGURE 4.2. Schematic diagram of the personnel during the technique as described in this chapter. Note that a very comfortable, ergonomically stable platform is established to perform the surgery. Note also that the surgeon is sitting down.

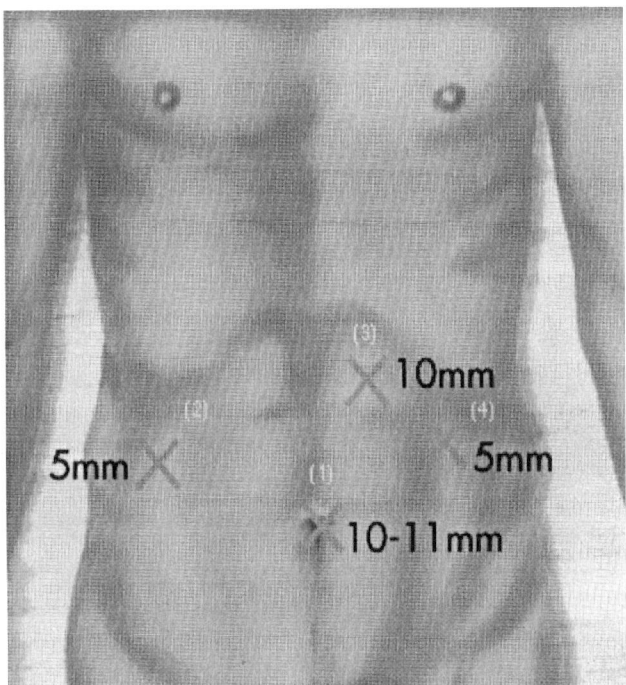

FIGURE 4.3. Schematic diagram of port placement in a laparoscopic cholecy-stectomy . The umbilicus is still a primary trocar site and the laparoscope is placed at this position. The lateral port is placed along the anterior axillary line two finger breaths from the costal margin. This represents the standard technique. The modi-fication of port placement involves the midclavicular port and xyphoid port. The xyphoid port, instead of being to the right of the midline is moved to the left. The midclavicular port is brought to the lateral edge of the left rectus muscle half way between the umbilical and xyphoid port.

rotating the patient 30 degrees toward the surgeon. Next, the height of the table positioned to its lower limit. The surgeon is seated on the left side of the patient (Fig. 4.2).

Unlike the traditional technique that features the surgeon occupying the xyphoid operating point and an assistant actually controlling the traction and countertraction, the surgeon is in total control with this operative strategy. The Hartman's pouch is grasped with the left hand and the dissec-tion is carried out with the right hand. Disaster is initiated quite frequently by an overzealous assistant who aggressively grabs the Hartman's pouch area and brings the common bile duct into harm's way. This technique also correlates with the two-handed operative strategy employed in open surgery.

Scenario 3

We will now use as our clinical demonstration platform a laparoscopic cholecystectomy performed in the face of acute cholecystitis. After the establishment of the pneumoperitoneum, the first challenge for the surgeon is to obtain proper exposure. This can be very difficult with an acute inflammatory situation. An omental phlegmon frequently envelops the entire gall bladder. This can be quite a nuisance because it does not fall away from the gall bladder with common maneuvers used for traditional exposure. There may also be adhesions that may exist because there is a dual process of acute cholecystitis superimposed on adhesions from chronic disease. Your first move should be to place a 5 mm blunt probe through the right lateral trocar site. This will help to determine if the omentum and any associated adhesions can be separated from the gallbladder easily. If the blunt probe proves not to be successful because of dense adhesions, then sharp dissection will be necessary to obtain separation of the gallbladder from the thickened omentum. When taking down adhesions try to remove them very close to the gallbladder wall. By staying in this place bleeding will be minimized. You should be prepared at this point to add an extra port in the upper right lower quadrant to insert a retractor. This helps in obtaining proper exposure especially when the patient is obese. Remember to make sure that all adhesions, including those between the omentum and the liver, are taken down. Maximum mobility of the liver must be achieved to obtain proper exposure (Fig. 4.4).

Next, you must inspect the tenseness of the gallbladder to decide how manipulation of the organ will be achieved. If the gallbladder is tense, then it is preferable to use a 5-mm ovarian aspiration needle in order to achieve decompression. The organ can then be grasped with greater ease. It is questionable whether or not the gallbladder should be totally decompressed. Some surgeons may choose to leave the gallbladder partially decompressed in order to achieve a more effective separation of the gallbladder from its normal resting place on the liver. If the gallbladder wall is thickened, then the regular 5-mm grasper will not be effective in achieving proper exposure; therefore, we suggest a 5- or 10-mm toothed grasper to provide a more secure manipulation of the organ (Fig. 4.5). If the proper aggressive graspers are not available, then exposure can be achieved by what we call "influence retraction." With this technique a blunt 5–10-mm instrument is placed into the abdomen. The gallbladder is not actually grasped; rather, it is bluntly manipulated and influenced into the proper position for exposure.

Once proper exposure has been accomplished, you are now ready to begin the most critical part of the procedure. The hepatoduodenal ligament may be thickened and edematous with no visible anatomical cues available to you. The proper technique in this clinical situation is to start your dissection superior and lateral and then work medially. By starting laterally,

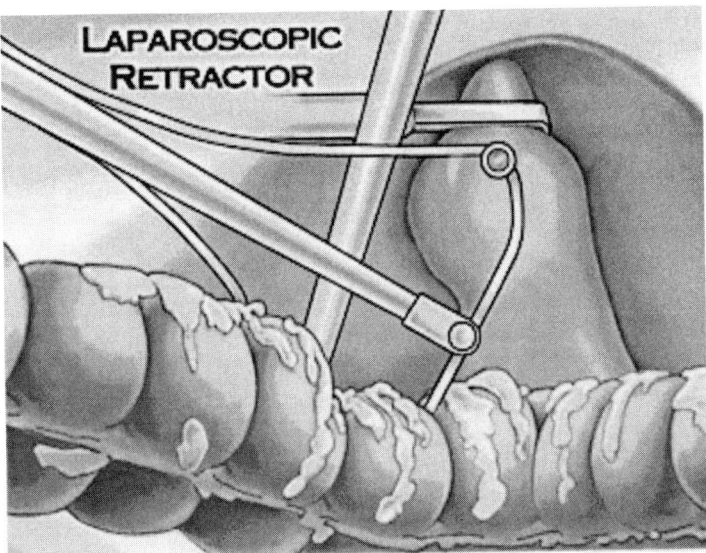

FIGURE 4.4. Schematic diagram of use of laparoscopic retractor. Maximum mobility of the liver must be achieved to obtain proper exposure. Caution must be used to retract the colon away from the gallbladder and liver beds gently.

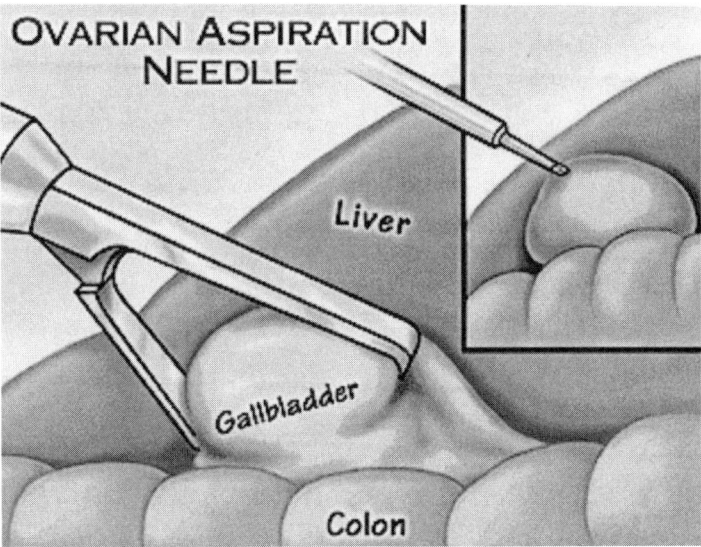

FIGURE 4.5. Schematic diagram demonstrating a tense gallbladder. If the gall bladder wall is thickened, then the regular 5-mm grasper will not be effective in achieving proper exposure. It may be necessary to aspirate the gallbladder contents.

you can establish very early whether or not the Hartman's pouch/common bile duct angle is open or closed. If the angle is closed, then this situation leads frequently to a common bile duct injury by misidentification of the common bile duct for the cystic duct. Avoid taking your dissection medially, before the lateral boundary of your dissection is established. By disciplining yourself to dissect lateral to medial the Hartman's pouch can be encountered first and your dissection can be directed to establish this important anatomical configuration. By documenting the Hartman's pouch/common bile duct angle and subsequently the cystic duct, then and only then should you proceed medially.

You can now proceed to perform the dissection of the triangle of Calot. A three-phase dissection strategy is used. The first phase is the *disclosure phase*. During this phase, very superficial dissection is performed in order to disclose the gross whereabouts of underlying structures. This requires a very meticulous dissection. With an acute inflammatory process, this can of course present a serious challenge; therefore, it may be very helpful to use liberal aquadissection to help to debride the tissues in the hepatoduodenal ligament (Fig. 4.6). In addition, a 5-mm atraumatic "peanut" can be very helpful in the disclosure phase (Fig. 4.7). Once this phase has been established, then and only then should you proceed with the *separation phase* of the dissection. Remember that this phase must proceed with the most lateral structure first and then the most medial structure. This will serve as

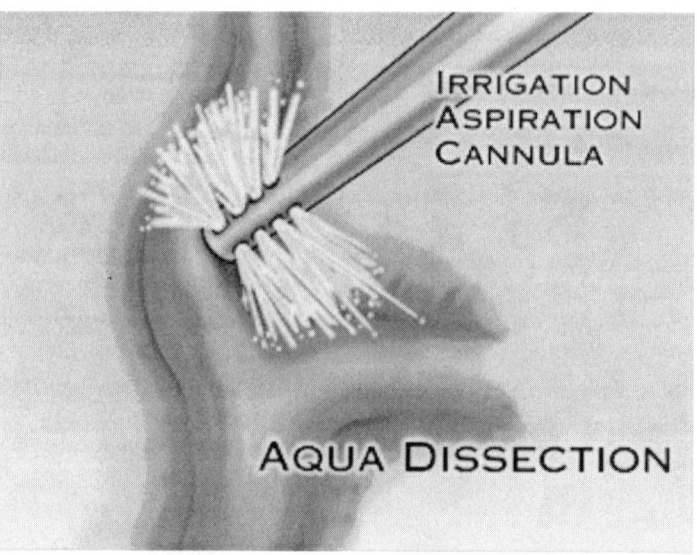

FIGURE 4.6. Schematic diagram of use of liberal aquadissection to help to debride the tissues in the hepatoduodenal ligament.

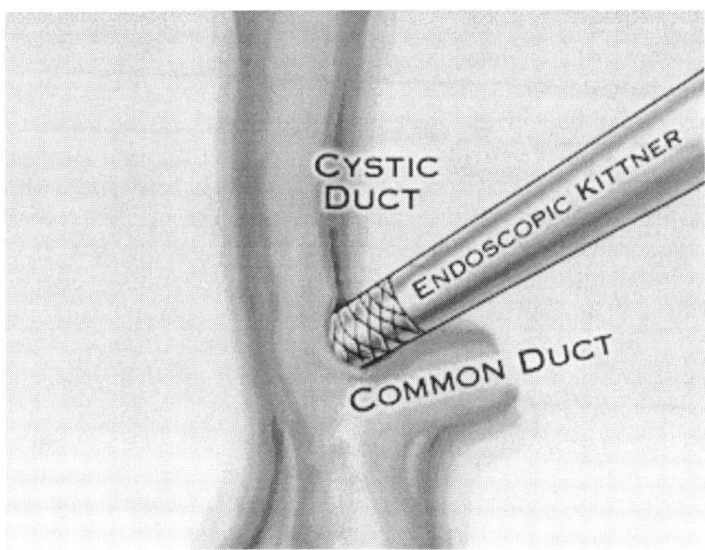

FIGURE 4.7. Schematic diagram of a 5-mm atraumatic "peanut." This is very useful in the disclosure phase (see text).

another checkpoint to verify the establishment of the Hartman's pouch/ common bile duct angle and the identification of the cystic duct.

It is important for you to inspect the posterior portion of the hepatoduodenal ligament before the ligation phase is established. Make sure that complete removal of the peritoneum and underlying tissues have been established in this frequently overlooked area. Check to see if you have a "positive horseshoe" sign. This sign relates to the common bile duct as it is retracted upward by the establishment of proper exposure. If the common bile duct is rendered in the shape of a horseshoe, then there is great danger that the common bile duct has been brought into the line of dissection and the cystic duct has not properly been identified.

During the separation phase, there must be establishment of a proper length of the structure to be ligated. It is preferable that 1–2 cm a segment of the structure to be ligated must be established before proper ligation can occur. This is important so that the clips placed have proper separation for safe division. Once the ligation and division of the proper structure has been achieved, inspect and identify all the important structures to make sure to your satisfaction that no injuries have been committed.

You are now ready for the *extraction stage* of the procedure, which involves the removal of the gallbladder from the gallbladder bed. Before this phase begins, you must inspect the areolar tissue at the gallbladder– liver interface. This is referred to as the "garbage can" area. The posterior cystic artery frequently resides within this tissue. Dissect this area with great caution in order to avoid a vascular mishap. Aquadissection with the special 5-mm irrigators injecting saline under 600 mmHg pressure is used in order to establish a saline-induced separation between the gallbladder and the gallbladder bed in the liver (Fig. 4.8). This also helps to establish hemostasis secondary to the hydrostatic pressures on smaller anterior vessels. In the face of edema, which is frequently associated with acute cholecystitis, separation of the gallbladder from the liver can be achieved quite frequently from aquadissection alone without the use of cautery, which is frequently ineffective in the face of a large amount of edema. If this is not effective in maintaining hemostasis, then the argon beam coagulator should be utilized to achieve hemostasis.

The gallbladder is always removed by placing it within an extraction bag. This is especially important in the face of acute cholecystitis with a large number of stones. In the literature it has been established that if these stones are lost in the abdomen they can cause remote postoperative sequelae; therefore, the extraction of this infected organ in an extraction bag is infected recommended. These infected organs are quite frequently packed full of stones, and the extraction through the umbilical port can prove to be quite difficult. If this situation is met, then we therefore suggest that the umbilical incision is extended and the gallbladder extracted effort-

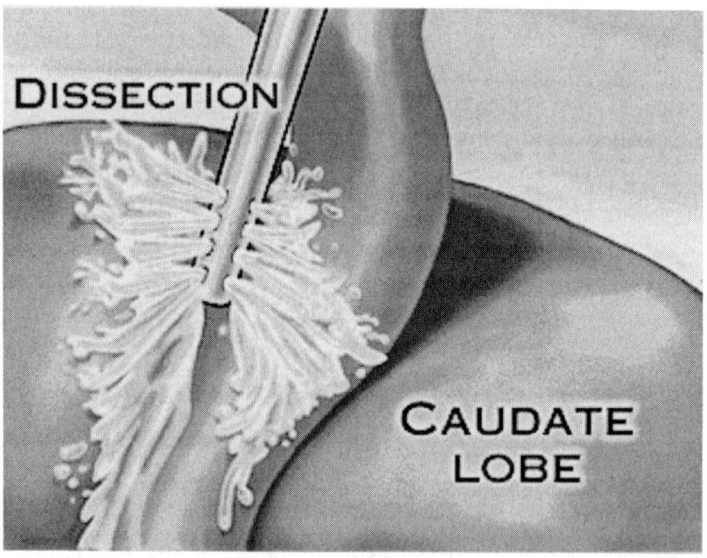

FIGURE 4.8. The extraction stage of the procedure involves the removal of the gallbladder from the gallbladder bed. Note the aquadissection with the special 5-mm irrigators to inject saline under 600 mmHg pressure in order to establish a saline-induced separation between the gallbladder and the gallbladder bed in the liver.

lessly. The slightly enlarged incision does not inversely affect the patient's recovery pattern.

If we are to decrease the incidence of common bile duct injuries that are committed in the United States each year, then many attributing factors must be accounted for and the proper technique waystations established to safeguard the patient. Many countermeasures have been identified in this chapter that can help establish a lower common bile duct injury rate. Because of the recognition of clinical conditions that predispose to injuries, the establishment of advanced laparoscopic skills, the adherence of a standardized operative strategy, and the maturation of clinical judgment, a minimized incidence of common bile duct injuries can be realized.

References

1. Asbun HJ, Rossi RL. Techniques of laparoscopic cholecystectomy: the difficult operation. Surg Clin N Am 1994;74:755–775.
2. Michels NA. Blood supply and anatomy of the upper abdominal organs with a descriptive atlas. JB Lippincott, Philadelphia, 1955.
3. Hunter JG. Commentary-techniques of laparoscopic cholecystectomy: the difficult Operation. Surg Clin No Am 1994;74:777–780.
4. Rosser JC, Rosser LE, Savalgi RS. Skill acquisition and assessment for laparoscopic surgery. Arch Surg 1997;132:200–204.

5
Bile Duct Injuries

Ioannis G. Kaklamanos and Dana K. Andersen

History

The majority of the injuries of the biliary tract is iatrogenic. They are usually associated with operations in the upper abdomen. More than 80% of the injuries occur during cholecystectomy, which is the most common operation of the digestive system. Langenbuch performed the first cholecystectomy in 1882, after which the number of cholecystectomies increased rapidly, inevitably increasing the number of complications. Iatrogenic bile duct injuries are unfortunately not rare and may have disastrous consequences and very significant long-term morbidity and mortality.[1,2] With adherence to well-established technical principles for open cholecystectomy, the incidence of bile duct injuries remained less 0.5% in most of the published retrospective series.[3-5]

The introduction of laparoscopic cholecystectomy in 1987 signified a new era in the surgery of the biliary tract. The frequency of laparoscopic cholecystectomy and other laparoscopic operations has rapidly increased since then, and the number of cholecystectomies performed annually has increased by 15–20%. Early series with large numbers of patients reported bile duct injury rates ranging between 0.5–1.5%,[6] significantly higher than with the open cholecystectomy (Table 5.1). Centers specialized in the repair of biliary injuries have experienced a dramatic increase in the number of referrals. There are several reasons why the incidence of injuries during laparoscopic surgery is higher: The monocular view that the conventional camera provides, the use of the electrocautery near Calot's triangle, and the surgeon's "learning curve," might all be contributing factors.

Bile duct injuries range from small postoperative bile leaks, with little clinical significance, to severe injuries and strictures of the intrahepatic ducts with devastating consequences. We will review the types and mechanisms of iatrogenic bile duct injuries after laparoscopic surgery and summarize the diagnostic modalities and options for surgical and nonsurgical management.

TABLE 5.1. Complications after open and laparoscopic cholecystectomy.

Complication	Open ($n = 6,538$)	Laparoscopic ($n = 13,159$)
Major vascular injury	0	4
Hematoma or hemorrhage	6	18
Major bile duct injury	2	31
Bile leaks (requiring surgery)	3	13
Bowel or bladder perforation	1	6
Incarcerated bowel, dehiscence, or small bowel obstruction	6	6
Other	5	12

Date reported by New York State hospitals for the period April to October 1992.
Source: Bernard HR, TW Hartman. Am J Surg 1993;165:533.

Types of Injury

Cystic Duct Injuries and Bile Leak

Bile leaks after cholecystectomy may arise from three sources: the cystic duct (50%), a subvesical or gallbladder bed bile duct (duct of Luschka) (25%), or an injury to a major bile duct (25%). The incidence of bile leak after laparoscopic cholecystectomy ranges between 1 and 2% in most series.[7–9]

Cystic duct leak is the most common biliary injury associated with laparoscopic cholecystectomy. The most common mechanism of bile leak is failure to ligate the cystic duct safely due to inadequate application of the endoscopic clips. The presence of a wide and friable cystic duct, as in cases of acute cholecystitis, may result in inadequate application of the clips. The closure of the cystic duct stump may be difficult if an intraoperative cholangiogram has been performed through a short and inflamed cystic duct. In this case, the application of clips only may be inadequate and ligation of the cystic duct with an "endo-loop" may be necessary.

Severe inflammation of the gallbladder and the cystic duct can cause ischemia necrosis of the stump with postoperative bile leak. Any doubts regarding the blood supply and the viability of the cystic duct stump should make a surgeon particularly cautious. Laparoscopic suture ligation of the cystic duct or conversion to open procedure may be necessary in these cases.

Bile leaks cause bile collections (bilomas) or biliary fistulas. Bilomas can become secondarily infected, causing localized infection or peritonitis, which are potentially life-threatening complications. Percutaneous drainage of a biloma of any significant size is indicated to avoid secondary infection and peritonitis. Most of the bile leaks secondary to inadequate ligation of the cystic duct stump resolve after endoscopic replacement of a biliary stent, which seals the site of the leak and allows healing of the stump. Reoperation with identification and ligation of the cystic duct stump is only infrequently necessary.

Excessive right upper quadrant pain or an elevated bilirubin in the immediate postoperative period should prompt examination for a bile leak. An ultrasound examination of the area may detect a fluid collection, and a radionuclide imaging study [e.g., hepatoiminodiacetic acid (HIDA) scan] may demonstrate extravasation of bile in the region. Endoscopic retrograde cholangiopancreatography (ERCP) is the procedure of choice to confirm a suspected bile leak, and it can quickly control the leak with placement of an endoscopic stent.

Extrahepatic Bile Duct Injuries

Injuries below the confluence of the two main hepatic ducts are extrahepatic, whereas injures above this level are essentially intrahepatic because the confluence is located deep in the porta hepatis. The majority of the injuries associated with laparoscopic cholecystectomy are extrahepatic. Most commonly the extrahepatic portion of the common hepatic duct is injured. Injuries of the extrahepatic biliary ducts occur during attempted dissection in the triangle of Calot. Inadequate identification of the structures results in injury of the common bile duct or the hepatic duct. One of these structures is most commonly misidentified as the cystic duct, and it is clipped and transected during the operation (Fig. 5.1). If the injury is not recognized at this stage of the procedure, the dissection continues superiorly, where the right hepatic artery may be mistaken as the cystic artery and divided. Dissecting sharply near the bile ducts or near the cystic duct–hepatic duct junction can also cause the injury. In this case, the leak of bile during the procedure alerts the surgeon and indicates the likelihood of an injury.

Injuries of the extrahepatic bile ducts are either partial lacerations or complete transections. If the injury is not recognized and the dissection continues, then excision of part of the duct and loss of tissue may occur, making the repair of the injury even more challenging. In a reported series from referral centers, simple lacerations are the minority, with most of the laparoscopic injuries being severe lacerations or transections.[10,11]

Intrahepatic Bile Duct Injuries

Injuries at or above the confluence of the two main hepatic ducts are essentially intrahepatic because this anatomic area is covered by liver parenchyma. These injuries occur most frequently during dissection of the gallbladder off the liver bed, especially in the presence of severe inflamma-

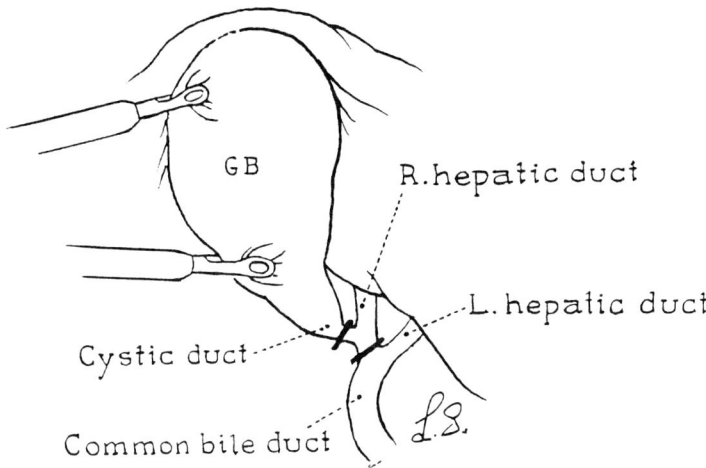

GB

R.hepatic duct

L.hepatic duct

Cystic duct

Common bile duct

FIGURE 5.1. Mechanism of injury. The misidentification of the cystic duct or mis-application of clips constitutes the most common errors, which lead to a major bile duct injury. (*Source*: Bailey, RW. Complications of laparoscopic general surgery. In Zucker KA (ed.) Surgical Laparoscopy Qual Med Publ, Inc., St. Louis, MO, 1991, p. 331.)

tion and scarring of the triangle of Calot. The right hepatic duct is far more commonly injured than the left. The duct is misidentified as the cystic duct or as "accessory" duct, clipped, and divided. Injury to the left hepatic duct occurs when misidentification of the structures results in dissection on the medial aspect of the common bile duct. Even experienced laparoscopic surgeons may encounter difficulties in dissection and identification of structures in the porta hepatis. Prompt cholangiography and a willingness to convert to open celiotomy if the dissection is difficult are essential to avoid injury. Inability to perform cholangiography or the appearance of an "incomplete" or inadequate cholangiogram are indications to convert to an open procedure.

Strictures of the Bile Ducts

Bile duct strictures following cholecystectomy occur either early or late after the operation. The severity of the stricture may vary according to the degree and the location. They can be classified in four types according to the system described by Bismuth[12] (Fig. 5.2). Grade I strictures are distal strictures located more than 2 cm from the confluence of the left and right hepatic ducts; grade II strictures involve the common hepatic duct, less than 2 cm from the confluence; grade III strictures are within 1 cm of the confluence; and grade IV strictures involve the confluence of the hepatic

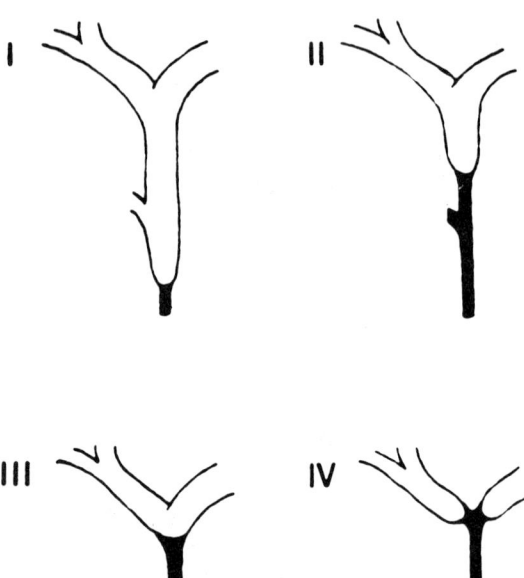

FIGURE 5.2. Classification of bile duct Strictures. I. Greater than 2 cm distal to confluence, II. Greater than 1 cm distal to confluence, III. Less than 1 cm to the confluence but not involving right or left ducts, IV. Involvement of the confluence with obstruction of right or left duct. (*Source*: Bismuth, H. Postoperative strictures of the bile duct, In: Blumgart, LH (ed.) The biliary tract. Churchill Livingstone, Edinburgh, 1982, p. 209.)

ducts. The chances of a successful repair and a satisfactory outcome vary inversely with the grade of stricture.

Mechanisms of postoperative strictures are direct injury to the duct, clipping of the duct, thermal injury, devascularization of the duct during dissection, or inflammation and scarring secondary to bile leakage. Application of a clip near the confluence of the cystic duct with the hepatic duct may cause partial or complete obstruction of the common hepatic duct. Strictures caused by this mechanism usually occur early, within days or weeks of the operation. Strictures caused by secondary inflammation or thermal injury may only become clinically obvious months or even years after the original operation.

Ischemia is an important etiologic factor for the formation of bile duct strictures. The hepatic duct and the common bile duct receive their blood supply from axial arteries located generally at 3 and 9 o'clock. Unnecessary dissection around the common bile duct during laparoscopic cholecystectomy and the excessive use of electrocautery can cause damage to the feeding vessels with subsequent formation of ischemic strictures.

Bile leak from the cystic duct or from small injuries of the common bile duct can cause an intense local inflammatory response, which may be intensified further in the presence of infection. The inflammation results in fibrosis and scarring, which contribute to stricture formation. Scar tissue may also result from a hematoma in the porta hepatis, if adequate hemostasis was not obtained during the operation.

Iatrogenic strictures of the major bile ducts after laparoscopic cholecystectomy can be potentially devastating complications that usually require surgical repair. Endoscopic and transhepatic stenting and dilation may offer useful temporary treatment of a stricture. These are frequently successful measures to alleviate infection, jaundice, and inflammation before definitive repair is embarked upon.

Mechanisms of Injury and Risk Factors

Anatomic Variations

The anatomy of the biliary ducts and blood vessels in the hepatoduodenal ligament can vary greatly, so anatomic variation is the rule and not an exception in this area. The cystic artery usually arises from the right hepatic artery, but it may arise from the left hepatic, common hepatic, gastroduodenal, or even the superior mesenteric artery (Fig. 5.3). Double or accessory cystic arteries are present in 8–12% of the cases. The course of the cystic artery may also vary, usually crossing behind, but sometimes anterior to, the common hepatic duct. If the cystic artery originates from the proximal portion of the right hepatic artery or from the common hepatic artery, then it may lie close to the common hepatic duct. In this case, the duct may be injured during the dissection or the clipping of the cystic artery.

Variations of the anatomic position of the cystic duct are also common. Accessory hepatic ducts are present in approximately 15% of cases. They usually drain a portion of the right lobe of the liver and join the right hepatic duct, the common hepatic duct, or the infundibulum of the gallbladder. The duct of Luschka is a small accessory duct that may drain directly from the liver into the body of the gallbladder (Fig. 5.4).

The plethora of anatomic variations in the area of the Calot's triangle makes the dissection during laparoscopic cholecystectomy technically demanding. All of the structures should be recognized with certainty before being ligated and divided. Recognition of the junction of the cystic duct with the gallbladder may be difficult in the presence of inflammation. Any doubts about the anatomic position of the structures should prompt intraoperative cholangiogram and conversion to open surgery, if necessary.

Complicated Pathology

Acute inflammation and scarring of Calot's triangle constitute risk factors for operative injury to the bile ducts. Acute edematous infiltration of the tissues, as in cases of acute cholecystitis or acute pancreatitis, obscures the

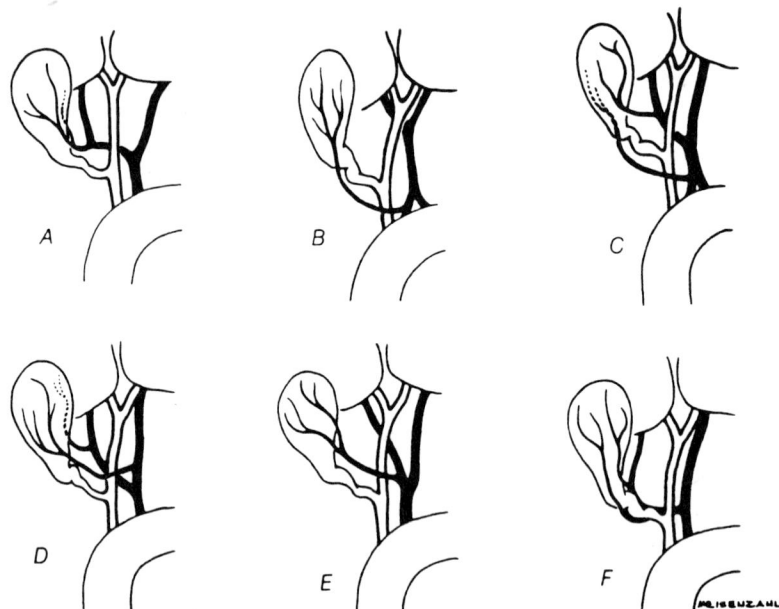

FIGURE 5.3. Arterial anomalies of the extrahepatic biliary system. (A) Cystic artery arises from right hepatic artery in 95% of cases. (B) Cystic artery arises from gastroduodenal artery. (C) Two cystic arteries, arising from right hepatic and common hepatic arteries. (D) Two cystic arteries, arising from left hepatic and right hepatic arteries. (E) Cystic artery coursing anterior to common hepatic duct. (F) Two cystic arteries arising from abnormally located right hepatic artery. (*Source*: Schwartz, SL. Gallbladder and extrahepatic biliary system. In: Schwartz, SL (ed.) Principles of surgery, McGraw-Hill, New York, 1984, p. 1310.) Reprinted with permission.

view of the surgeon during laparoscopic cholecystectomy and makes the recognition of the structures difficult. In cases of long-standing chronic cholecystitis, the gallbladder becomes small and fibrosed (scleroatrophic gallbladder). As a result of the fibrosis in the porta hepatis, the recognition of the structures and dissection during laparoscopic cholecystectomy may be extremely laborious, predisposing to injuries.

Involvement of the common bile duct may occur in cases of severe inflammation of the gallbladder, as it does in the Mirizzi syndrome or in cholecystobiliary fistula.[13] Any attempt to continue the procedure laparoscopically may cause severe injury to the common bile duct. Typical cholecystectomy may not be feasible in these cases. Conversion to an open procedure is usually necessary in order to perform cholecystectomy, chlocystostomy, or repair of the common bile duct, as needed. Distortion of the anatomic relationship of the common bile duct with the duodenum may be also caused by the presence of a penetrating duodenal ulcer. The

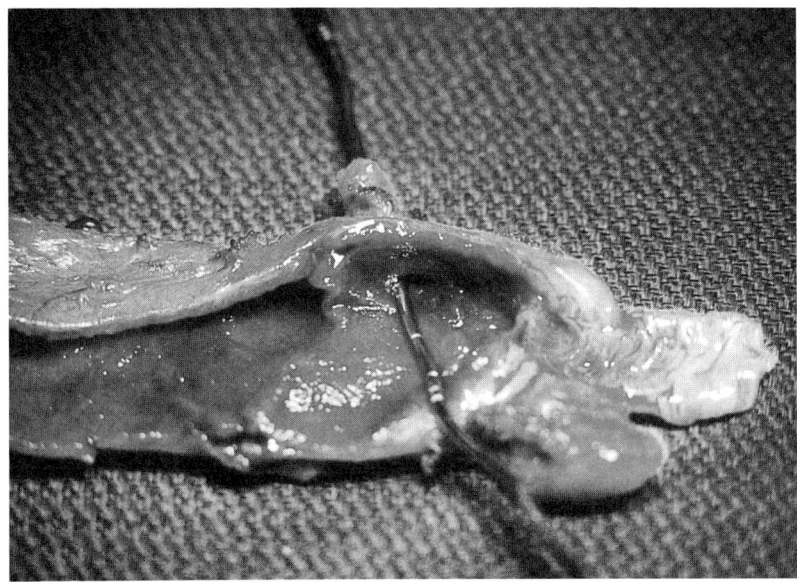

FIGURE 5.4. Duct of luschka. Operative photograph of gallbladder with probe in accessory duct of luschka.

inflammation present in cases of acute or chronic pancreatitis can also cause difficulty in recognition of the structures of Calot's triangle. Thorough preoperative investigation minimizes the possibility that these conditions are unexpectedly discovered during laparoscopic cholecystectomy. If this is the case, however, then laparoscopic dissection may be unsafe, and conversion of the procedure to open celiotomy is prudent.

Technical Errors

With the accumulation of experience and upon review of multiple complications, it has been shown that inappropriate operative technique is also a predisposing factor for bile duct injuries. In this section we will present the so-called technical errors that have been identified to contribute to bile duct injury.

In order to expose structures and facilitate dissection during laparoscopic cholecystectomy, cephalad and lateral retraction of the gallbladder is necessary. Errors in the retraction technique may predispose to bile duct injuries. Excessive retraction of the gallbladder may cause common bile duct injury by avulsing the cystic duct off of the common bile duct. The assistant should be cautious, especially in the presence of acute inflammation or a gangrenous gallbladder where inflamed bile ducts become friable. Inadequate or medial retraction of the gallbladder predisposes to injury by closing the space between the common bile duct and the cystic duct.

Application of the cystic duct clip too close to the cystic duct–common bile duct junction may cause partial obstruction of the common bile duct with subsequent scar tissue formation and stricture. This type of injury can be avoided by clearly identifying the cystic duct–common bile duct junction before clipping. Strenuous dissection too close to the common bile duct may jeopardize its blood supply with secondary formation of a stricture. Dissection should be avoided at the 3 and 9 o'clock positions of the axial vessels providing the blood supply to the duct. Vigorous dissection close to the common bile duct wall should also be avoided, again because of risk of direct injury of the duct, especially if inflammation is present. The dissection should be done close to the cystic duct–gallbladder junction, and not near the common bile duct.

The "blind" application of clips to obtain hemostasis is another frequent error. When the view of the surgeon is obscured by blood, irrigation of the area and cleaning of the laparoscope provides adequate view for identification of the bleeding vessel and hemostasis. If laparoscopic control of the bleeding is not possible, then the procedure should be converted to open celiotomy before significant blood loss occurs. Technical errors have been identified to be the cause of most of the cases of bile duct injuries.[14] Although these are more likely to occur early in the surgeon's "learning curve,"[15,16] major duct injuries continue to occur, even after clinical competence is achieved.

Thermal and Laser Injuries

Hemostasis and dissection during laparoscopic cholecystectomy are greatly facilitated by using the electrocautery. Penetration of the thermal energy depends on the relative conductivity of the tissue, which varies with the content in water and lipids. The depth of penetration into the surrounding tissues cannot precisely be controlled. Excessive use of high-intensity electrocautery may cause burn injuries to the bile ducts or late strictures by coagulating the vessels and jeopardizing the blood supply. The use of electrocautery during dissection near the common bile duct should be avoided. If the use of electrocautery is necessary for obtaining hemostasis, then it should be of very short duration and low intensity. Bipolar electrocautery, which delivers the current between two points in a more controlled fashion, may be a safer technique of hemostasis.

The initial enthusiasm for the use of laser during laparoscopic cholecystectomy collapsed after the observation that laser can cause severe injuries with loss of tissue.[17] The use of both electrocautery and laser should be avoided near metallic clips, which conduct the temperature and can cause thermal injury to surrounding tissues.

Diagnosis of the Injury

Presentation of the Patient

If the injury is not recognized intraoperatively, signs and symptoms vary according to the type and severity of the injury. Patients with small leaks from the cystic duct usually present with right upper quadrant pain, which is due to the intraperitoneal collection of bile. Fever and leukocytosis are common findings if infection is present. Lacerations of the common bile duct result in large accumulations of bile in the sub-hepatic area, which causes significant peritoneal irritation with severe pain, nausea, and vomiting. Physical examination reveals tenderness and guarding in the right upper quadrant. Absorption of bile from the peritoneal cavity results in elevation of total and direct bilirubin. Biliary peritonitis can be caused from suprainfection of the initially sterile bile collection. In these cases, the patient may present with a septic picture, including high fever, elevated white blood cell (WBC) count, and positive blood cultures.

Patients with postoperative bile duct strictures present with a picture of biliary obstruction. The time of presentation varies, but nearly 70% of patients are diagnosed within the first 6 months.[18] If the injury is suspected at the time of the surgery and the patient is regularly followed, then the first finding is progressive elevation of the liver function tests, particularly alkaline phosphatase and bilirubin. The patient may also present with jaundice or episodes of cholangitis caused by cholestasis.

The most valuable laboratory investigation is a complete liver profile, which will show evidence of cholestasis. The total and direct bilirubin may be elevated, alkaline phosphatase is usually elevated, and the amino-trasferases may be normal or slightly elevated. If long-lasting obstruction is present, then the synthetic function of the liver may be impaired, as shown by elevated prothrombin time and low albumin.

Imaging Studies

If a bile collection in the right upper quadrant is suspected, then ultrasonography (u/s) or computed tomographic (CT) scanning of the ab-domen will visualize the collection and assess the size of the common bile duct. The same studies can be used for guidance if percutaneous drainage of the collection is necessary. If the collection is small, then it may be difficult to differentiate from postoperative changes or small hematomas in the subhepatic area. In these cases, hepatobiliary scintigraphy may be helpful in visualizing an active bile leak or in demonstrating a complete duct obstruc-tion. Scintigraphy, however, cannot provide adequate anatomic definition of the injury, and further investigation will be necessary.

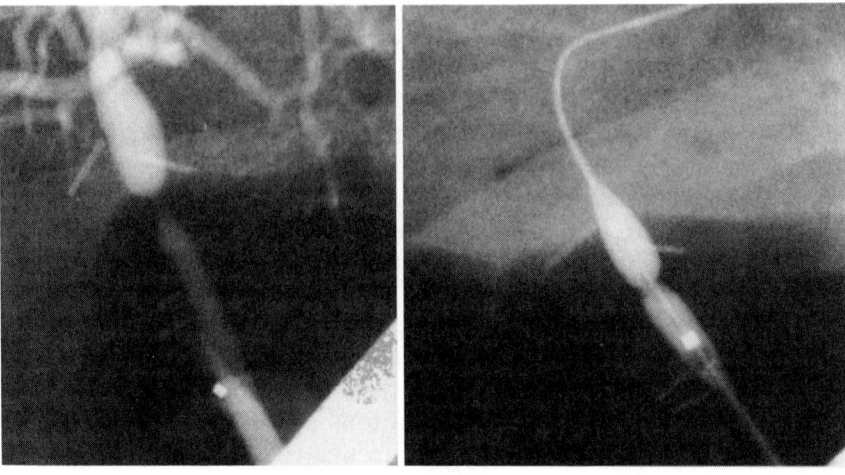

A   B

FIGURE 5.5. Endoscopic management of bile duct injury. (A) Short segment bile duct stricture following laparoscopic cholecystectomy with proximal dilatation. (B) Balloon dilatation of the stricture is performed through endoscope. (*Source*: Smith, MT, GA Leighman. Endoscopic management of benign biliary strictures. In: Braasch, JW, RK Tompkins. Surgical disease of the biliary tract and pancreas, Mosby, St. Louis, MO, 1994, p. 292.)

The study of choice in patients with suspected bile duct injury is the endoscopic retrograde cholangiopancreatoghphy (ERCP). ERCP can detect bile leaks from the cystic duct or from a lacerated common hepatic duct, bile duct strictures or retained stones (Fig. 5.5). The use of ERCP also offers some therapeutic options in the management of bile duct injuries, which are discussed below.

Percutaneous transhepatic cholangiography (PTC) is a valuable tool in assessing the proximal extent of the injury and in identifying the proximal biliary stump (Fig. 5.6). In cases of complete obstruction it can also visualize injured segmental ducts or it can be used for drainage of the proximal biliary tree. The information obtained from direct visualization of the biliary tree with ERCP or transhepatic cholangiography is essential before any surgical repair of the injury is attempted.

Management of Bile Duct Injuries

The strategy in the management of bile duct injuries depends upon two major factors: the type of injury and the time elapsed from the original operation until the injury is recognized. Advances in endoscopic and interventional techniques now offer more options in the treatment of complex injuries. The treatment of choice is surgical reconstruction of the injury or the strictures, combined, if necessary, with endoscopic or percutaneous techniques.

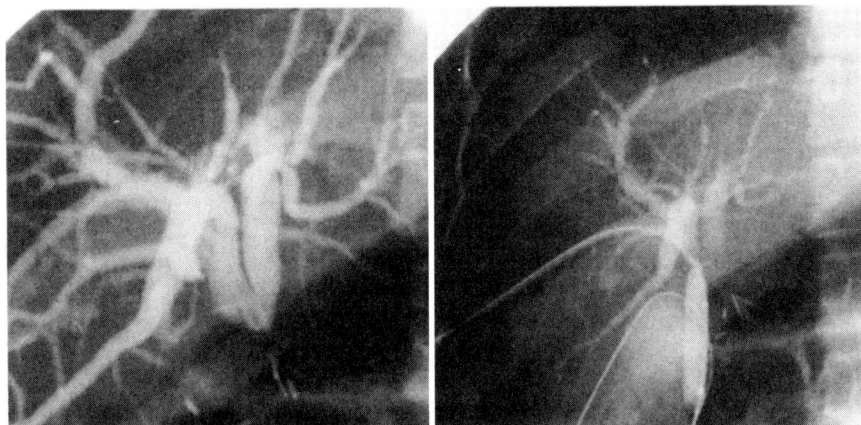

A   B

FIGURE 5.6. Percutaneous management of bile duct Injury. (A) Percutaneous transhepatic cholangiogram shows complete occlusion of choledochojejunostomy anastomosis, performed to repair injury sustained at laparoscopic cholecystectomy. (B) After percutaneous biliary drainage and passage of 8-mm diameter angioplasty balloon with dilatation of stricture. (*Source*: Kaufman, SL, Percutaneous dilatation of benign biliary strictures. In: Braasch, JW and RK Tompkins (eds.), Surgical disease of the biliary tract and pancreas, Mosby, St. Louis, MO, 1994, p. 281.)

Nonsurgical Methods

Interventional radiologic methods applied in the management of bile duct injuries include PTC and the CT- or u/s-guided drainage of collections. Bacteriologic examination of the fluid indicates the appropriate antibiotic coverage in cases of infection. Percutaneous catheter drainage of an infected collection is advisable before any surgical reconstruction is attempted. The transhepatic approach offers the option of draining the proximal biliary tree in cases of complete biliary obstruction. After the identification of the proximal extent of the injury, a transhepatic catheter can be placed over a guide wire, which can be left in place until the operation. Percutaneous techniques also have been used in the management of biliary strictures. Balloon dilators of various sizes are passed transhepatically over a guide wire to dilate biliary strictures. A stent is then left in place to maintain patency of the duct. Short-term results of this technique seem to be satisfactory.[19–21]

ERCP is a valuable tool in the diagnosis and management of bile duct injuries. Bile leaks from the cystic duct can be managed entirely endoscopically. After the site of the leak has been identified, a sphincterotomy is performed in order to lower the pressure in the common bile duct. Bile flow is pressure dependent and bile will take the path of least resistance. By lowering the pressure in the common bile duct, bile will flow preferentially distally into the duodenum and not through the cystic duct stump. Placement of a stent at the level of the leaking cystic duct may seal the leak and facilitate the healing. The stent is usually removed after 3–4 weeks. The report results of this technique in the management of bile leaks from the cystic duct are quite satisfactory.[22,23] Endoscopic dilatation of bile duct strictures can be attempted in cases of low-grade strictures and in patients who are poor surgical candidates. After a sphincterotomy is performed, a balloon catheter is advanced to the level of the stricture, and dilatation is attempted by inflating the balloon. After successful dilatation, a stent is left in place, which is removed after several weeks. The short- and medium-term results of this technique are good.[24,25] Interventional radiologic and endoscopic techniques may be used alone or in combination with surgery for the management of postoperative bile duct injuries, in selected groups of patients. Due to the fact that there are few long-term results with these methods, surgical reconstruction remains the gold standard in the management of iatrogenic injuries of the bile ducts.

Surgical Treatment

Mayo performed the first reconstruction of a post cholecystectomy injury in 1905 by anastomosing the hepatic duct with the jejunum. The number of reconstructive operations on the biliary tract is increasing as a result of the increasing number of bile duct injuries. The goal of the operative reconstruction is to restore the continuity of the biliary tree or to reestablish normal flow of bile in the gastrointestinal tract. Two main categories of operations exist: (1) reestablishment of the continuity of the biliary tract by directly reanastomosing the injured bile duct, and (2) creating an anastomosis between the bile duct and the gastrointestinal tract. The type of operation depends on the type of injury, the timing of the repair, and the experience of the surgeon.

Repair of Injuries Recognized at the Time of Initial Surgery

Repair of Small Lacerations

Small partial lacerations of the bile ducts or small injuries that result from avulsion of the cystic duct can be repaired directly over the T-tube. The defect of the bile duct wall should be minimal, and the blood supply preserved in order to safely attempt this approach. More significant defects should be repaired with one of the procedures described in the following sections.

End-to-End Repair

If bile duct injury is suspected at the time of the laparoscopic cholecystectomy, then an intraoperative cholangiogram should be performed to confirm the injury and to delineate the anatomy of the bile ducts. The procedure is converted to open celiotomy and the injury is reassessed. If the injury involves the common bile duct or the common hepatic duct, then an end-to-end anastomosis of the duct may be attempted. This type of repair should be avoided, however, in cases of high injury, near the confluence of the two hepatic ducts. Absolute requirements for performing this procedure are: (1) no loss of bile duct tissue, (2) enough length of the duct to allow a tension-free anastomosis, (3) a bile duct adequate size, (4) preserved blood supply to the two stumps, and (5) absence of infection in the right upper quadrant. The duodenum is mobilized with a Kocher maneuver to facilitate the approximation of the two segments. The segment of the duct that has sustained a sharp injury or has been clipped should be excised to well vascularized viable tissue. A single layer anastomosis is constructed in an end-to-end fashion by using monofilament absorbable or nonabsorbable suture material. A T-tube is usually placed in the duct with the long limb exiting through a separate site. The T-tube is removed after a few weeks. A closed system or a sump catheter can be left in place to drain any bile leaks.

Repair of Biliary Strictures and Injuries Recognized Postoperatively

The majority of bile duct injuries are recognized postoperatively; therefore, reconstruction takes place several days or even weeks after the initial operation. In a similar way, operations for biliary strictures are undertaken after a significant time period has lapsed since the initial operation. As a result, inflammatory reaction or fibrosis may be found at the time of reconstruction. Drainage of bile collections and control of infection is essential before any attempt at reconstruction. The goal of the operation is to create an anastomosis of the bile duct with the gastrointestinal tract. The segment of the GI tract used for the anastomosis is either the duodenum (choledochoduodenostomy) or the jejunum (roux-en-Y choledocho- or hepaticojejunostomy). Using the duodenum for the anastomosis offers the advantage of endoscopic accessibility if a postoperative anastomotic stricture develops. Creation of a choledochoduodenostomy for repair of a bile duct injury is not feasible most of the time because of the distance between the segment of the duct proximal to the injury and the duodenum. The anastomosis is also prone to stricture formation, due to the small size of the injured bile duct, or the presence of crush or thermal injury to the duct.

Hepaticojejunostomy and Choledochojejunostomy

The operation begins with dissection of the area of the porta hepatis and identification of the bile ducts. The injury or stricture is identified and any devitalized or fibrosed tissue is excised. Placement of an endoscopic or transhepatic stent in the biliary duct before the operation may facilitate the recognition of the structures and the dissection. The distal bile duct is oversewn and the proximal segment is debrided to healthy tissue. A Roux-en-Y loop of jejunum is used to create an end-to-side mucosa-to-mucosa anastomosis (Fig. 5.7). The anastomosis can be performed in one or two layers using absorbable or nonabsorbable monofilament suture material. The use of transanastomotic stents is controversial. The use of the stent is not necessary when the distal hepatic duct or the common bile duct is used for the anastomosis, if a wide mucosa-to-mucosa anastomosis has been created.[26] For intrahepatic anastomosis near the confluence of the hepatic ducts, the placement of the stent may facilitate the creation of the anastomosis,[27] as a stent, a T-tube, or a silastic transhepatic tube can be used. The timing of removal of the stent depends on the quality of the segment of the bile duct used. If the proximal segment of the duct was fibrosed or adequate length was not available for a mucosa-to-mucosa anastomosis, then a long-term stent may be necessary. A horseshoe-shaped matallic marker or a coronary bypass type "O" ring can be sewn to the antimesenteric border of the Roux limb and secured to the anterior abdominal wall to allow for a transjejunal biliary intervention in the future.[28] The use of a Roux-en-Y limb of jejunum is preferable because it prevents the reflux of intestinal contents into the bile duct and minimizes the risk of cholangitis.

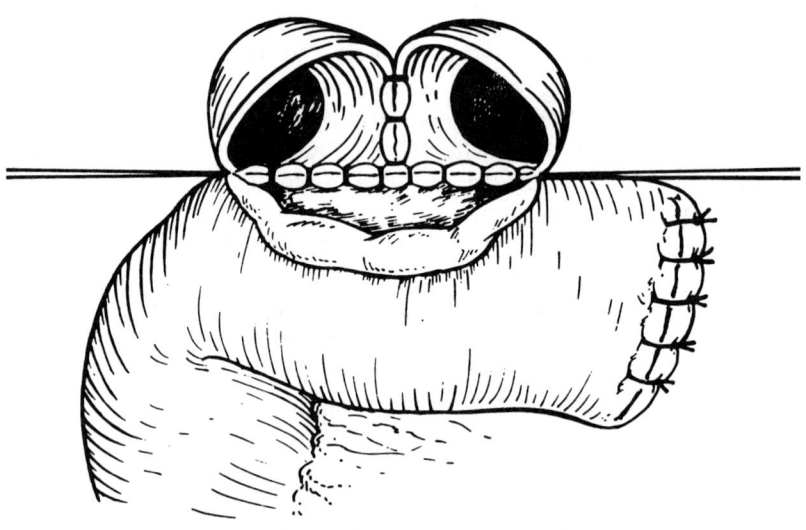

FIGURE 5.7. Technique of high hepaticojejunostomy anastomosis. An end-to-side anastomosis is created to the roux limb of jejunum. The right and left hepatic ducts are joined to form a single large anastomosis. (*Source*: Cuschieri, A. Sclerosing Cholangitis. In: Schwartz SI, Ellis H (eds) Maingot's Abdominal Operations, 8th ed. Appleton-Century Crofts, Norwalket.)

Repair of High Biliary Strictures: The Hepp-Couinaud Technique

Biliary strictures located just below the confluence of the hepatic ducts or which involve the confluence (Bismuth type III and IV) are technically difficult to repair. Often the confluence has to be debrided and an anastomosis of both the hepatic ducts and the jejunum is created. In cases where severe inflammation of the region of the bifurcation prevents adequate dissection or visualization of the confluence, the use of the left hepatic duct for an anastomosis proximal to the bifurcation may be preferable because (1) the anatomic consistency of the left hepatic duct and its branches, and (2) the left duct is more accessible than the right in the hilum of the liver.

Based on the anatomic works of Couinaud, Jacques Hepp redescribed the operative technique of exposure and dissection of the intrahepatic segment of the left hepatic duct and the creation of anastomosis of the left hepatic duct with a limb of jejunum for the repair of high biliary duct strictures.[29] The left hepatic duct lies outside the liver parenchyma, between the caudate and the quadrate lobes of the liver. The left duct is the most anterior element of the portal triad, and dividing the hilar plate ("la plaque hilair") which Couinaud described as a "thickened part of Glisson's capsule," can expose it. The operation begins by dissecting the area of the hilum and recognizing the confluence of the hepatic ducts. The use of a 25 G needle to aspirate bile facilitates the identification of the ducts. An intraoperative cholangiogram is performed to delineate the anatomy of the bile ducts. The ligamentum teres is divided and retracted cephalad to expose the inferior aspect of the liver. The Glisson's capsule is incised between the caudate and quadrate lobes, and the hilar plate is separated from the liver parenchyma with blunt dissection. The left hepatic duct is opened after it has been exposed, and a wide side-to-side hepaticojejunostomy with a Roux-en-Y limb of jejunum is created (Fig. 5.8). The use of a stent is optional and depends on the technicalities of each particular anastomosis and the preferences of the surgeon. The stent may be a "U"-shaped tube or a straight tube exiting through the liver or through the jejunum. The subhepatic area is drained with a closed suction or a sump drain, which is removed postoperatively, if there is no biliary drainage.

Mucosal Graft: Rodney Smith Technique

If the creation of a mucosa-to-mucosa anastomosis is not feasible, due to inability to dissect the hilar structures, then the mucosal graft technique can be used to create a communications of the left hepatic duct with the jejunum. The left hepatic duct is cannulated transhepatically. The tube is advanced to the hilum of the liver and pulled out at the level of the hepatic duct confluence. The tube is subsequently introduced in the jejunal loop through an opening and sutured to the jejunum. The transhepatic tube is pulled to bring the jejunum into the hilum of the liver. The serosa of the

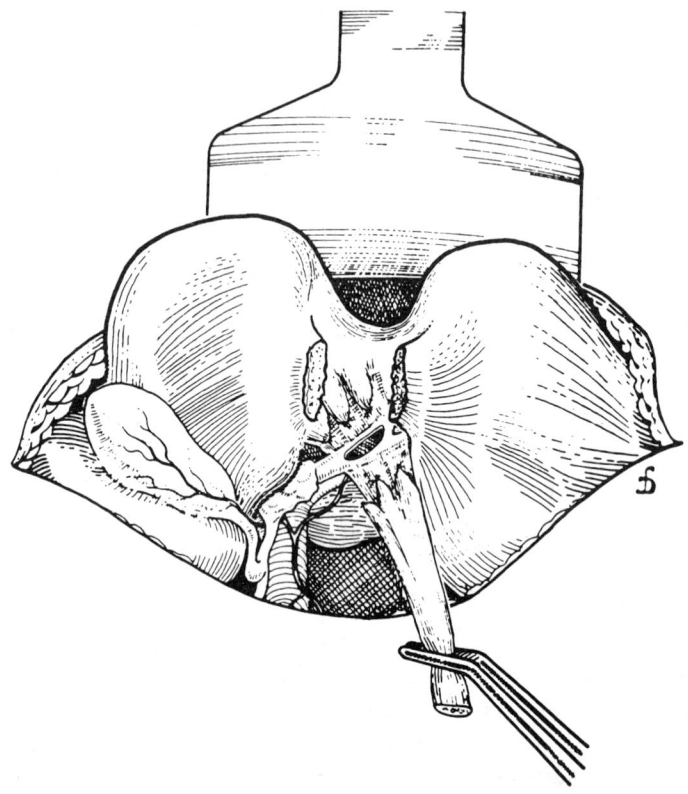

FIGURE 5.8. Approach to left hepatic duct for biliary enteric anastomosis. Left hepatic (segment III) duct is exposed beneath the hilar plate after dissection through the ligamentum teres. A long choledochotomy can be made to allow an ample anastomosis to a Roux-en-Y limb of jejunum. (*Source*: Blumgart, LH, CJ Kelly. BR J Surg 1984;71:257, Blackwell Science LTD.)

jejunum is sutured to the Glisson's capsule with interrupted sutures. The reported long-term results of this technique are good.[30]

Long-Term Results

The operative mortality for repair of bile duct strictures is significant. In a cumulative review of 7,643 procedures performed in 5,586 patients since 1900, an overall mortality rate of 8.3% was reported.[31] More recent reviews, however, report mortality less than 5%.[12,32] The number of previous attempts at repair and the type of the stricture significantly influence the operative mortality. Operations for repair of type III and IV strictures, as well as operation performed for repair of recurrent strictures, have significantly higher mortality.[1] The operative morbidity is also significant and it is influenced by the same factors.[1,32] The most common postoperative complications for operations performed for biliary reconstruction are: anastomotic leak, cholangitis, and hepatic failure.

The high incidence of recurrent stricture in patients who undergo biliary reconstruction for an iatrogenic injury to the bile ducts makes the long-term follow up of these patients necessary. Patients with recurrent strictures usually present with abdominal pain, liver failure, jaundice, and recurrent episodes of cholangitis. Some patients present with mild elevation of liver function tests, but remain asymptomatic. Grading systems have been developed to evaluate the outcome of patients undergoing operations for a benign biliary stricture (Table 5.2).

Mild elevation of liver enzymes is not uncommon after biliary reconstruction. Progressive elevation of liver enzymes even in the absence of symptoms should alert the surgeon to further investigate the possibility of a recurrent stricture. Ultrasound examination of the liver may show intrahepatic ductile dilatation. If the bile ducts are dilated or if the patient experiences episodes of cholangitis, then imaging of the biliary tree is necessary. If the patient has had Roux-en-Y hepaticojejunostomy, then detailed imaging of the bile ducts and the anastomosis can be achieved with percutaneous transhepatic cholangiography.

Good long-term results can be achieved in 70–80% of patients.[18,33] The success of the repair is inversely proportional to the number of previous operations for reconstruction.[12] Other factors influencing the outcome are: the type of the injury, the type of the repair, and the experience of the surgeon. Operations for repair of higher type II and IV injuries have a higher incidence of recurrent strictures. For proximal strictures, especially type IV strictures, superior results have been reported with the Hepp-Couinaud technique.[34] The long-term results of end-to-end primary repair of the bile duct seem to be inferior overall to the results of the hepaticojejunostomy. A failure rate of 40–50%, for end-to-end repair, has been reported in series with long patient follow up.[35,36]

The experience of the surgeon is an important factor influencing the outcome of the operation. The success of the initial repair is crucial in the

TABLE 5.2. Grading system for evaluation of patients undergoing operation for benign biliary stricture.

Grade A:	Normal LFTs, asymptomatic.
Grade B:	Mild elevation LFTs, asymptomatic.
Grade C:	Abnormal LFTs, cholangitis, pain.
Grade D:	Surgical revision or dilatation required.

From McDonald ML, Farnell MB, Nagorney DM, et al. Benign biliary strictures: repair and outcome with a contemporary approach. Surgery 1995;118:582–591.

long-term patency of the anastomosis. If the surgeon is not experienced in performing high hepaticojejunostomies, he or she should ask for assistance or refer the patient to a center with experience in this type of operation.

Long-term follow up of patients is necessary because recurrent strictures may appear months or even years after the initial repair. Approximately two-thirds of the recurrent strictures will appear within 2 years, and 90% within five years of the initial operation.[18] If a recurrent stricture occurs, then transhepatic balloon dilatation and stent placement may be effective. Percutaneously placed angioplasty balloon catheters are used to progressively dilate the stricture. A stent is left in place after the procedure. Most of the patients with recurrent strictures, however, will require reoperation. Reoperations for repair of recurrent bile duct strictures are generally more laborious, due to the significant amount of fibrosis present and the difficult dissection of hilum of the liver. In this case, the utilization of the left hepatic duct for the anastomosis is an effective approach.

References

1. Moossa AR, Mayer AD, Stabile B. Iatrogenic injury to the bile duct. Who, how, where. Arch Surg 1990;125:1028–1031.
2. Smith EB. Iatrogenic injuries to extrahepatic bile duct and associated vessels: a 25-year analysis. J Natl Med Assoc 1982;74:735–738.
3. Roslyn JJ, Binns GS, Hughes EFX, et al. Open cholecystectomy. A contemporary analysis of 42,474 patients. Ann Surg 1993;218:129–137.
4. Route M, Podlech P, Jaschke W, et al. Management of bile duct injuries and strictures following cholecystectomy. World J Surg 1993;17:553–562.
5. Gouma DJ, Go PM. Bile duct injury during laparoscopic and conventional cholecystectomy. J Am Coll Surg 1994;253:229–233.
6. Deziel DJ, Millikan KW, Economou SG, et al. Complications of laparoscopic cholecystectomy: a national survey of 4,292 hospitals and an analysis of 77,640 cases. Am J Surg 1993;165:9–14.
7. Peck JJ. Endoscopic cholecystectomy: an analysis of complications. Arch Surg 1991;126:1197.
8. Wolfe BM, Gardiner BN, Leary BF, et al. Endoscopic cholecystectomy: an analysis of complications. Arch Surg 1991;126:1192–1198.
9. Bonatsos G, Leandros E, Dourakis N, et al. Laparoscopic eholesystectomy. Intraoperative findings and postoperative complications. Surg Endosc 1995; 9:889–893.
10. Rossi RL, Schirmer WJ, Braasch JW, et al. Laparoscopic bile duct injuries. Risk factors, recognition and repair. Arch Surg 1992;127:596–602.
11. Asbun HJ, Rossi RL, Lowell JA, et al. Bile duct injury during laparoscopic cholecystectomy: mechanism of injury, prevention and management. World J Surg 1993;17:547–552.
12. Blumgart LH, Kelley CJ, Benjamin IS. Benign bile duct strictures following cholecystectomy: critical factors in management. Br J Surg 1984;71:836–843.
13. Csendes A, Diaz JC, Burdiles P, et al. Mirizzi syndrome and cholecystobiliary fistula: a unifying classification. Br J Surg 1989;76:1139–1143.

14. Davidoff AM, Pappas TN, Murray EA, et al. Mechanisms of major biliary injury during laparoscopic cholecystectomy. Ann Surg 1992;21593:196–202.

15. Southern Surgeons Club. A prospective analysis of 1,518 laparoscopic cholecystectomies. N Engl J Med 1991;324:1073–1078.

16. Larson GM, Vitale GC, Casey, et al. Multipractice analysis of laparoscopic cholecystectomy in 1,983 patients. Am J Surg 1992;163:221–226.

17. Easter DW, Moossa AR. Laser and laparoscopic cholecystectomy: a hazardous union. Arch Surg 1991;126:423.

18. Pitt HA, Miyamoto T, Parapatis SK, et al. Factors influencing outcome in patients with postoperative biliary strictures. Am J Surg 144:14–21.

19. Lee MJ, Mueller PR, Saini S, et al. Percutaneous dilatation of benign biliary strictures: single-session therapy with general anesthesia. AJR 1991;157:1263–1266.

20. Maccioni F, Rossi M, Salvatori FM, et al. Metallic stents in benign biliary strictures: three-year follow-up. Card Interv Radiol 1992;15:360–366.

21. Trambert JJ, Bron KM, Zajko AB, et al. Percutaneous transhepatic balloon dilatation of benign biliary strictures. AJR 1987;149:945–948.

22. Rezieg M, Barkun JS, Barkun AN. The management of bile leaks in the era of laparoscopic cholecystectomy. Gastrointest Endosc 1993;39:330.

23. Howell DA, Bosco JL, Sampson LN, et al. Endoscopic management of cystic duct fistulas after laparoscopic cholecystectomy. Endoscopy 1992;24:796–798.

24. Davids PHP, Rauws EAJ, Coene PPLO, et al. Endoscopic stenting for postoperative biliary strictures. Gastrointest Endosc 1992;38:12–18.

25. Berkelhammer C, Kortan P, Haber GB. Endoscopic biliary prosthesis as treatment for benign postoperative bile duct strictures. Gastrointest Endoc 1989; 35:95–101.

26. Lillemoe KD, Pitt HA, Cameron JL. Postoperative bile duct strictures. Surg Clin N Am 1990;70:1355–1379.

27. Rossi RL, Tsao JL. Biliary reconstruction. Surg Clin N Am 1994;74:825–841.

28. Branum G, Schmitt C, Baillie J, et al. Management of major biliary complications after laparoscopic cholecystectomy. Ann Surg 1993;217:532–542.

29. Hepp J. Hepaticojejunostomy using the left biliary trunk for iatrogenic biliary lesions: the French connection. World J Surg 1985;9:507–511.

30. Wexler MJ, Smith R. Jejunal mucosal graft: a sutureless technique for repair of high bile duct strictures. Am J Surg 1975;129:204–211.

31. Warren KW, Christophi C, Armendari ZR. The evolution and current perspectives of the treatment of benign bile duct strictures: a review. Surg Gastroenterol 1982;1:141–154.

32. Genest JF, Ganon E, Grunfest-Broniatowski S. Benign biliary stricutres: an analytic review (1970–1984). Am Surg 1986;99:409–413.

33. Innes JT, Ferrara JJ, Carey LC. Biliary reconstruction without transanastomotic stent. Am Surg 1988;54:27–30.

34. McDonald ML, Farnell MB, Nagorney DM, et al. Benign biliary strictures: repair and outcome with a contemporary approach. Surgery 1995;118:582–591.

35. Pellegrini CA, Thomas MJ, Way LW. Recurrent biliary stricture: patterns of recurrence and outcome of surgical therapy. Am J Surg 1984;147:175–180.

36. Csendes A, Diaz JC, Burdiles P, et al. Late results of immediate primary end-to-end repair in accidental section of the common bile duct. GO 1989;168:125–130.

Part II
Gastric and Esophageal Surgery

6
Endogastric Surgery

MARGRET ODDSDOTTIR

Lesions of the gastric wall and the gastric mucosa usually require removal either because of symptoms or for diagnosis. Wedge resections are sometimes possible for small lesions on the anterior wall of the body of the stomach; however, a careful excision via gastrotomy or partial gastrectomy have been required for lesions on the posterior gastric wall and those close to either the pylorus or the gastroesophageal junction. For a trained laparoscopic surgeon, a laparoscopic wedge resection of an anterior gastric wall lesion can usually be accomplished. Laparoscopic endogastric surgery has been gaining popularity. Endogastric surgery was first described by Way et al. using special trocars for intraluminal surgery to do pancreatic cystgastrostomy.[1] Several reports have been published subsequently that use similar techniques to remove gastric lesions.[2–8] The method has been given several different names, such as endoluminal surgery, endogastric surgery, laparoscopic intragastric surgery (LIGS), and transgastric surgery. The techniques vary slightly, but along with a gastroscope all involve a laparoscopic approach with special trocars passed through the abdominal wall and the anterior gastric wall into the stomach.

Preoperative localization of a gastric lesion is often inaccurate. When dealing with a gastric lesion that requires excision, the surgeon therefore needs to be prepared to do endogastric surgery or a laparoscopic wedge resection, as well as a laparoscopic gastrotomy and excicion of the lesion from within the stomach. Neither wedge resection nor gastrotomy and excision are by definition endogastric surgery; however, both are techniques that the laparoscopic surgeon needs to be ready to perform when planning endogastric surgery to remove a gastric lesion.[9–15] A brief description of thesc techniques will therefore be included in this text.

Indications

Pancreatic cystgastrostomy was the first procedure described using laparoscopic endoluminal surgery.[1,8] It is feasible because one can create a nice window with good hemostasis and an excellent view of the interior of

TABLE 6.1. Endogastric surgery—indications.

- Cyst-gastrostomy
- Gastric polyps
- Submucosal gastric tumors
- Bleeding gastric ulcers
- Dieulafoy's
- (Early gastric cancer)

the cyst. Any type of benign gastric lesion that needs excision is an indication for laparoscopic endogastric surgery. Table 6.1 shows the indications published so far.

Patient Preparation and Position

The work-up of each patient varies, depending on the lesion and/or the underlying disease (Fig. 6.1). A CT-scan and/or endoluminal ultrasound may help to delineate the size and depth of a submucosal mass or a pseudocyst, but an esophagogastroduodenoscopy is performed in all of these patients.

The patient is prepared for general anesthesia as well as possible laparotomy. Gastroscopy equipment with a video-screen needs to be in

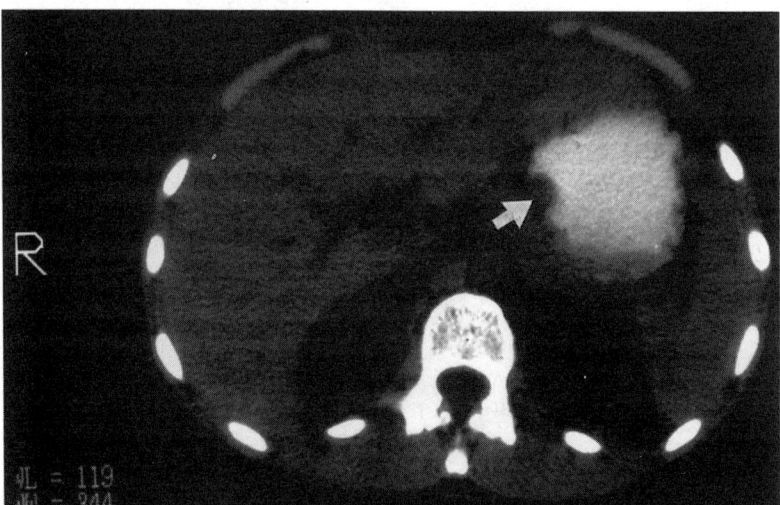

FIGURE 6.1. CT-scan of a submucosal lesion on the lesser curvature of the stomach. The lesion was successfully excised, using endoluminal techniques. The lesion turned out to be a pancreatic rest.

the room (or, if using the OR video screens, the possibility of doing a split screen picture). It will facilitate the procedure if a skilled endoscopic surgeon drives the gastroscope. It is possible, but cumbersome, to have the operative surgeon or an assistant brake the field and do the gastroscopy. It varies from one case to the other how much the gastroscope is used, but it is always needed for localization of the lesion. In addition, the gastroscope can be very helpful with the placement and the introduction of trocars into the stomach and with insufflation of the stomach, and it can also be used to retreive the specimen with an endoscopic basket.

Technique

The patient is placed supine on the operating table. For many lesions in the stomach, especially in the upper part and at the gastroesophageal junction, it is convenient for the surgeon to stand between the patients legs. For endogastric surgery there are basically two techniques used for access. They vary slightly and will be described separately. Wedge resection and excision via gastrotomy will be described briefly because they are an option that may prove more feasible when the lesion has been properly localized intraoperatively. In general, when a submucosal tumor is removed, the mucosal defect can be left open if it is small (<3–4cm) and it is only a mucosal defect. If large or deep, then the defect needs to be oversewn with either running or interrupted absorbable stitches.

Endogastric Surgery I

After insufflation the first 10-mm trocar for the laparoscope, is placed in the umbilicus. A 5-mm trocar is placed in the epigastrium. The gastroscope is advanced into the stomach, the stomach insufflated, and the lesion identified. With a grasper in the epigastric port, one can now localize the lesion exactly. If endogastric surgery seems appropriate, three Radially Expanding Dilators 5-mm trocars (R.E.D.) (from InnerDyne Inc., 1244 Reamwood Ave, Sunnyvale, CA 94089) are passed through the abdominal wall and the anterior gastric wall and into the stomach (Fig. 6.2). If possible, at least 3cm should be between each trocar. If the trocars are placed too closely to one another, bimanual work will be difficult. Both the laparoscopic view and the gastroscopic view guide the trocar placement. For the first R.E.D. trocar it may be necessary to grasp the anterior stomach wall while inserting it into the stomach. Once the trocars are placed, a 5-mm, 30-degree forward oblique viewing laparoscope is passed into the stomach. The intra-abdominal pressure is lowered to below 8mmHg, and the stomach insufflated to 15mmHg. It is usually not necessary to obstruct the duodenum with a balloon to prevent air leak. With working instruments in the two remaining R.E.D. ports, the lesion is excised, bleeding is oversewn, or the

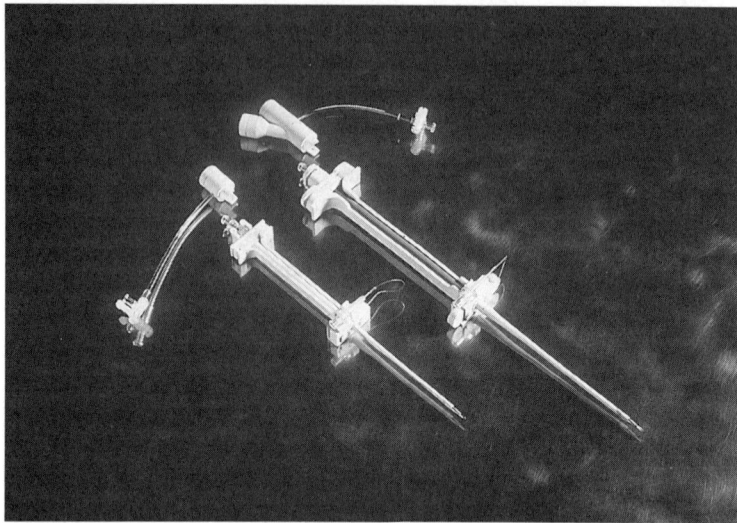

FIGURE 6.2. Radially expanding dilators trocars (R.E.D.). These trocars have a sharp core needle for introduction. The outer sheath is radially expanded, once the trocar is in place. The balloon at the end is then insufflated.

pancreatic pseudocyst is fenestrated. Regular 5-mm laparoscopic instruments are used. If a specimen needs to be retrieved, it can be placed in a wire basket passed via the gastroscope, and pulled out through the esophagus. The trocars are pulled back into the abdomen when the intragastric procedure is finished. Because these trocars are radially expanding, the holes in the gastric wall are small and one interrupted 2-0 stitch is enough to close each of them.

Endogastric Surgery II

The second technique begins with gastroscopy. The stomach is insufflated and the lesion is identified. While observing the image from the gastroscope, the abdominal wall is compressed to select the sites for the trocars. Skin incisions are made and three trocars with balloons on the shaft, are introduced through the abdominal wall directly into the distended stomach. With the balloons inflated the stomach is pulled against the abdominal wall (Fig. 6.3). Again, if possible, the trocars should be at least 3 cm apart. Any size of trocars can be used. A laparoscope and standard laparoscopic instruments are passed directly into the stomach. If a specimen is obtained, then it can be retrieved either with the gastroscope using a wire-basket or through the laparoscopic cannula. If a malignancy is suspected, then the specimen is placed in a bag before retrieval. Using this technique, the trocar

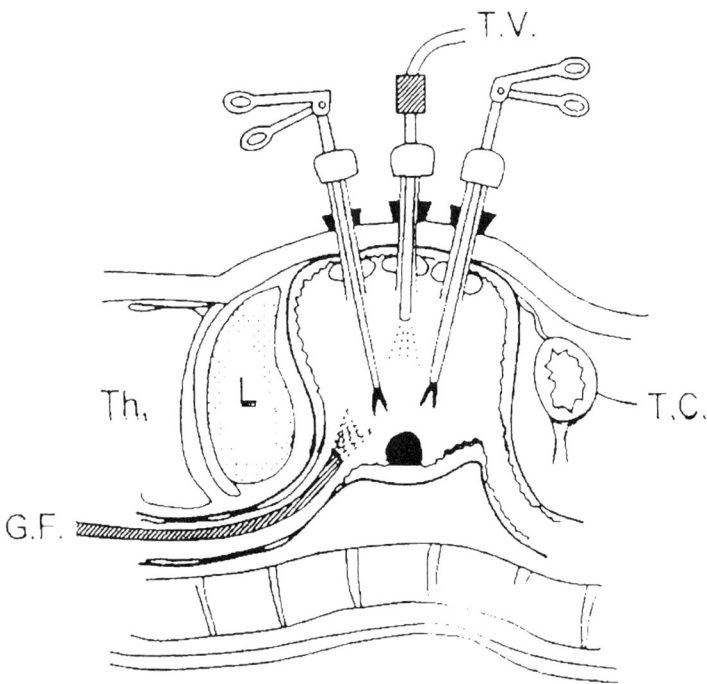

FIGURE 6.3. Trocars with ballons on the shaft have been introduced into the stomach. With the balloons inflated, the stomach is pulled up against the abdominal wall. (From Ohashi S: Laparoscopic intraluminal (intragastric) surgery for early gastric cancer: A new concept in laparoscopic surgery. Surg Endosc 9: 169–171, Springer-Verlag, 1995; with permission.)

size allows an ultrasonically activated shears or a laparoscopic stapler to be used inside the stomach. When the intragastric surgery is done, the trocars are pulled out of the stomach and a pneumoperitoneum established. The trocar stab wounds in the gastric wall are closed with interrupted stitches.

Wedge Resection

If the location and the size of the lesion is such that a wedge resection is possible, then wedge resection is usually the simplest option. One still needs a gastroscope to localize the lesion and guide the resection. Three trocars are placed, but one needs to be placed in a convenient position and be big enough for a laparoscopic stapler. Several applications of the stapler may be necessary (Fig. 6.4). The wedge resection can similarly be done with scissors and diathermy or the ultrasonically activated shears, leaving a gastrotomy to be closed.

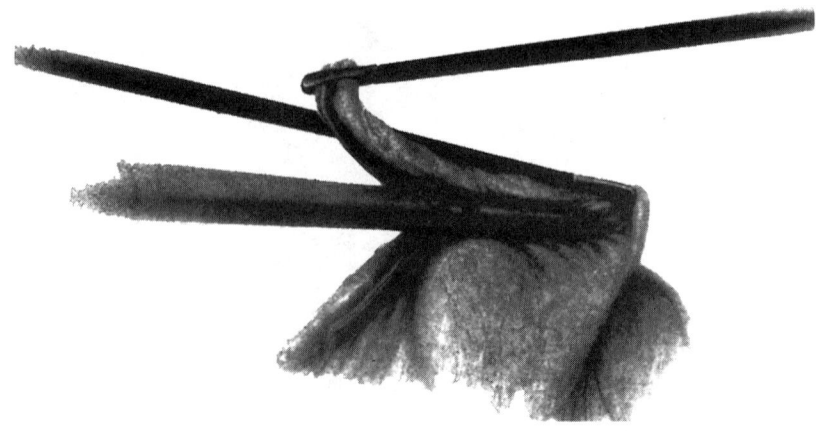

FIGURE 6.4. Wedge resection being done using a laparoscopic stapler.

Gastrotomy and Excision

Excision of a gastric lesion via laparoscopic gastrotomy can be used for any of the indications listed for endogastric surgery independant of the location. Gastroscopy is helpful here to localize the lesion and guide the gastrotomy placement. A significantly smaller gastrotomy is needed for laparoscopic procedures than for open procedures. The gastrotomy can done using electrocautery and scissors, the ultrasonically activated shears, or a laparoscopic stapler. The edges of the gastrotomy are pulled apart. This gives an excellent view and access to most sites of the stomach. The laparoscopic intragastric procedure is performed using standard laparoscopic instruments. The gastrotomy can be closed with stitches or a stapler. There is obviously more risk of spillage of gastric secretions with a gastrotomy than with the techniques described earlier; however, spill can be minimized with good gastric suctioning before and during the gastric procedure. Postoperative infection because of peritoneal contamination has not been a problem in the reported cases.[10,11,13,15]

Results

The reported results of endogastric surgery are good. No complications are reported in the litterature, except for a postoperative fever for 24 hours in one patient;[8] however, reported series are small, and some only case reports.

At the University Hospital of Iceland, seven patients have had laparoscopic gastric surgery for benign gastric lesions. Table 6.2 lists the indications and the procerdures performed for each of these seven patients. The one complication thus far occured after a gastrotomy and excision of a

TABLE 6.2. Laparoscopic gastric surgery, University Hospital Iceland.

Endogastric
- cyst-gastrostomy
- adenomatous polyps
- submucosal tumor (*pancreatic rest*)
- bleeding ulcer (*cardia*)

Gastrotomy
- submucosal tumor (*pancreatic rest*)

Wedge resection
- adenomatous polyp
- gastric ulcer with dysplasia

Note: Technique applied in seven patients.

subucosal lesion. A 32-year-old male with intermittent epigastric pain and vomiting was found on gastroscopy to have a submucosal lesion in the distal corpus near the greater curvature, and a wedge resection was planned. When localized intraoperatively with gastroscopy and laparoscopy, however, it was obviously too close to the pylorus for a wedge resection. Because we were out of the special balloon trocars, an anterior gastrotomy was made and the lesion was excised. The defect was oversewn and the gastrotomy was closed with a running stitch. He began taking liquids by mouth on the first postoperative day but on the following day, he developed severe epigastric pain with guarding and rebound tenderness. When taken to the operating room for laparoscopy a few hours later, he was found to have a leak at the proximal end of the sutured gastrotomy. There was no spill in the abdomen. The leak, which seemed to be between the last few running stitches, was oversewn without further sequela. Except for this one patient, who stayed in the hospital for 7 days, the patients were discharged on postoperative day 2 or 3.

Comments

Endogastric surgery combines laparoscopic and endoscopic techniques. It provides minimally invasive access to lesions in the gastric wall or cysts behind the stomach that would otherwise be difficult via the laparoscope alone. In addition, it often provides a better view of the field than observed during laparotomy. This is especially true for lesions in upper part of the stomach.

For lesions on the anterior gastric wall, wedge resection may be feasible if the lesions are not too close to the pylorus or the gastroesophageal junction. It may be difficult to decide on what will be the best approach until in the operating room because gastroscopy alone does not always provide good localization. Laparoscopic gastrotomy and excision of the lesion may be preferred if the lesions are big or the exposure difficult using endoluminal techniques. When planning a laparoscopic approach to a gastric lesion, it is therefore important to be ready to perform any of the previously mentioned techniques. The exact localization of the lesion will determine which technique will be appropriate. Finally, if there is any suspicion of malignancy, then these techniques should be used with caution and the specimen placed in a bag before retrieval. Size, depth of penetration, histology, and possible dissemination have to be outlined prior to resection.

References

1. Way LW, Legha P, Mori T. Laparoscopic cystgastrostomy: the first operation in the field of intraluminal laparoscopic surgery. Surg Endosc 1994;8:448.
2. Taniguchi E, Kamiike W, Yamanishi H, et al. Laparoscopic intragastric surgery foor gastric leiomyoma. Surg Endosc 1997;11:287–289.
3. Kanehira E, Mori A, Watanabe T, et al. A technique of laparoscopic intragastric surgery in the treatment of gastric carcinoma in situ. Surg Endosc 1994;8:547.
4. Hashimoto S, Munakata Y, Hayashi K, et al. Laparoscopic intraluminal resection for the submucosal tumor in the cardia. Surg Endosc 1994;8:547.
5. Murai R, Ando H, Mitsumori N, et al. Laparoscopic intragastric mucosal resection. Surg Endosc 1994;8:599.
6. Kitano S, Kawanaka H, Tomikawa M, et al. Bleeding from gastric ulcer halted by laparoscopic suture ligation. Surg Endosc 1994;8:405–407.
7. Ohashi S. Laparoscopic intraluminal (intragastric) surgery for early gastric cancer. A new concept in laparoscopic surgery. Surg Endosc 1995;9:169–171.
8. Gagner M. Laparoscopic transgastric cystogastrostomy for pancreatic pseudocyst. Sages Manual, 1994; p 73.
9. Gurbuz AT, Peetz ME. Resection of a gastric leiomyoma using combined laparoscopic and gastroscopic approach. Surg Endosc 1997;11:285–286.
10. Ibrahim IM, Silvestri F, Zingler B. Laparoscopic resection of posterior gastric leiomyoma. Surg Endosc 1997;11:277–279.
11. Siu WT, Leong HT, Li MKW. Laparoscopic resection of bleeding gastric polyps. Surg Endosc 1997;11:283–284.
12. Otani Y, Ohgami M, Hoshiya Y, et al. Laparoscopic wedge resection of the stomach for carcinoid tumor using a lesion lifting method. Surg Endosc 1997; 8:546.
13. Basso N, Silecchia G, Pizzuto G, et al. Laparoscopic excision of posterior gastric wall leiomyoma. Surg Laparosc Endosc 1996;6:65–67.
14. Yamashita Y, Bekki F, Kakegawa T, et al. Two laparoscopic techniques for resection of leiomyoma in the stomach. Surg Laparosc Endosc 1995;5:38–42.
15. Petelin JB, Renner P. Laparoscopic pancreatic pseudocyst-gastrostomy. Surg Endosc 1994;8:448.

7
Anatomy and Clinical Outcomes in Surgery for Esophageal Reflux

RIFAT LATIFI, JAMES C. ROSSER JR., and HAROLD BREM

Anatomy of Laparoscopic Antireflux Surgery

Performance of laparoscopic antireflux surgery requires mastery of pertinent anatomy as seen through the laparoscope. Important landmarks include the left lobe of the liver, the left triangular ligament, the gastrophrenic ligament the phrenoesophageal ligament, the caudate lobe of liver, the anterior vagus with its hepatic branch, the right posterior vagus nerve, the distal esophagus, the left and right crura of the diaphragm, the stomach, spleen, and short gastric vessels. In addition to the preceding structures detailed familiarity with the lesser omentum, aortic hiatus, vessels and lymphatics of the hiatal region as well as the diaphragm, transverse colon, and pancreas are essential. Understanding the normal and pathological anatomy and its variants as seen in laparoscopic dissection will minimze or help avoid misadventures such as bleeding, liver injuries, gastric perforation, splenic injuries, pneumomediastinum, dysphagia and vagal injuries. Examples of important anatomical structures[1,2] are found in Figures 7.1 to 7.4.

Clinical Studies

Although long-term clinical outcomes of laparoscopic fundoplication (LFP) will not be known for several decades, the short-term success of this operation has been established.[3] Outcomes of laparoscopic Nissen fundoplication (LNF) and open Nissen fundoplication were similar in 81 patients (47 open, 34 LNF) graded by functional parameters.[4] There was no mortality in either group and no difference in morbidity, but lower esophageal sphincter pressures (LES) in LNF were markedly higher. In another study 132 patients underwent laparoscopic fundoplication with overall morbidity of 7.5%, and good-to-excellent results were achieved in 94% of patients.[5]

Three hundred patients underwent LFP (252 Nissen fundoplication [NFP] and 48 Toupet technique) for gastroesophageal reflux (GER) associ-

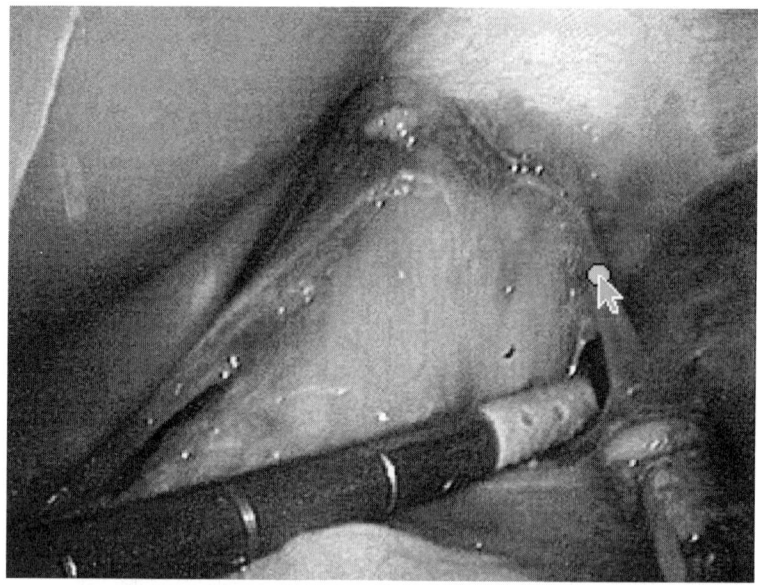

FIGURE 7.1. Photograph demonstrating the left anterior vagus nerve. Arrow points to nerve. It is of critical importance to avoid dissection near the vagus nerves.

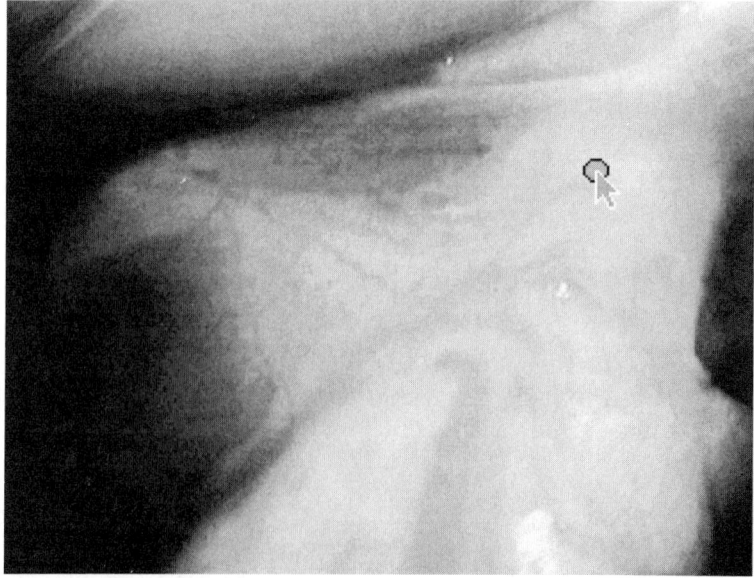

FIGURE 7.2. Photograph demonstrating the phrenoesophageal ligament.

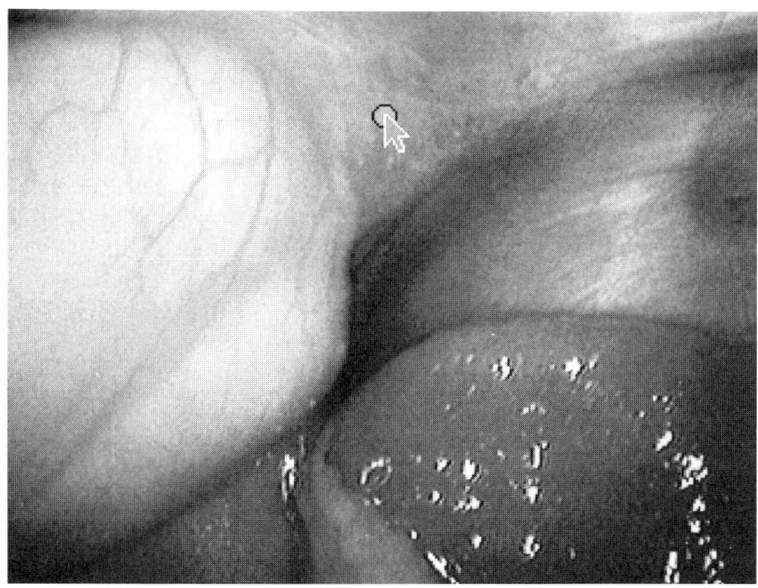

FIGURE 7.3. Photograph demonstrating the gastrophrenic ligament.

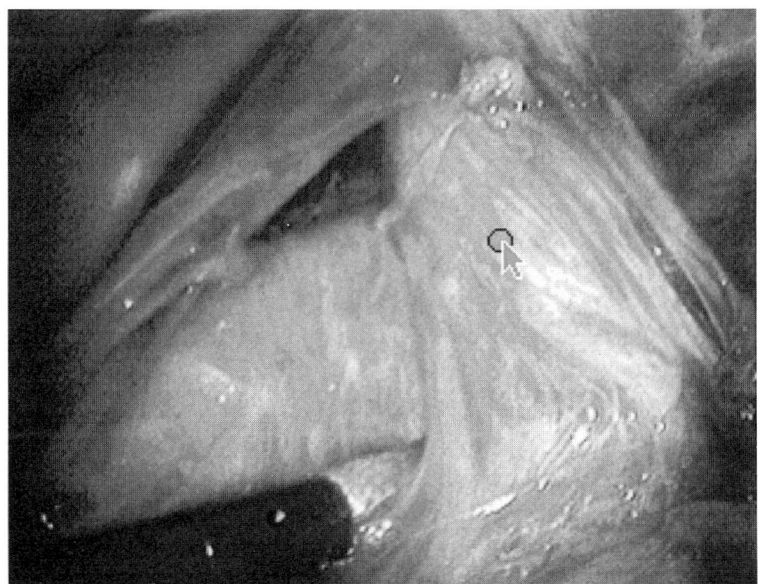

FIGURE 7.4. Photograph demonstrating the distal esophagus.

ated with atypical reflux symptoms, erosive esophagitis, or Barrett's esophagus, as well as an abnormal 24-hour pH probe. Ninety-three percent of patients at 1 year following the operation were free of heartburn. Furthermore, atypical reflux symptoms (e.g., asthma, hoarseness, chest pain, cough) were eliminated or improved in 87% of patients.[6] Three of the four patents in this series who had a recurrence of regurgitation and abnormal esophageal pH had a slipped fundoplication detected with barium swallow, and required reoperation. Overall patient satisfaction in this study was excellent at 97%. A follow-up satisfaction survey at 1 year was 91%, whereas esophageal motility and esophageal pressure was improved in 75% of patients, but worse in 10%.[6] Two percent of patients (five patients) developed postoperative dysphagia or reflux as a result of an intact fundoplication herniating into the chest. They required repeat operation. Major and minor complications were reported to be 6% and 2%, respectively.[6]

A variation of Nissen fundoplication is laparoscopic Nissen-Rossetti fundoplication. This type of fundoplication was reported in 148 patients.[7] Sixteen percent (19 of 117) of the patients that were followed from 3 to 31 months had adverse symptoms, four of which required laparoscopic reoperation, and five who needed endoscopic dilatation. Overall 18 (12.5%) had intraoperative complications, with bleeding as the most common (12 patients), followed by pleural opening (five), whereas 14 (9.5%) patients had various postoperative complications (e.g., bleeding, dysphagia, pleural effusion, wound infection, diarrhea, and tachycardia). Nonetheless, these authors suggest that this procedure can be carried out safely and effectively, with similar results to the open technique.

LNF was successful in 207 patients in another series of 230 patients.[8] Twenty-three (10%) of the patients underwent reoperation, with 10 of those for paraesophageal hernia and persistent dysphagia. There was one death in this series, due to superior mesenteric thrombosis and celiac artery thrombosis, and four cases of pulmonary embolism. In order to decrease the rate of complications these authors suggested routine repair of the posterior paraesophageal hernia, reduction of diathermy usage around the hiatus when possible, and avoidance of vigorous retraction of stomach. Overall relief of GER symptoms was reported in 98% of patients with a follow-up ranging up to 40 months (median 16 months), and 88% in those undergoing single operation respectively.[8] Laparoscopic FP has also been proven to be applicable with good outcome in infants and children.[9]

Partial or Complete Fundoplication: Does It Matter?

Fundoplication for GER has undergone multiple modifications. The results of each technique appear to depend on the surgeon's level of comfort performing the chosen technique.[10] The issue of partial or complete laparoscopic fundoplication, which is similar to an open technique, continues to generate debate.[11] In a study of 231 patients, short-term results were similar when laparoscopic partial fundoplication (PFP) was compared with laparoscopic Nissen-Rosetti fundoplication (NRFP).[2] It is interesting that these authors reported fewer side effects with PFP than they did with NRFP as demonstrated by an earlier return to normal diet, a lower dysphagia rate and overall higher satisfaction.[2] Other studies have reported better results with Toupet FP when compared with NRFP when short gastric vessels were not divided, although esophageal pH measurements were similar.[12] In this study postoperative LES pressures were higher in NRFP. Complete FP without short gastric division was also associated with a higher degree of dysphagia and gas-bloating. In a randomized, prospective study comparing NFP with Toupet fundoplication,[13] no advantages were found when complete or partial FP (modified Toupet) after the division of short gastric vessels, was performed. Laparoscopic NRFP was also associated with higher rates of failure, recurrent disease, or severe dysphagia.[14] In a study of 503 patients, seventeen of 19 patients who failed antireflux surgery had NRFP.[14]

Larger scale studies and long-term follow-up do not allow us to draw clear cut conclusions of the superiority of partial versus complete fundoplication or dividing or not dividing short gastric vessels. Some regard partial posterior FP and total FP, with division of short gastric vessels, to be associated with better outcome when patients are selected appropriately;[14] however, it is clear that which ever technique is used it must last a life time.[11]

Perioperative Complications

Complications of laparoscopic fundoplications are grouped into intraoperative, postoperative, and long-term complications. Specific intraoperative complications in NFP are bleeding from the liver, pneumothorax, and perforation of the esophagus or the stomach. Intraoperative bleeding from the site of trocar insertion, left lobe of the liver, retroesophageal mobilization, pleural opening, and gastric perforation was reported in (12.5%) patients.[7] A retrospective review of short-term results of 2,453 patients showed that 1% had an esophageal or gastric perforation and 1.1%[15] had bleeding complications that required blood transfusion, whereas 0.2% required further surgery for persistent bleeding, 0.4% for a missed perforation, and 0.9% for crural perforation, paraesophageal herniation, or gastric volvulus.[15] The mortality of patients in this large series was 0.2%. The causes of death were missed duodenal perforation, a missed esophageal perforation, ischemic bowel with mesenteric thrombosis, or myocardial infarction.[15] Perforations of the viscus and bleeding from trocar-induced injuries are avoidable by strict application of well-learned techniques of inducing proper pneumoperitonenum and direct visualization of the trocars as they enter.[1] Injuries from the placement of the Veress needle are abdominal wall vascular injuries such as epigastric artery lacerations, rectus muscle hematomas, visceral organ injuries, or major vascular injuries in the abdomen.

These complications should become very rare with experience gained in the laboratory and in the operating room. Although it is alarming, subcutaneous emphysema is of no clinical value and is usually self-limited. On the other hand, massive subcutaneous emphysema may be complicated with hypercarbic acidemia, which may be a cause for prolonged intubation and ventilatory support in a patient with underlying pulmonary disease. Mediastinal emphysema is more common in patients with large hiatal hernia that require extensive dissection, but it might also occur in the absence of mediastinal dissection.

Pneumothorax occurs in up to 5% of cases[16] and is usually caused by dissection into the mediastinum and pleura. Chest tube placement is rarely required because the majority of these patients will be asymptomatic. Air embolism is a potentially deadly complication if it is not identified and treated promptly. It may happen when there is a major venous injury, which allows the access of carbon dioxide to central circulation. Careful monitoring of the patient by the anesthetist and monitoring of end-tidal CO_2 will identify this complication early and allow prompt treatment.

Other perioperative laparoscopic complications are pulmonary. These complications are similar to but are less frequent than those with the open technique (e.g., atelectasis, pleural effusion, and pneumonia). Wound infections are also reported at a significantly lower rate. Most early, large clinical series of LFPs reported that incidence of superficial wound infection is lower than it is with open technique.[1] Analysis of 758 patients that underwent LFP revealed that wound infection was present in 0.1%.[17]

Postoperative Complications

Dysphagia is the most common postoperative complication of this operation with incidence of up to 24%.[3] The failure of this operation is defined as the inability to swallow normally, experience of upper abdominal discomfort during after meals and has persistent or recurrence of symptoms. Other complications include gas bloating, inability to belch, increased flatulence, early satiety, nausea, dietary restriction, diarrhea, and delayed gastric emptying.

In most cases dysphagia is related to edema in the area of GE junction and hypomotility. Late postoperative dysphagia occurred in 5.5% of 2,453 patients.[15] In most cases this complication resolves within several days, but it may persist for up to 2–4 weeks. A liquid diet may mitigate the symptoms of persistent dysphagia; however, some patients may require esophageal dilatation. This dilatation, however, should be avoided for at least 6 weeks because complete disruption of the wrap may occur. Patients with poor esophageal motility and emptying in addition to dysphagia will eventually require reoperation. In a large series of patients reported, reoperation for dysphagia was required in less then 1%. In addition, patients who continue to have persistent dysphagia or evidence of aspiration for more than 1 year should also be considered for operative revision. Other postoperative complications within 30 days include acute paraesophageal herniation, gastric perforation, and mesenteric thrombosis.[8] Early reoperation (i.e., within 3 months) in this series[8] was performed for paraesophageal hernia (2.2%), dysphagia (1.7%), gastric obstruction (0.9%), and other reasons, including recurrent reflux, bleeding, and mesenteric thrombosis.

Summary

Where do we really stand with laparoscopic fundoplication? The results of studies in laparoscopic fundoplication show that safety is comparable and favorable when compared to an open technique.[18] Furthermore, the incidence of complications, morbidity, and mortality are similar to an open technique; however, LFP has other significant advantages over the open technique: less postoperative pain, shorter hospital stay, and earlier return to normal activities. This technique certainly has a great potential for further refinement and improvement of reflux disease. It is becoming a procedure of choice when surgical treatment of GER is indicated.

References

1. Rosser CJ. Laparoscopic Nissen fundoplication. CD rom. Springer-Verlag, New York 1997.
2. Coster DD, Bower WH, Wilson VT, et al. Laparoscopic partial fundoplication vs. Nissen-Rosetti fundoplication. Short-term result of 231 cases. Surg Endosc 1997;11:625–631.
3. Richardson WS, Trus TL, Hunter JG. Laparoscopic antireflux surgery. Surg Clin N Am 1995;76:437–450.
4. Peters JH, Heimbucher J, Kauer WKH, et al. Clinical and physiologic comparison of laparoscopic and open Nissen fundoplication. J Am Coll Surg 1995; 180:385–393.
5. Weerts JM, Dallemagne B, Hamoir E, et al. Laparoscopic Nissen fundoplication: detailed analysis of 132 patients. Surg Laparosc Endosc 1993;5:539–364.
6. Hunter JG, Trus TL, Branun GD, et al. A physiologic approach to laparoscopic fundoplication for gastroesophageal reflux disease. Ann Surg 1996;223:673–687.
7. Fountaumard E, Espalieu P, Boulez J. Laparoscopic Nissen fundoplication. Surg Endosc 1995;9:869–873.

8. Watson A, Spychal RT, Brown MG, et al. Laparoscopic "physiological" antireflux procedure: preliminary results of a prospective symptomatic and objective study. Surg Endosc 1995;82:651–656.

9. van der Zee DC, Bax NMA. Laparoscopic Thal fundoplication in menatlly retarded children. Surg Endosc 1996;10:659–661.

10. Patti MG, De Bellis M, De Pinto M, et al. Partial fundoplication for gastroesophageal reflux. Surg Endosc 1997;11:445–448.

11. Crookes PF, DeMeester TR. Complete and partial laparoscopic fundoplication for gastroesophageal reflux disease (editorial). Surg Endoscop 1997;11:613–614.

12. Bell RCW, Hanna P, Powers B, et al. Clinical and manometric results of laparoscopic partial (Toupet) and complete (Rossetti-Nissen) fundoplication. Surg Endosc 1996;10:724–728.

13. Laws HL, Clements RH, Swillie CM. A randomized, prospective comparison of the Nissen fundoplication versus the Toupet fundoplication for gastroesophageal reflux disease. Ann Surg 1997;225:647–653.

14. Dallemangne B, Weerts JM, Jehaes C, et al. Causes of failures of laparoscopic antireflux operations. Surg Endosc 1996;10:305–310.

15. Perdikis G, Hinder RA, Lund RJ, et al. Laparoscopic fundoplication: where do we stand? Surg Lap Endosc 1997;7:17–21.

16. Hallerback B, Glise H, Johanson B, et al. Laparoscopic Rosseti fundoplication. Surg Endosc 1994;8:1417–1422.

17. Collet D, Cadiere GB, The Formation for the Development of Laparoscopic Surgery for Gastroesophageal Reflux Disease Group. Conversions and complications of laparoscopic treatment gagstroesophageal reflux disease. Am J Surg 1995;169:622–626.

18. Eypasch E, Neugebauer E, Fischer F, et al. Laparoscopic antireflux surgery for gastroesophageal reflux disease (GERD). Results of a Consensus Development Conference (Fourth International Congress of the European Association for Endoscopic Surgery, 1996). Surg Endosc 1997;11:413–426.

8
Pathophysiology of Esophageal Reflux

JAMES C. ROSSER JR., RIFAT LATIFI, and HAROLD BREM

Gastroesophageal reflux disease (GERD) is a common condition that affects approximately 40 million Americans.[1] Although most episodes of acid reflux are asymptomatic, up to 36% of otherwise healthy Americans suffer from heartburn at least once per month. Of that group, 7% experience heartburn as often as once per day. It has been estimated that approximately 2% of the adult population suffers from GERD, based on objective measures such as endoscopic (Figs. 8.1 to 8.3) or histological examination. The incidence of GERD increases markedly after the age of 40, and it is not uncommon for patients experiencing symptoms to wait years before seeking medical treatment.

The clinical spectrum of GERD ranges from the symptomatic post-prandial heartburn to significant morbid and pathological processes such as anemia, ulcerative esophagitis (2–7%), strictures of the esophagus (4–20%), and Barrett's esophagus (10–15%) (2%).[1] Furthermore, Barrett's esophagus often progresses to esophageal carcinoma.

Etiology of GERD

GERD is attributed to a combination of conditions that increase the actual or relative presence of acid reflux in the esophagus. These conditions include transient lower esophageal sphincter (LES) relaxation, decreased LES resting tone, impaired esophageal clearance, delayed gastric emptying, decreased salivation, and impaired tissue resistance.

Lifestyle factors can also cause increased risk of reflux. Smoking, large meals, fatty foods, caffeine, pregnancy, obesity, body position, drugs, hormones, and paraplegia may all exacerbate GERD. Hiatal hernia also frequently accompanies severe GERD. The hernia may prolong transient LES relaxation and delay acid clearance due to impaired esophageal emptying. Thus, hiatal hernia may contribute to prolonged acid exposure following reflux, resulting in GERD symptoms and esophageal damage. Approximately half of the patients with GERD have some relief of their symptoms by modifying their diet and other life-style changes.

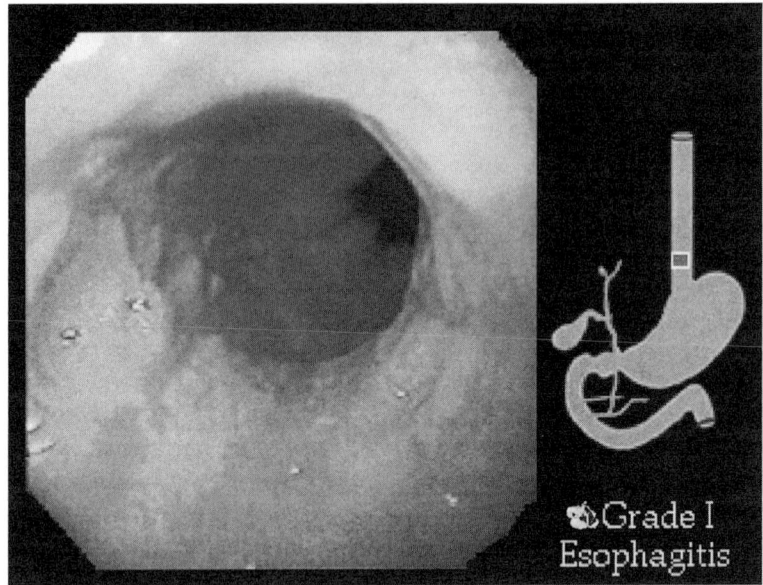

FIGURE 8.1. An endoscopic view of mild esophagitis or grade 1 esophagitis.

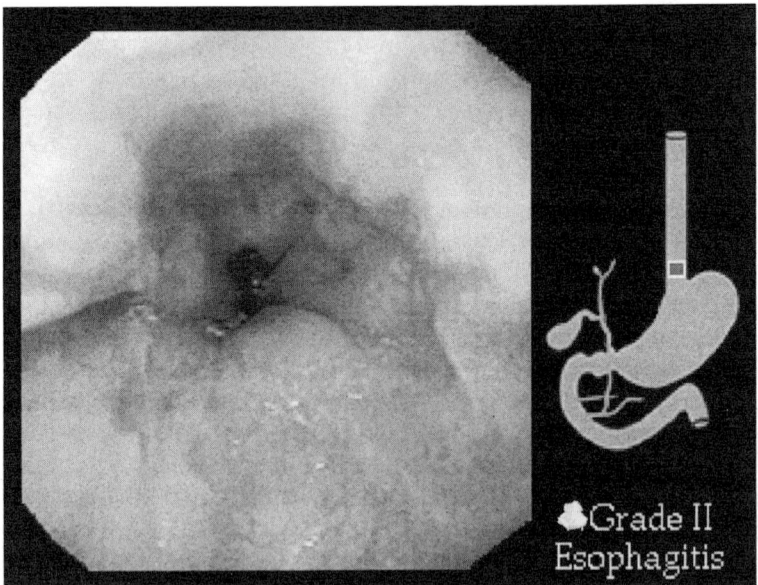

FIGURE 8.2. An endoscopic view of moderate esophagitis or grade 2 esophagitis.

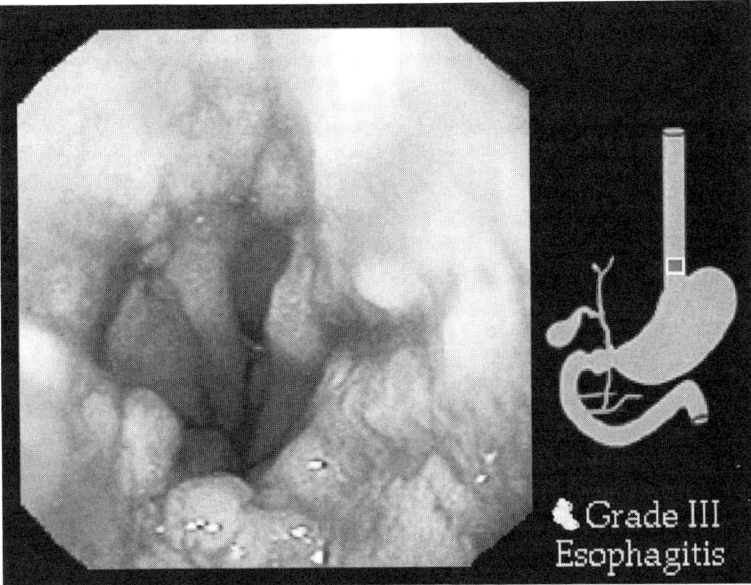

Grade III
Esophagitis

FIGURE 8.3. An endoscopic view of severe esophagitis or grade 3 esophagitis.

A careful history will often show what factors are important for individual patients. Whereas avoidance of exacerbating factors may be helpful, there are relatively little data to support lifestyle modification alone for the long-term relief of symptoms among patients with GERD.

The majority of symptomatic patients will necessitate medical therapy with acid-reducing agents. Many of these patients will have inadequate control of GERD as well as recurrent symptoms upon discontinuation of medical therapy.[2] Some 5–10% of patients who have evidence of severe esophagitis are the subgroup in which antireflux therapy should be considered.[3] Operative intervention has received renewed interest despite highly effective medical treatment because of the low morbidity of minimally invasive approaches, complications, cost concerns, and problems of compliance in protracted medical therapy for a life-long condition.

Pathophysiology of GERD

Gastroesophageal reflux is both a normal physiologic response that occurs in the general population and a pathophysiological response that can result in mild to severe symptoms. GERD can be described as any symptomatic clinical condition or change in tissue structure that results from the reflux of stomach or duodenal contents into the esophagus.

Heartburn, which is a burning sensation or discomfort behind the sternum, is the most common symptom of GERD. It is in part secondary to regurgitation of gastric contents into the esophagus.

Among patients with significant GERD, dysphagia is common and may denote stricture in the esophagus. The etiology of GERD can be attributed to such factors as transient lower esophageal sphincter (LES) relaxation, decreased LES resting tone, delayed stomach emptying, ineffective esophageal clearance, and diminished salivation. Other contributing factors include the potency of the refluxed material and the ability of the esophageal mucosa to resist injury and repair itself.

Most episodes of GERD occur during the day, usually after eating; however, some sufferers also experience reflux during sleep. Nocturnal reflux is commonly associated with a higher risk and a higher degree of esophagitis. Acid remains in the esophagus for prolonged periods because there is less swallowing at night and less saliva produced to neutralize the acid. The symptoms and severity of esophageal mucosal damage are proportional to the acidity of the refluxate and the duration of esophageal acid exposure. With rare exceptions the development of esophagitis requires the presence of acid in the refluxate.

Almost everyone experiences a little acid reflux, particularly after meals. Acid reflux irritates the walls of the esophagus, inducing a secondary peristaltic contraction of the smooth muscle, and may produce the discomfort or pain known as heartburn. Most of the reflux episodes of the normal population are transient. After a meal, the LES usually remains closed. When it relaxes at an inappropriate time, it allows acid and food particles to reflux into the esophagus. Secondary peristalsis returns approximately 90% of the acid and food to the stomach. The LES closes again once peristalsis ends. The remaining acid in the esophagus is neutralized by successive swallowing of alkaline saliva. As long as these mechanisms remain in place the patient will not progress to gastroesophageal reflux disease.

Mechanisms of Gastroesophageal Reflux Disease

After swallowing, the LES should remain closed. Relaxation allows acid and food particles to reflux into the esophagus from the higher pressure intragastric stomach to the lower pressure intrathoracic esophagus. Among patients with GERD, gastric distention increases the frequency of transient LES relaxation, the frequency of reflux episodes, and amount of time gastric acid spends in the esophagus.

Another factor that increases esophageal acid exposure time among patients with GERD is ineffective esophageal clearance. Although peristalsis occurs, esophageal clearance is ineffective because of decreased amplitude of secondary peristaltic waves.

Patients with pathologic reflux often experience many episodes of short-duration reflux and/or several prolonged episodes where the acid may stay in the esophagus for up to several hours. Although the duration of esophageal acid exposure correlates with the frequency of symptoms, as well as with the extent and severity of esophageal mucosal injury, the degree of mucosal damage can be markedly accelerated if luminal pH is less than 2, or if conjugated bile salts are present in the refluxate.

Impaired Esophageal Clearance

Esophageal acid clearance is normally a two-step process. Peristalsis clears gastric fluid from the esophagus, and swallowed saliva neutralizes any remaining acid. Decreased amplitude of secondary peristaltic waves and segmental contractions can be demonstrated in some patients with GERD. Impaired esophageal clearance may be caused by an increase in the volume of refluxate and/or an irritant effect from a preceding reflux event. In rare cases, impaired esophageal clearance may be due to an underlying disease such as scleroderma, which combines poor tissue response with abnormal motility and abnormal sphincteric function.

Decreased Salivation

Saliva, which has a pH of 7.8–8.0, is rich in bicarbonate and can normally neutralize the residual acid coating the esophagus after a secondary peristaltic wave. Decreased salivation, therefore, can contribute to the duration of esophageal acid exposure.

Impaired Tissue Resistance

The ability of the esophageal mucosa to withstand injury can predict reflux damage. It seems to be influenced by the age and nutritional status of the individual. Tissue resistance in the esophagus consists of the membranes and intercellular junctional complexes that protect against acid injury by limiting the rate of hydrogen ions diffusing into the epithelium. The esophagus also produces bicarbonate, to buffer the acid, and mucus, which forms a protective barrier on the epithelial surface. The resistance of the esophageal mucosa to acid damage is much less than that of the stomach lining. When esophageal damage occurs, resident acid overwhelms or exceeds the local tissue resistance to digest epithelial protein.

Transient LES Relaxation

Transient LES relaxation (TLESR) is the mechanism by which reflux occurs in healthy people. Most patients with GERD have a normal resting LES tone. TLESRs are the dominant cause of reflux in these patients, occurring in up to 82% of reflux episodes. TLESRs can be induced by gastric or subthreshold pharyngeal stimulation, which initiates a vagally mediated noncholinergic inhibitory reflex in the LES. TLESRs are short-lived, usually lasting less than 30 seconds. No agent is indicated to treat GERD by preventing transient LES relaxation.

Decreased Resting Tone of LES

The lower esophageal sphincter is the primary barrier to reflux. A constantly weak, low-pressure LES allows reflux every time the pressure in the stomach exceeds that in the LES. This condition is present in a minority of GERD cases, and is usually associated with severe esophagitis.

Delayed Gastric Emptying

If gastric emptying is delayed, then the gastric fluid volume and pressure are increased. Delayed gastric emptying is believed to contribute to a small proportion of GERD cases by increasing the amount of fluid available for reflux.

Pulmonary and Wound Complications of GERD

Complications of GERD should be thought of in two categories. The first is pulmonary. These patients often present with respiratory complaints, such as shortness of breath and wheezing, and are often misdiagnosed as having asthma. Pulmonary manifestations, such as asthma, coughing, or intermittent wheezing, as well as vocal cord inflammation with hoarseness, may occur in some patients. These complications are as a result of acid reflux into the laryngeal and bronchial passages that trigger significant local inflammation. These patients' respiratory difficulties usually resolve after laparoscopic surgery.

   The second series of complications after reflux disease should be thought of as wounds. These patients suffer the morbidity from a local wound in the distal esophagus. The majority of patients with GERD will have a normal appearing and histologically normal distal esophagus upon endoscopy and biopsy. Nevertheless, the appearance of mild to severe esophagitis can be readily visualized grossly in many patients and grossly one can see that these are local wounds (Figs. 8.1 to 8.3). These wounds in patients with GERD are manifested by erythema, isolated erosions, confluent erosions, circumferential erosions, deep ulcers, esophageal stricture, or replacement of normal esophageal epithelium with abnormal (Barrett's) epithelium. In clinical terms this sequale is esophageal erosion, esophageal ulcer, esophageal stricture, or replacement of normal esophageal epithelium with abnormal (Barrett's) epithelium.

Surgical Therapy of GERD

Nissen fundoplication was reported in 1956.[4] Surgical treatment of gastro-esophageal reflux and gastric fundoplication since then, have undergone numerous technical modifications and changes in attempt to reduce recurrence of GERD, and diminish side effects and complications of these operations.[5]

Although this operation has been performed for decades, it was a long-term, controlled, randomized trial of 247 patients with complicated GERD (i.e., peptic esophageal ulcer, stricture, erosive esophagitis, or Barrett's esophagus) that showed that surgical therapy was far more efficacious than medical therapy in improving the symptoms and endoscopic findings of esophagitis.[6] Furthermore, this study concluded that antireflux surgical therapy, when performed by an experienced surgeon, is a valid alternative to protracted and cumbersome medical therapy.

The first laparoscopic Nissen fundoplications (LNFP) were reported in 1991.[7,8] These reports were followed by many published small series of LNFP that gave great impetus to surgical therapy of GER and proved to have all the advances of minimally invasive surgery. The goals of laparoscopic antireflux surgical intervention remain similar to those of an open technique[9] and include: positioning and lengthening of the LES in the abdominal cavity, increasing the pressure of LES, and narrowing the crura to hold LES. These goals must be achieved, however, without jeopardizing the patients' swallowing ability.

Indications for Laparoscopic Antireflux Surgery

Although the mechanism by which antireflux surgery affects GERD is not entirely clear,[10] its effectiveness in treating a select group of patients suffering from GERD has been clearly established. Furthermore, although the indications for antireflux surgery did not change significantly in the last years, the initial success and the popularity of laparoscopic treatment, fear by the patients of long-term side effects and cost containment concerns have decreased the threshold of patients and gastroenterologists in seeking definitive treatment of GERD. This is manifested by an increased number of these procedures performed by general surgeons.[11]

Antireflux surgery is traditionally reserved for patients who have been refractory to medical therapy.[3] Other current indications for operative intervention include noncompliance with medical therapy, recurrent strictures, laryngeal and pulmonary complications (laryngitis, bronchitis, aspiration pneumonia or asthma) and bleeding. Although antireflux procedure will arrest the reflux of acidic of alkaline gastric content into the esophagus and thus arrest the progression of metaplasia, heal ulceration, and resolve the stricture, its use in the face of Barrett's esophagus has been controversial.[12] Another group of patients where antireflux surgery is gaining momentum is in young patients who prefer surgery instead of a lifetime of exposure and the expense of medical therapy and life-style changes. Other diseases that are associated with GERD that require fundoplication include reflux-induced motility disorders, reflux after myotomy, and reflux in the severely neurologically impaired.[13] In addition to the preceding indications, the prerequisites for a successful antireflux surgery are careful patient selection, appropriate technique, and understanding of the principles of antireflux operation. Above all, the anatomy, physiology, and pathology of GERD should be mastered and integrated into the decision-making process when treating these patients surgically.[14,15]

Indications for Antireflux Surgery

In general, antireflux surgery is indicated in patients with increased esophageal exposure to gastric content, as documented by 24-hour esophageal pH studies, in patients with mechanically defective lower esophageal sphincter based on manometric studies, and in those patients with adequate esophageal contractility and peristalsis.[16] The basic indications for antireflux surgery are:

1. Failure of medical therapy
2. Noncompliance with treatment
3. Barrett's metaplasia
4. Aspiration with asthma or recurrent infection
5. Recurrent bleeding or anemia secondary to persistent esophagitis
6. Symptomatic children after 2 years of age with the GER. Antireflux surgery should be done sooner in infants who have significant morbidity from their reflux (e.g., failure to thrive or respiratory insufficiency).
7. Patients who have reflux as a consequence of their abdominal surgery. The pH of this reflux may be acidic, neutral or alkaline.
8. Reflux after esophageal myotomy
9. Motility disorders that result in reflux
10. Reflux that results in motility disorders
11. Stricture

Contraindications for Antireflux Surgery

The contraindications to laparoscopic Nissen fundoplication should be considered absolute, relative, or procedure specific. Absolute contraindications include those that would preclude laparotomy. The absolute contraindications to a laparoscopic antireflux surgery are:

1. Mechanical and paralytic ileus
2. Severe cardiac conduction abnormality
3. Myocardial infarction within the previous 6 months
4. Inability to tolerate general anesthesia
5. Severe pulmonary insufficiency
6. Cardiac ischemia
7. Cardiac failure
8. Coagulopathy
9. Peritonitis
10. Shock

Relative contraindications include to laparoscopic antireflux procedure include splenomegaly, an enlarged caudate lobe, an enlarged left lobe of the liver, multiple previous laparotomies, or a large portion of the stomach being tethered in the thoracic cavity. Procedure-specific contraindications include esophageal shortening, previous vagotomy, or previous gastrectomy. It must be emphasized that if there is esophageal shortening, then it will be extremely difficult to wrap the esophagus in the abdominal cavity, thereby negating the effectiveness of the procedure; therefore, if a patient has a shortened esophagus, or any of the previously mentioned surgical procedures, then a laparoscopic Nissen fundoplication should not be attempted.

Preoperative Studies

The decision for surgical antireflux procedure should not be based solely on symptoms of GERD because many upper gastrointestinal complaints are common and nonspecific, and they may accompany a variety of conditions including achalasia, diffuse esophageal spasm, cancer, peptic ulcer disease, gallstones, and coronary artery disease. Furthermore, asthma, chronic cough, chest pain, wheezing, and hoarseness may also be nonspecific, or they may represent different pathologic entities. The importance of objectively identifying which symptoms are the consequence of GERD is mandatory before any procedure is scheduled.

The evaluation of patients for antireflux surgery is independent of the choice of open versus laparoscopic technique. Many patients will have had with an upper gastrointestinal series (i.e., barium esophagram). Although this test is useful to evaluate other pathologic processes, the esophagram is highly unspecified for GERD that will require surgical intervention. However, a lateral video esophagram, however, does provide useful information about the length of the esophagus. Nevertheless, we do not routinely recommend an esophagram for a patient with GERD.

All patients undergoing an antireflux procedure should have an esophagogastroduodenoscopy (EGD) and manometry. If a symptomatic patient has esophagitis proven by biopsy, then a 24-hour pH probe is not necessary. The degree of reflux and mucosal damage should be graded using the Savory-Miller classification.[17] If the patient does not have esophagitis on EGD, however, then a 24-hour pH probe is necessary. If the DeMeester score[16] on the 24-hour probe is greater than 30, then antireflux surgery will have greater than 90% success rate of eliminating the preoperative symptoms. If the DeMeester score is less than 30 after objective evaluation, however, then, an exhaustive work up must be completed to rule out other pathological processes. Furthermore, if the DeMeester score is less than 30 or normal, then the symptom index portion of the pH evaluation can be useful to establish candidacy for antireflux surgery. To be specific, the symptom index[18] is an objective evaluation of the percentage of the subjective symptoms compared with the objective drop in pH. This emphasizes the importance and relevance of the pH probe and 24 hour test. This has replaced the provocative Bernstein test.[19] When there is occasionally a concern of gastric emptying, radionuclide imaging should be done. This will give an indication of the ability of the stomach to empty.[12]

Manometry is necessary in all patients for two distinct reasons. First, it is required to rule out other disease processes, such as achlasia and scleroderma. Second, the results of manometry will influence the specific type of antireflux surgery. For example, patients with normal peristaltic amplitude and reflux disease are ideal candidates for a Nissen fundoplication. On the other hand, patients with weak distal esophageal contractions benefit from a partial fundoplication such as the Toupet procedure.

Summary

The widespread use of H2 blockers and the long-term use of proton pump inhibitors predicted the end for surgical procedures to correct acid reflux. Less invasive procedures employed through the laparoscope, however, have made permanent physiologic correction more worthy of consideration. No one should be enthusiastic to call a patient who has not yet really tried a course of omeprazole a medical failure. The operations are in the realm of reasonable relative to medical therapy, but they have not acquired the lead position. Most patients with GERD are perfectly managed and kept safe from harm by medical management. In the course of managing patients with GERD, however, the conditions and complications discussed in this chapter may intervene to make the continued medical therapy unreasonable. In this regard it is a happy occasion for the GERD patient that the operations for this disease are now associated with low morbidity and superb results. The newer operations apply the same stringent scientific basis as do the more radical predecessors and for the meantime represent a powerful resource to patients and their gastroenterologists.

References

1. Spechler SJ. Epidemiology and natural history of gastro-esophageal reflux disease. Digestion 1992;51(Suppl 1):24–29.
2. Hinder RA, Filipi CJ. The technique of laparoscopic Nissen fundoplication. Surg Laparosc Endosc 1992;2:265–272.
3. Richter JE. Surgery for reflux disease-reflections of a gastroentreologist. N Engl J Med 1992;326:825–827.
4. Nissen R. Eine einfache operation zur beeinflussung der refluxoesophagitis. Schweiz Med Wochenschr 1956;86:590–592.
5. Jamieson GG, Duranceau A. What is Nissen fundoplication? Surg Obstr Gyn 1984;159:591–593.
6. Spechler SJ, The Department of Veterans Affairs Gastroesophageal Reflux Disease Study Group. Comparison of medical and surgical therapy for complicated gastroesophageal reflux disease in veterans. N Engl J Med 1992;326:786–792.
7. Geagea T. Laparoscopic Nissen fundoplication: preliminary report of ten cases. Surg Endosc 1991;5(4):170–173.
8. Dallamagne B, Weerts JM, Jehaes C, et al. Laparoscopic Nissen fundoplication: preliminary report. Surg Laparosc Endosc 1991;1:138–143.
9. Hinder RA, Laparoscopic Nissen fundoplication. Curr Tech Gen Surg 1993;2: 1–6.
10. Litle AG. Mechanism of action of antireflux surgery: theory and Fact. World J Surg 1992;16:320–325.
11. Hunter JG, Trus TL, Branum GD, et al. A physiologic approach to laparoscopic fundoplication for gastroesophageal reflux disease. Ann Surg 1996;223:673–687.
12. Richardson WS, Trus TL, Hunter JG. Laparoscopic antireflux surgery. Surg Clin North Am 1995;76:437–450.
13. Rosser CJ. Laparoscopic Nissen fundoplication. CD-Rom. Springer-Verlag, 1997.
14. Siewert JR, Feussner H, Walker SJ. Fundoplication: how to do it? Peri-esophageal wrapping as a therapeutic principal in gastro-esophageal reflux prevention. World J Surg 1992;16:326–334.
15. Hinder RA, Filipi CJ, Wetscher GJ. Management of gastroesophageal reflux. In: MacFadyen BV, Jr, Ponsky JL, eds. In Operative laparoscopy and thoracosopy, Lippincott-Raven Publishers, Philadelphia 1996:597–617.
16. Bremner RM, Bremner CG, DeMeester TR. Gastroesophageal reflux: the use of pH monitoring. Curr Probl Surg 1995;6:425–568.
17. Ollyo JB, Lang F, Fontolliet C, et al. Savary's new endoscopic grading of reflux-oesophagitis: a simple, reproducible, logical, complete and useful classification. Gastroenterology 1990;89:A100.

18. Jonston BT, McFarland RJ, Collins JS, et al. Symptom index as a marker of gastro-oesophageal reflux. Br J Surg 1992;79:1054–1055.
19. Berstein LM, Baker LA. A clinical test for esophagitis. Gastroenterology 1958;34:760–781.

9
Technique of Laparoscopic Nissen Fundoplication

JAMES C. ROSSER JR. and HAROLD BREM

This Nissen fundoplication technique has been successfully employed in more than 350 patients. It was designed with the knowledge that there are many technical variations in a laparoscopic Nissen fundoplication. The following specifics, however, were designed to provide maximum exposure and technical ease for the surgeon. It must be emphasized that this procedure can be done equally well whether the surgeon is right handed or left handed. This surgery however, can only be initiated if the surgeon is facile with the simultaneous use of both hands.

Room and Patient Setup

After general anesthesia is induced, the patient is placed in the modified lithotomy position with Allen stirrups and pneumatic compression boots are applied. Positioning is similar to that of a low anterior resection. An 18-gauge nasogastric tube and a 16-gauge bladder catheter are inserted.

As in all laparoscopic procedures optical correctness must be established. *Optical correctness* is defined as proper alignment of all of the visualization equipment such that there is no "operative site/video monitor directional discrepancy." Optical correctness is established by having the surgeon, camera, operative site, and a monitor in a direct line (Fig. 9.1). In addition, surgeon must never operate with the monitor over his/her shoulder. Nothing is more frustrating or potentially harmful as moving the tip of an instrument to the right and seeing it move to the left on the monitor. This provides maximum flexibility and exposure during the procedure; furthermore, it means that surgeons will never be looking over their shoulder.

Trocar Placement

Table 9.1 and Figure 9.2 demonstrate the specific placement of each trocar. The first four are 10-mm trocars, but ports #5 and #6 are 5-mm trocars. With new instrumentation as well as advance miniaturized optics and hand

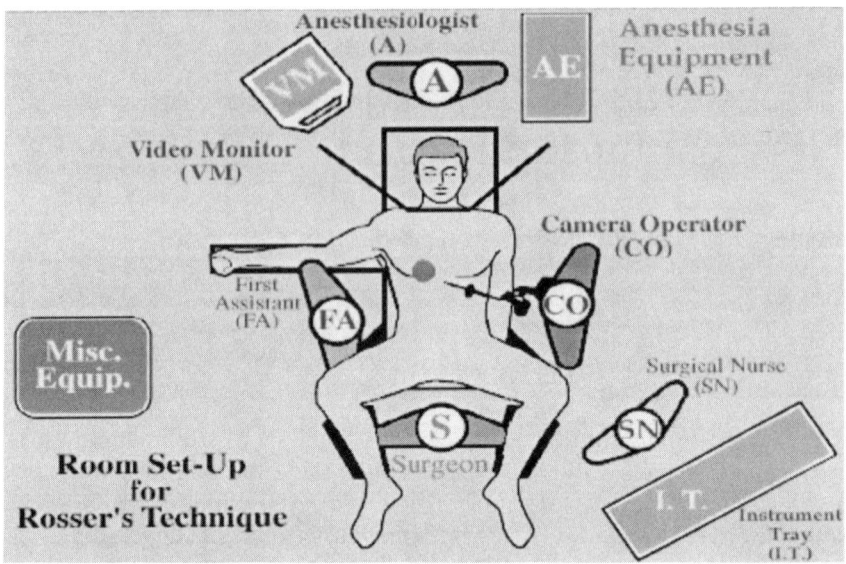

FIGURE 9.1. Schematic illustration of optical correctness in a laparoscopic Nissen fundoplication. In all laparoscopic procedures when the surgeon moves to the right, the image should move to the right on the television monitor; similarly, when the surgeon moves to the left, the image on the television screen should move to the left. Specific placement of all the operating room personnel and equipment. This facilitates optical correctness. Note that only one video screen is necessary in this orientation.

instruments, nearly all of these ports can be 5-mm trocars. Prior to all incisions, 2 ml of 0.5% bupivicaine is injected subcutaneously at the trocar site. A #11 blade is utilized for the incisions. Each incision must be at least the size of the diameter of the trocar to avoid an uncontrolled entry into the abdominal cavity.

After the camera is placed through trocar #1, the 30-degree laparoscope is rotated in an upward direction so that the anterior abdominal wall can be easily visualized.

We emphasize that all of the trocars should be placed through the abdominal wall in a perpendicular fashion. This facilitates ease of entry and avoids "bunching" of the trocars intraabdominally.

Pneumoperitoneum

A 10-mm transverse incision is made in the right upper quadrant, two fingerbreaths medial to the anterior axillary line and two fingerbreaths from the costal margin. The superior and inferior edges of the skin and subcutaneous tissue are lifted upward (e.g., with a towel clip), and an extra long Veress needle (150mm) is inserted. The long needle prevents dislodgment when lifting up on the skin.

After the Veress needle is placed, a 10-ml syringe is used to aspirate to check for blood or bile. Next, the drop test is performed. Three milliliters of saline are injected into the hub of the Veress needle. If the saline flows in easily, then the tip of the needle is usually in a proper location. It should be remembered that you obtain a false positive "drop test" if the needle is in the subcutaneous tissues.

After a positive drop test, the insufflation tubing is connected to the needle. The pressure should be 6mmHg or less; however, if the "critical opening pressure" is ≥10mmHg, then the needle should be repositioned and the abdominal wall lifted up, and the drop test repeated. If the pressure is still high, and you feel comfortable with the needle position, then it may be necessary to use 25mmHg for the first 1 L of insufflation (this is because it is not rare for a piece of omentum to impede flow of CO_2 in the right upper quadrant). After 1 L of CO_2 has been introduced, all four quadrants should be percussed to ascertain that an symmetrical and diffuse "global pneumoperitoneum" is present. A second test to ascertain a global pneumoperitoneum is to place direct pressure in the left lower quadrant

TABLE 9.1. Optimal placement of trocars.

Trocar#	Location of trocar	Purpose of trocar
1.	Two fingerbreadths below the costal margin & two fingerbreadths medial to the right anterior axillary line.	Initially for the veress needle & camera. After all trocars are placed, the liver retractor is inserted.
2.	Two fingerbreadths below the costal margin & two fingerbreadths medial to the left anterior axillary line	After all trocars are placed, the camera is inserted.
3.	Below the xiphoid process	Suction, irrigation, retraction, ultrasound coagulation.
4.	Two finger breadths below and two finger breadths lateral to trocar #2.	Retraction of stomach
5.	1/2 the distance between the xiphoid process and the umbilicus immediately to the right of the rectus abdominus muscle	Dissection & retraction. 5mm ultrasound coagulation.
6.	1/2 the distance between the xiphoid process and the umbilicus immediately to the left of the rectus abdominus muscle	Dissection & retraction.

Note: Six trocars are usually utilized. They appear here as they are placed sequentially, 1–6. The right-hand column lists the surgical use of each of these trocars.

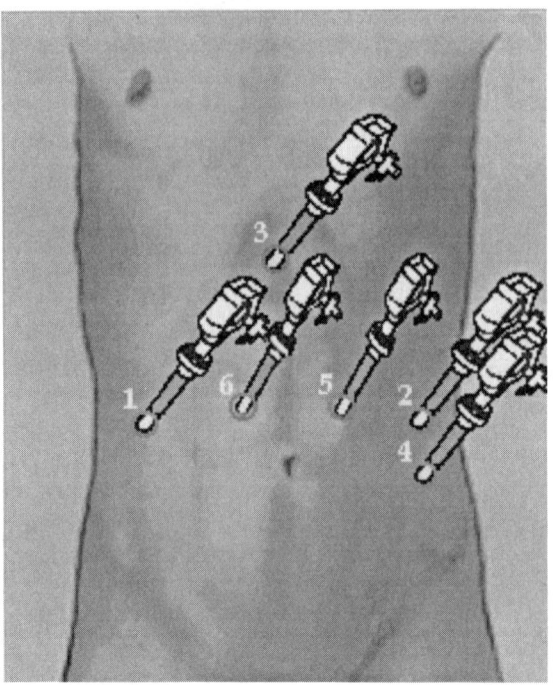

FIGURE 9.2. Schematic diagram of markings on the abdomen of all six ports after all six trocars are placed. Trocars #1–4 are 10-mm ports; trocars #5 and 6 are 5-mm ports (see text and Table 3.1).

and ascertain that the intraabdominal pressure reading increases by at least 5 mmHg. If the patient has any scar in the right upper quadrant (e.g. from a previous cholecystectomy), then an alternative site is chosen in the left upper quadrant. If this is not acceptable, then the pneumoperitoneum is established by the Hasson or Rosser technique.[1] The usual pressure of the working pneumoperitoneum is 15 mmHg.

After a pneumoperitoneum is established, the Veress needle is removed and a 10 mm port is placed. This allows the insertion of a 30-degree laparoscope. It is rotated upward to provide visualization of the anterior abdominal wall. The #2 port site is a mirror image of the first, but it is placed in the left upper quadrant. This is the port used for the camera. Port #4 may not be necessary in some patients when the greater omentum is not massive and exposure can easily be obtained. The #5 and #6 trocars are placed immediately lateral to the rectus abdominus muscles while avoiding the superior epigastric vessels, usually halfway between the xyphoid and umbilicus. If the patient is particularly tall or large, then it may be necessary to place trocars #5 and #6 several centimeters more cephalad. After all six trocars are placed the camera is switched to the left upper quadrant port (e.g., port #2). Figure 9.5 is a photograph of the abdominal wall of a patient after all six trocars were placed.

After all of the trocars are secured, the camera is moved to port #2 and the patient is placed in at least a 30-degree reverse Trendelenburg. The 30-degree laparoscope is rotated in a downward direction to view the operative field (Fig. 9.3).

Anterior Retraction of the Liver

The liver retractor is placed in the #1 port in the right upper quadrant. It is important to place the retractor under the left lobe of the liver when it is fully closed. The retractor is then deployed to an open position. The assistant retracts the liver with the right hand. The left hand is utilized for irrigation and suction through the #3 port (subxiphoid).

Inferior Retraction of the Stomach

The deployment of the retractor does not by itself establish proper exposure. The stomach usually must be retracted in a inferior and lateral direction. This is accomplished by placement of a Babcock retractor through port #4. This completes the exposure of the gastroesophageal region.

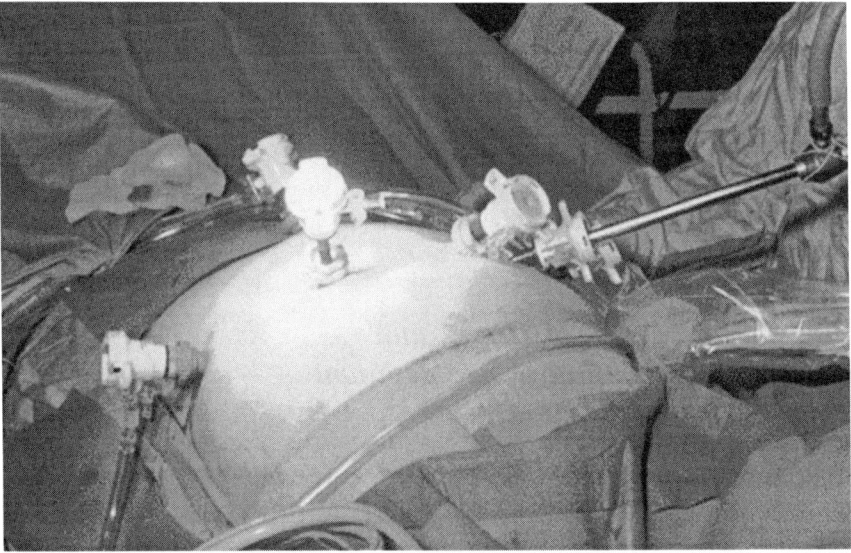

FIGURE 9.3. Photograph of appearance of abdominal wall in patient undergoing laparoscopic Nissen fundoplication after all six ports were placed.

The goal in steps 5–7 is to expose the distal esophagus. Approximately 90% of this dissection should be done without cautery. This helps in decreasing the chance of esophageal injuries; however, cautery should be used without hesitation in the appropriate situations. The control for the coagulation is usually by a foot pedal. Because hemostasis is so critical in this procedure and to avoid inappropriate use of the cutting current, the cut setting should be set to zero.

Maturation of the Horseshoe Dissection Pattern to Expose the Lower Esophagus and the Esophageal Hiatus

A layered approach must be emphasized because it promotes the orderly and safe progression of the dissection phase of the procedure. Immediately identify the gastrohepatic ligament, the phrenoesophageal ligament, and the gastrosplenic ligament. The surgeon must first be aware of two anatomical structures in harm's way: the caudate lobe of the liver and an aberrant hepatic artery.

Division of the Gastrohepatic Ligament

This step initiates a horseshoe (∩) dissection configuration that begins on the right side of the esophagus and ends on the left side. The gastrohepatic ligament is retracted to the patient's left by using a grasper through the #5 port. The caudate lobe of the liver can usually be seen through this somewhat transparent structure. Endoshears are used through port #6 to cut the mostly avascular gastrohepatic ligament.

Twelve percent of patients will have an aberrant left hepatic artery, which comes in various sizes. It is found in the cephalad portion of the gastrohepatic ligament. This aberrant vessel should be spared. If it is less than 3 or 4mm in diameter, however, then it can be sacrificed without fear of complications.

Dissection of the Superficial and Deep Phrenoesophageal Attachments

This area represents the closed portion of the horseshoe dissection pattern. The dissection initially takes down the peritoneum only with Endoshears through the #6 port. Then, the deeper dissection is accomplished with a blunt technique utilizing a peanut through the #5 port. Some cautery may be necessary in this area, which is usually vascular (secondary to the esophageal branches of the left gastric artery). Great caution must be used, however, because the underlying esophagus is prone to thermal injury.

Dissection of the Superficial Gastrophrenic Attachments

Mostly blunt dissection is utilized to divide the gastrophrenic attachments, which start in the area anterior and to the left of esophagus. A grasper is placed through port #5 and a peanut and/or Endoshears are used through port #6. Cautery is not used in this part of the dissection, but it can be used when necessary. Be careful not to extend your dissection into the gastro-splenic ligament. You may be met with uncontrolled bleeding from the short gastric vessels.

Separation of the Esophagus from the Right and Left Crus

Initial separation of the esophagus and the right crus is obtained with a grasper through the #6 port and a Maryland dissector through the #5 port. The Maryland is spread parallel to the fibers of the right crus along a white line denoting the anatomic separation point of the two structures. After initial separation, two blunt dissectors (peanuts) are inserted into the #5 and #6 ports. They are simultaneously thrust in opposite directions (cephalad and caudad). This maneuver completes the separation.

Maturation of the Retroesophageal Window

Only blunt dissection is used to complete the retroesophageal dissection. This is necessary to decrease the possibility of esophageal or gastric perforation. The dissection is continued by using the "SWIM TECHNIQUE." The right-hand instrument is used to elevate the esophagus, whereas the left hand bluntly dissects. As the esophagus is liberated the right hand is progressively repositioned with an instrument over instrument motion until the retroesophageal window is completed. In order to further mature the retroesophageal window, blunt dissection is continued with the two peanuts in a cephalad to caudal direction. This is known as "walking the dog." If there is any difficulty in breaking through the gastrophrenic ligament and completing the maturation of the retroesophageal window, then proceed directly to division of the short gastric vessels. Ligation and division of the short gastrics facilitates the retroesophageal dissection.

It is important to avoid excessive dissection into the mediastinum to prevent pleural entry, and to avoid a pneumomediastinum or pneumo-thorax. Another potential hazard are vessels emanating from the left crus. Hook cautery may be necessary to coagulate these vessels. If they are large vessels, then clips should be utilized. Finally, limit posterior dissection because of the aorta.

Ligation of the Short Gastric Vessels

It is almost always necessary to ligate the short gastric vessels to assure adequate mobilization of the fundus. In order to accomplish this, the gastrosplenic peritoneum (e.g., the superficial peritoneum from the left curs of the diaphragm to the splenic capsule) must be divided. The vessels can be ligated with clips, bipolar, stapling device, or an ultrasonic coagulation and division device. This device moves ≥55,000 cycles per second, which coagulates proteins and ligates the vessels. It is emphasized that this ultrasonically activated instrument can either be placed through a 5-mm United States Surgical Corporation (USSC) port or a 10-mm (Ethicon) port. If the 10 mm instrument is used, then the #3 port will be used as the working site. The #5 port is used if the 5-mm instrument is used. The advantages include (1) minimal risk to adjacent tissue thereby negating the risk of propagation of a monopolar coagulation and (2) elimination of the suturing obstacles that clips present.

Specific technical details of take down of the short gastrics are as follows:

i. The Babcock through the #4 port is repositioned and removes the greater omentum from the operative area.

ii. A 5-mm grasper is placed through the #6 port to retract the fundus to the patient's right and place the gastrosplenic ligament under stretch.

iii. A Maryland dissector is placed through the #5 port in order to create the initial entry into the lesser sac.

iv. Use the Maryland dissector to spread parallel to the short gastrics, prior to ligation and division. Parallel dissection to the short gastrics is essential in order to avoid inadvertent shearing and subsequent bleeding of these blood vessels.

v. Place a peanut or blunted grasper through the #3 port to retract the spleen in a lateral direction, if the 5-mm harmonic device is to be used. Place it through the #5 port, if the 10-mm devise is used.

vi. Use the #3 port to bring in the 10-mm harmonic device to coagulate and divide the short gastric vessels. If a 5-mm ultrasonic coagulation and division device (USSC Norwalk, Connecticut, USA) is used, then it is brought through the #5 port. Place a grasper through the #3 port to retract the cardia of the stomach in a medial direction and place the 5-mm ultrasonic coagulation and division device through the #5 port.

Placement of the Bougie Prior to Closure of the Hiatal Hernia

If the esophageal hiatus is greater than two times the width of the esophagus, then at least one suture is used to close it. A 0-nonabsorbable is recommended. Before suturing, a #50 French lubricated Bougie is passed into the proximal stomach. It may be necessary to remove the nasogastric tube in order to facilitate passage of the Bougie. It is emphasized that in order to prevent perforation, a skilled and experienced anesthesiologist or surgeon must perform this potentially dangerous maneuver. After the Bougie reaches the level of the cricopharyngeus muscle, final placement is accomplished with visualization. Passage of the Bougie is facilitated by straightening the distal esophagus with gentle traction on the esophagus utilizing graspers through ports #5 and #6.

Closure of the Hiatal Hernia

An extracoporal suture technique is used to close the hiatus. The crura are approximated to each other with 0 nonabsorbable sutures. A Surgiwhip (122-cm extracoporal suturing appliance from USSC, Norwalk, Connecticut, USA) is used to facilitate this. Intracorporal suturing is not used because of the need to tie the knot under great tension.

A Rosser needle assist device (Cabot) grasps the nonabsorbable 122-cm whip stitch® (USSC Norwalk, Connecticut, USA) and places it through the #3 port. A Rosser needle holder (Cabot) is placed with the right hand through the #5 port and grasps the needle.[3] The suture is placed either anteriorly or posteriorly to the esophagus depending on the natural anatomical configuration of the hiatus. The needle is passed through the left and right crus of the diaphragm with a "two-step" technique. In order to avoid trauma by pulling the suture through the tissue, the "pulley technique" is employed. The left-hand needle assist instrument is placed through the #3 port and picks up the suture 5 cm above the needle. The right hand guides the Rosser needle holder through the #5 port and pulls down the suture connected to the appliance. As the right hand pulls down the suture the left hand withdraws the needle until it exits from the number three port. When 15 cm of suture has been acquired, a fisherman's knot is then executed. Break off the proximal end of the Surgiwhip® and the knot is pushed down to the operative site with the plastic portion of the appliance. Place the needle holder and assist devise through the #5 and #6 ports. Gently tug on the two cut ends of the suture to further secure the knot. This is known as the "Cahow tug."

Positioning of the Fundus Around the Esophagus

i. The Bougie is removed and a blunt instrument is placed through the #5 and #6 ports to reestablish the retroesophageal space with the "swim technique".
ii. An aggressive grasper is placed through the #6 port and passed through the retroesophageal window.

iii. The Babcock retractor is placed through the #4 port and used to position the stomach so that the cardiac portion can be passed to the aggressive grasper.
iv. The stomach is then pulled through the window with the #6 port instrument and pushed with the #4 instrument. The Babcock is then used to grasp the posterior fundic portion of the wrap.
v. Be careful not to twist the wrap. Make sure that the fundic wrap is floppy by bringing both portions of the wrap together. This is called the "Cahow Kiss." This helps to document adequate looseness and mobility of the wrap.

Fundoplication

The length of the fundoplication should be 23 cm. An increased length of the wrap will increase the incidence of postoperative dysphagia. A 50–60 F Bougie must be in place in the esophagus before the extracorporeal sutures are placed. The lower aspect of the fundoplication is established first. This helps to avoid constructing a "slipped Nissen." This is accomplished by the extracoporeal technique described earlier. The esophagus is included in the suturing process. Two of these sutures are placed about 2 cm apart. Visualize the anterior vagus nerves and be certain that the needle does not pass through them.

Transabdominal Fixation Suture

After the Bougie is removed, a suture is placed between the posterior fundic wrap and the central tendon of the diaphragm. This suture is placed in order to maintain the wrap in the abdominal cavity. As previously described a single 0 nonabsorbable suture utilizing a Surgiwhip® (USSC Norwalk, Connecticut, USA) is placed.

Closure

Irrigation and inspection are meticulously accomplished. The fascia of all four 10-mm ports are closed with a 0 absorbable suture. The skin is approximated with 5-0 absorbable suture in interrupted subcuticular fashion, and steristrips are placed. The nasogastric tube and bladder catheter are removed while the patient is anesthetized.

Postoperative Care

On average, sips of liquids are initiated on the first postoperative day. A programmable analgesic intravenous distributor is utilized the first 24 hours. The diet is advanced rapidly to a soft diet and the patient is usually discharged home on the second or third postoperative day. We often do not admit the patient to the hospital; rather, the patient is admitted to an adjacent special postoperative recovery facility. This is known as the "Recovery Hotel."[4]

References

1. Rosser J. CD-ROM: Laparoscopic nissen fundopliaction: surgical procedure. Springer-Verlag, 1997. New York.
2. James "Butch' Rosser, personal series.
3. Rosser J. CD-ROM: The art of laparoscopic suturing. Radcliffe Medical Press, New York, 1995.
4. Rosser J. Laparoscopic surgical procedures at the "recovery hotel." Bull Am Coll Surg 1997;82:29–32.

10
Laparoscopic Esophageal Surgery in Achalasia

MARGRET ODDSDOTTIR

Achalasia is a primary esophageal motility disorder of unknown etiology. It is a rare disorder (1/100,000) that affects males and females equally. Achalasia is characterized by progressive loss of peristalsis in the body of the esophagus and failure of a normal or hypertensive lower esophageal sphincter (LES) to relax in response to swallowing.[1,2] No form of therapy returns esophageal peristalsis or LES function to normal. Therapy is aimed instead at relieving the functional obstruction at the gastroesophageal junction. Medical efforts to relieve the distal esophageal obstruction have been largely unsatisfactory. Surgical cardiomyotomy, introduced by Heller in 1913, provides excellent relief of dysphagia in 85–95% of patients with achalasia, with minimal complications.[1-4] Thoracotomy or laparotomy, however, has been required, which results in significant pain and prolonged recovery period. Pressure-controlled balloon dilatation and, more recently, botulinum toxin (Botox) injection of the lower esophageal sphincter have therefore become the primary treatment for achalasia.[5-7] This is in spite of lower success rate, frequent retreatment, and, for pneumatic dilatation, a perforation rate of 3–5%.[3,5,7]

Laparoscopic cardiomyotomy for achalasia was first reported in 1991 by Shimi et al.[8] The patient had complete relief of dysphagia and no untoward symptoms. Several reports on laparoscopic cardiomyotomy have been published since then.[2,6,8-11] Today, laparoscopic cardiomyotomy has proven to be safe, effective, and associated with minimal discomfort.[2,6,8-11]

Preoperative Evaluation and Preparation

It is important to establish the correct diagnosis prior to treatment because other disorders can present in a similar fashion. These include malignant obstruction (especially when the sphincter is infiltrated), gastroesophageal reflux with stricture formation, diffuse esophageal spasms, and nutcracker esophagus. Diagnostic work-up therefore includes an endoscopic examination with biopsies as necessary, a barium swallow, and esophageal manometry. If a peptic stricture is suspected, then a 24-hour pH study is indicated. A CT scan is obtained if a malignant obstruction is suspected.

Patients with proven achalasia who can tolerate general anesthesia are candidates for cardiomyotomy. Prior balloon dilatation and/or botulinum toxin injection is not a contraindication for cardiomyotomy. In these patients, however, the periesophageal dissection and the myotomy may become difficult because of scarring in the area.

The Procedure

The surgeon needs to stand between the patient's legs, facing the monitors to maintain coaxial alignment with the gastroesophageal junction and the video-laparoscope (Fig. 10.1).

The hiatal exposure and the mobilization of distal esophagus and cardia is the same as that for laparoscopic fundoplication. The dissection begins by incising the avascular area of the gastrohepatic omentum above the hepatic branch of the vagus. This exposes the caudate lobe of the liver and the right crus. The right and left crura of the diaphragm are identified and separated from the esophagus. The posterior esophageal attachments are divided under direct vision. A Penrose drain is passed around the esophagus, and used for traction. The periesophageal dissection is completed by dissecting both crura free of all epiphrenic tissue, mobilizing an adequate length of the esophagus, and developing a posterior window large enough for a loose partial fundoplication (270-degree). The epiphrenic fat pad is dissected off the anterior surface of the gastroesophageal junction and the cardia.

The myotomy is started on the anterior surface of the esophagus, to the left of the anterior vagus nerve, just proximal to the gastroesophageal junction. The longitudinal fibers are separated using the twin action of a pair of scissors. The transverse fibers are separated from the underlying mucosa with blunt dissection, and then divided with hook-cautery or scissors (Fig. 10.2). Once in the submucosal plane, the mucosa bulges up. This is clearly seen in the magnified laparoscopic view. The myotomy is now carried proximally for 5–6 cm above the gastroesophageal junction. The myotomy is carried distally across the gastroesophageal junction and on to the stomach for about 1 cm. On the stomach site, the separation of the muscle layers from the mucosa is more difficult to achieve than it is on the esophagus. This may result in more bleeding than that encountered during the esophageal myotomy, as well as increased risk of perforation. Once the myotomy is completed, the muscle edges are separated from the underlying mucosa for approximately 40% of the esophageal circumference. The orogastric tube, which is placed at the beginning of the procedure, is pulled back into the distal esophagus, and about 100 ml of diluted methylene blue solution is infused down the tube. This will clearly

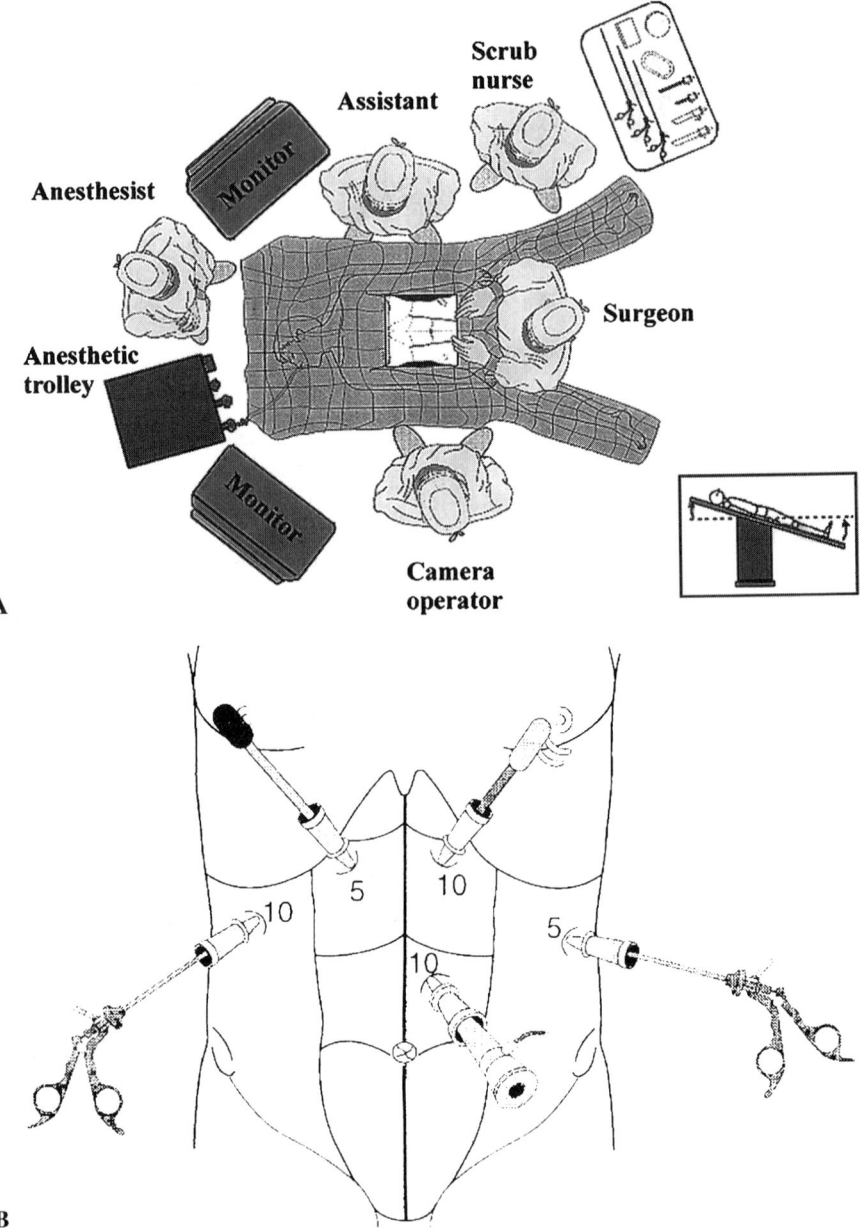

FIGURE 10.1. (A) The operating room set-up. (B) The trocar placement. The supraumbilical trocar and the right subcostal trocar are placed 15 cm from the xiphoid. The left subcostal trocar about 10 cm from the xiphoid. The epigastric trocar is placed as high as the liver edge allows and as lateral as the falciform ligament allows. The left flank port is about 7-cm lateral to the left subcostal trocar.

demonstrate any mucosal perforation. If a perforation is encountered, then it can be closed with a stitch. Some surgeons prefer to have a flexible endoscope or a dilator in the esophagus as they do their myotomy. I prefer not to place anything but an orogastric tube in the esophagus. With the gastroesophageal junction mobilized as described, one can control the tension and freely move the distal esophagus and the cardia by pulling the Penrose drain. Finally, the mucosa is easily identified as it bulges out, when not stretched by a dilator or an endoscope.

An antireflux procedure—either a posterior fundoplication (Toupet) or an anterior fundoplication (Dor)—is recommended in conjunction with the myotomy (Fig. 10.3).[12] Both can be accomplished with the laparoscopic approach.[2,6,9–14] I prefer a Toupet, except for very dilated esophagi. In those instances, an anterior fundoplication is more appropriate because a posterior fundoplication may cause a relative outlet obstruction by angling the gastroesophageal junction anteriorly.

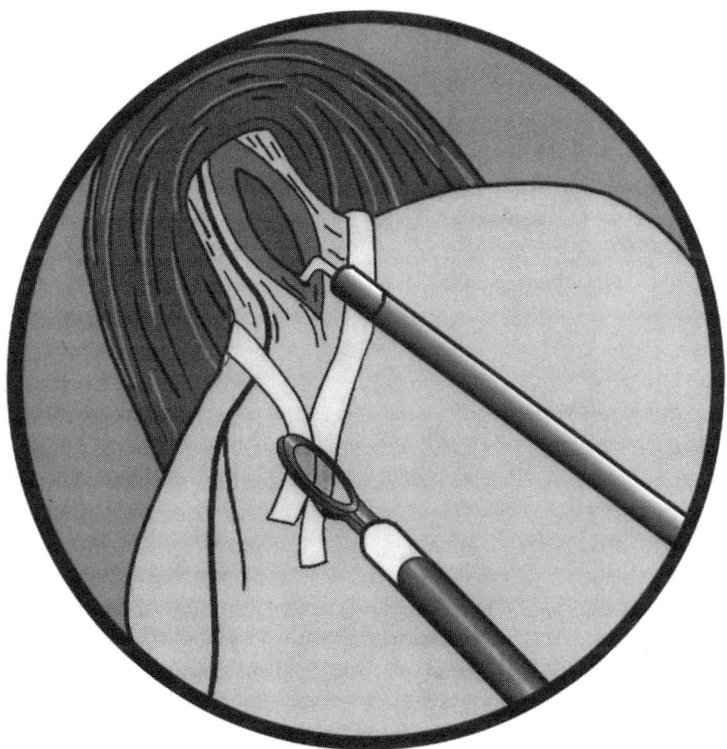

FIGURE 10.2. The myotomy being carried proximally, using hook electrocautery. Care must be taken to elevate the muscle fibers away from the mucosa before the electrocautery is applied.

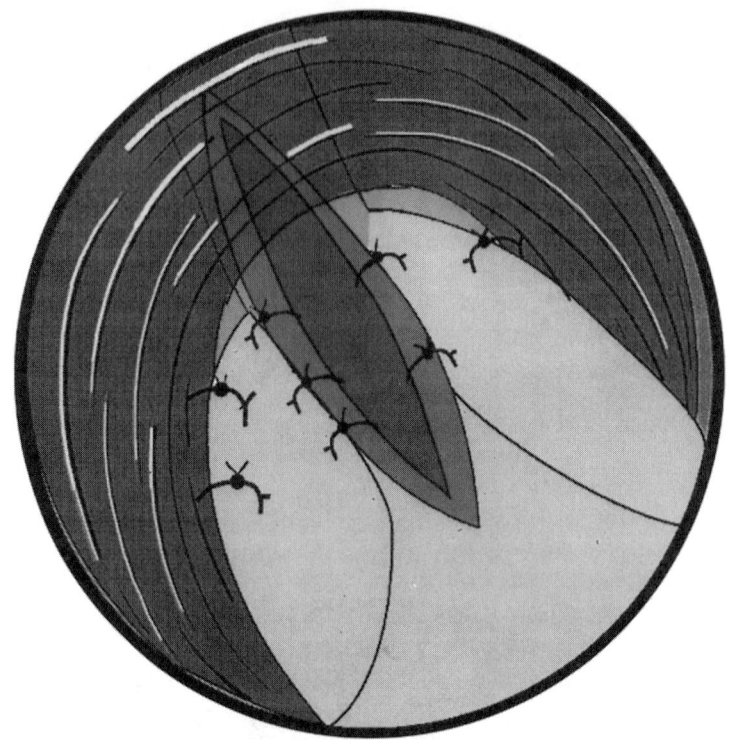

FIGURE 10.3. Completed abdominal myotomy with Toupet hemi-fundoplication. (From Swanstrom LL, Pennings J. Laparoscopic esophagomyotomy for achalasia. Surg Endosc 1995;9(3):286–292, Springer-Verlag; with permission.)

The posterior fundoplication is performed by suturing the fundus on each side of the esophagus to the cut edge of the muscularis, as well as tacking it to the crura posteriorly. It is a personal choice whether or not the greater curvature is mobilized for the fundoplication, but I prefer to do so to ensure a loose and tension-free fundoplication. An anterior fundoplication is done by rolling the fundus over the exposed mucosa and suturing it to the cut edge of the muscularis on each side, as well as to the anterior crural arch.

Complications

The most common complication is a small perforation of the mucosa.[2,6,9,10,14] This is usually easily recognized; if not at once, then during an infusion of methylene blue dye into the esophagus or, if using an endoscope, by insufflating air. These lacerations are clean and are easily repaired with a stitch. Recognized mucosal lacerations that are repaired during laparoscopic cardiomyotomy carry a low risk of infection.

Late perforations are rare. One of my patients presented with a perforation on postoperative day 5. When explored laparoscopically (less than 6 hours later) he was found to have a clean-cut, 1-cm laceration in the middle of the exposed mucosa. It was sutured and he had an uneventful postoperative course.

Bleeding can occur from several sites. The muscle-edges of the myotomy may bleed, especially on the stomach side. Most of these stop spontaneously. Care should be taken when using coagulation in this area because of risk of thermal injury and perforation. Blood loss that requires transfusion is not reported for laparoscopic cardiomyotomy. Even a small amount of bleeding, however, can be annoying because it absorbs the light and obscures the view.

Up to 5% of postoperative chest films show a small pneumothorax.[2] These pneumothoraces rarely require intervention for respiratory compromise and the lungs reexpand quickly as the CO_2 is rapidly absorbed.

Results

Several reports on laparoscopic cardiomyotomy have been published recently. The largest one, which had 85 patients and a mean follow-up for 20 months, shows excellent and good results in 82 patients (96.4%); however, two required reoperation (laparoscopic) for dysphagia.[9]

In a report from Hunter et al., 36 of 40 patients (90%) with achalasia had alleviation of dysphagia following laparoscopic cardiomyotomy.[6] An additional two were improved. Of the four patients who did not have elimination of dysphagia following cardiomyotomy, two had previous transthoracic cardiomyotomy, one had sigmoid esophagus, and one had moderate esophageal dilation.

In 12 patients followed for the mean of 16 months, Swanstrom and Pennings observed good to excellent relief of dysphagia in all twelve patients.[10] Manometry in 11 of these 12 patients showed a mean decrease in the lower esophageal sphincter pressure from 33.4 mmHg preoperatively to 19.3 mmHg postoperatively.

The longest follow-up in the literature for laparoscopic cardiomyotomy is about 6 years, but most are 1–3 years.[2,6,8–11,14] Dysphagia is relieved in 90–98% of patients in these reports (combined, over more than 200 patients).

Comments

Reflux is a common problem after conventional (open) cardiomyotomy. The literature clearly indicates that an antireflux procedure should be added to a conventional abdominal cardiomyotomy.[2,6,12,13] The same arguments can be applied for the laparoscopic approach. The Dor procedure requires less mobilization of the fundus and the gastroesophageal junction and therefore is easier to perform.[15] The Toupet fundoplication, however, is a proven, effective antireflux procedure. When it is performed in conjunction with cardiomyotomy, it helps to keep the edges of the myotomy apart.[2,6,10,13,16] If the gastroesophageal junction is not dissected circumferentially, then one can argue that an antireflux procedure is only needed if the patient has a hiatal hernia or if a sutured mucosal perforation needs to be buttressed. Minimal dissection, however, consists of taking down the phrenoesophageal membrane and mobilizing the esophagus for at least 5 cm anterolaterally. In addition, the LES is completely disrupted by the myotomy. By mere disruption of the LES by forceful balloon dilatation, reflux becomes a common problem.[5] A partial fundoplication at the time of the myotomy adds about 30 minutes to the procedure, but a disabling reflux is prevented.

Esophageal myotomy for achalasia can be performed either via the chest or the abdomen. Thoracoscopic cardiomyotomy does not allow the same alignment between the operating instruments and the esophagus as does the laparoscopic approach. The instruments come in almost perpendicular to the esophagus, making dissection and suturing difficult. This is particularly of concern at the distal part of the dissection, which is the most difficult section and is not well visualized during thoracoscopic cardiomyotomy. In addition, the thoracoscopic approach requires double lumen endotrachial intubation and pulmonary collapse for exposure of the esophagus.[17,18] For the conventional (open) thoracic cardiomyotomy, the consensus on antireflux procedure is not as clear as that for abdominal cardiomyotomy.[1,4] Thoracoscopic antireflux procedures have been described, but they are not routinely performed.[19] Finally, should a conversion to an open procedure be necessary, the morbidity of the thoracic incision is significantly higher than is that of the abdominal one.

Conclusion

Cardiomyotomy for achalasia is one of the ideal procedures for the videoendoscopic approach. Magnification of the operative field during laparoscopic surgery allows for a precise division of the muscle fibers with excellent results. The number of reports on cardiomyotomy performed with minimal access surgery is growing.[2,6,8–11,14] They all show the same excellent results as conventional (open) myotomy, with minimal morbidity, short hospital stay, and early return to routine activity.

References

1. Ellis FH. Functional disorders of the esophagus. In: Zuidema GD, Orringer MB eds. Shackelford's surgery of the alimentary tract. Third ed. WB Saunders Company, Philadelphia, 1991, p. 146.

2. Oddsdottir M. Laparoscopic management of achalasia. Surg Clin N Am 1996; 76:451–457.
3. Csendes A, Braghetto I, Henriquez A, et al. Late results of a prospective randomized study comparing forceful dilatation and oephagomyotomy in patients with achalasia. Gut 1989;30:299–304.
4. Ellis FH. Oesophagomyotomy for achalasia: a 22-year experience. Br J Surg 1993;80:882.
5. Sauer L, Pellegrini CA, Way LW. The treatment of achalasia. Arch Surg 1989; 124:929–932.
6. Hunter JG, Trus TL, Branum GD, et al. Laparoscopic Heller myotomy and fundoplication for achalasia. Ann Surg 1997;225:655–664.
7. Abid S, Champion G, Richter JE, et al. Treatment of achalasia: the best of both worlds. Am J Gastroenterol 1994;89:979.
8. Shimi S, Nathanson LK, Cuschieri A. Laparoscopic cardiomyotomy for achalasia. J R Coll Surg Edin 1991;36:152–154.
9. DePaula AL, Hashiba K, Bafutto M. Laparoscopic approach to esophageal achalasia. Surg Endosc 1995;9:220.
10. Swanstrom LL, Pennings J. Laparoscopic esophagomyotomy for achalasia. Surg Endosc 1995;9:286–292.
11. Rosati R, Fumigalli U, Bonavina A, et al. Laparoscopic Heller-Dor procedure with intraoperative balloon dilatation of the cardia. Surg Endosc 1994;8:463.
12. Andreollo NA, Earlam RJ. Heller's myotomy for achalasia: is an added anti-reflux procedure necessary? Br J Surg 1987;74:765–769.
13. Crookes PF, Wilkinson AJ, Johnston GW. Heller's myotomy with partial fundoplication. Br J Surg 1989;76:98.
14. Ancona E, Peracchia A, Zaninotto G, et al. Heller laparoscopic cardiomyotomy with antireflux anterior fundoplication (Dor) in the treatment of esophageal achalasia. Surg Endosc 1993;7:459.
15. Dor J, Humbert P, Paoli JM, et al. Traitement du reflux par la technique dite de Heller-Nissen modifiee. Presse Med 1967;75:2563.
16. Toupet A. Technique d'oesophago-gastroplastie avec phreno-gastropexie applique dans la cure radicale des hernies hiatales et comme complement de l'operation de Heller dans les cardiospasmes. Acad Chir 1963;89:394.
17. Pellegrini CA, Leichter R, Patti M, et al. Thoracoscopic esophageal myotomy in the treatment of achalasia. Ann Thorac Surg 1993;56:680–682.
18. Monson JRT, Darzi A, Carey PD, et al. Thoracoscopic Heller's cardiomyotomy: a new approach for achalasia. Surg Laparosc Endosc 1994;4:6.
19. Champion JK, McKernan JB. Thoracoscopic Belsey fundoplication for complicated gastroesophageal reflux disease. Scientific Session manual, SAGES 1997, 1997;74.

11
Laparoscopic Transhiatal Esophagectomy

JOSEPH B. PETELIN

Transhiatal esophagectomy (THE) was first successfully performed by Turner in 1933.[1] As anesthetic methods improved, the transthoracic approach to esophageal resection became the preferred modality. Nevertheless, the morbidity of the transthoracic approach eventually led to a reintroduction of the transhiatal approach by Orringer in 1978.[2] Institution-specific and multiinstitution studies since that time have failed to provide a consistent picture of the preferred approach to esophagectomy. While some studies suggest that transthoracic esophagectomy (TTE) provides better outcomes, others indicate that THE is associated with lower morbidity and equivalent respectability rates.[3–6] Thus, esophageal surgeons continue to be challenged to improve the surgical treatment of esophageal disorders, even in the 1990s.

This situation led some groups to use newer minimally invasive techniques to improve the treatment of esophageal disease. Krasna et al. demonstrated that thoracoscopic and laparoscopic exploration are more accurate than other less invasive staging methods of esophageal cancer.[7] Sadanaga and colleagues have reported that the use of a laparoscope, placed through an upper midline laparotomy, improved the accuracy of otherwise blind blunt dissection of the esophagus through a transhiatal approach.[8] Cuschieri demonstrated a thoracoscopic approach to subtotal esophagectomy in 1994.[9] Coosemens and associates reported on Belgian experience of 20 thorascopic esophagectomies.[10]

Finally, in 1995 DePaula reported successful results of his first 12 laparoscopic transhiatal esophagectomies.[11] He noted an impressive postoperative course in most of his patients. No patients required ICU admission. All patients were extubated in the recovery room. Patients had fewer pulmonary complications than those undergoing other techniques. Ambulation occurred sooner; hospital stay was decreased; and patients resumed normal activities sooner. He concluded that this approach should be considered for patients harboring lesions in the distal third of the esophagus, but that a thorascopic approach should be considered for mid- and upper-third lesions.

Indications for and Advantages of Laparoscopic Transhiatal Esophagectomy

The indications for laparoscopic transhiatal esophagectomy (LTHE) are essentially the same as those for open transhiatal esophagectomy. These include advanced achalasia, severe reflux stenosis, and neoplasia. Whereas DePaula recommends an alternative approach for middle third esophageal tumors, the transhiatal approach also appears appropriate for tumors of the cervical esophagus.

Avoidance of the complications and morbidity associated with a transthoracic open approach is the primary theoretical advantage of the LTHE approach. Decreased likelihood of uncontrolled mediastinal bleeding, avoidance of tracheobronchial injury, decreased postoperative pulmonary insufficiency, absence of ICU admission, shorter hospital stay, more rapid resumption of normal activity, and decreased mortality appear to be the primary benefits of this approach.

Unlike open THE, the laparoscopic approach provides excellent visualization of posterior mediastinum, which allows a more precise dissection and avoidance of injury to surrounding structures. Intraoperative hypotension, which is commonly seen in open THE,[12] and which has been shown to be secondary to impaired venous return during the blunt dissection, appears to be nearly completely avoided with LTHE.

Techniques of Laparoscopic Transhiatal Esophagectomy

The technique of LTHE essentially evolved from that used for laparoscopic antireflux surgery. As more aggressive laparoscopic attempts to treat patients with paraesophageal herniae and intrathoracic stomach led surgeons further cephalad into the mediastinum through a naturally widened hiatus, it was natural to consider performing more proximal esophageal dissection in patients without an enlarged hiatus as well.

The operating theater is arranged so that both monitors are located at the head of the table. The patient is placed in low lithotomy position, with the patient's head turned to the right. The entire neck, chest, and abdomen are prepped and draped into the operative field. The surgeon stands between the patient's lower extremities (Fig. 11.1).

Laparoscopic access is gained through the intended initial port site location, which is located approximately 4–5 cm superior to the umbilicus. The laparoscope will be inserted through this port, and will need to travel all the way into the lower mediastinum. The port may therefore need to be placed more superiorly in tall individuals. Secondary ports are placed under direct laparoscopic visualization in locations similar to those used for

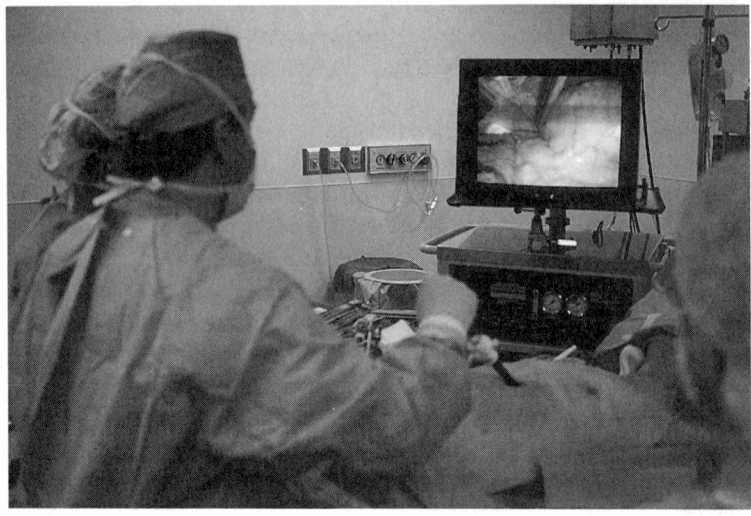

FIGURE 11.1. Patient–surgeon position for laparoscopic transhiatal esophagectomy.

antireflux surgery. Two are placed in the right upper quadrant and two are placed in the left upper quadrant. It is more important to keep these at least one hand-breadth apart so that instrument conflict does not occur (Fig. 11.2).

Exploration

The abdomen is explored to determine the extent of the disease process, the presence of concomitant pathology, the presence of metastatic disease, the potential mobility of the stomach and duodenum, and the resectability of the lesion. Prior gastric resection or duodenal ulcer surgery would present relative contraindications to the procedure and would necessitate intestinal interposition. Because the stomach might not prove to be suitable for mobilization to the neck, preoperative mechanical and antibiotic colon preparation should be considered.

Gastric and Duodenal Mobilization

The lateral attachments of the duodenum are divided to facilitate gastric mobility toward the esophageal hiatus. This may be accomplished with

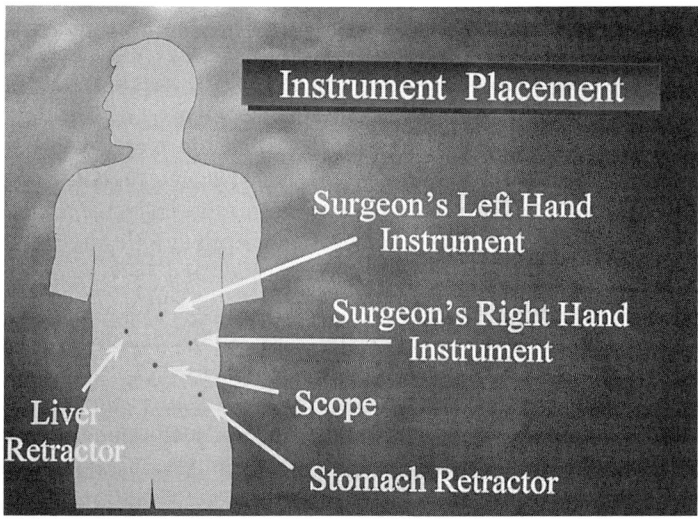

FIGURE 11.2. Port site locations for laparoscopic transhiatal esophagectomy.

scissors or a hook diathermy probe. The gastrocolic omentum is divided along with the left gastroepiploic artery. Great care is taken to avoid injury to the right gastroepiploic artery. The short gastric vessels are controlled and divided without injury to the spleen. The pars flaccida is incised and the left gastric artery and vein are divided. The right gastric artery is preserved. Both the right gastric and gastroepiploic arteries provide blood supply to the stomach tube. If the resection is being done for malignancy, then the celiac nodes are included with the specimen. At this time the crural dissection is usually started posteriorly. The phrenoesophageal membrane is incised and the esophagogastric junction mobilized. As this occurs, the hiatus will usually dilate enough to permit subsequent proximal dissection. At this juncture, the stomach is then inspected anteriorly and posteriorly to insure viability, absence of injury, and free mobility toward the mediastinum.

Gastric Outlet Treatment

Because vagal interruption accompanies esophagectomy, the gastric outlet must be manipulated to allow for adequate gastric emptying. Both the author and DePaula favor pyloromyotomy, although pyloroplasty is an option. This is accomplished with hook diathermy or a harmonic scalpel.

Mediastinal Dissection

The mediastinal dissection is carried cephalad to the aortic arch (Figs. 11.3 to 11.5). Blunt techniques are usually effective for most of this dissection, but some vessels that may be encountered will require control with either clips, diathermy, or harmonic energy. The latter two modalities present more risk of injury to surrounding structures and should be used cautiously. Although the author has not yet experienced pneumothorax during this maneuver, it is a potential complication and should be considered as a possible cause for otherwise unexplained intraoperative cardiorespiratory instability. Communication between the anesthesiologist and the surgeon, therefore, is mandatory during this part of the procedure.

As the dissection approaches the aortic arch, considerable pressure may be applied to the heart as it is in the open blunt technique. The surgeon should be aware of this potential problem and limit the duration of anterior retraction on the pericardium. Communication with the anesthesiologist is again essential. At the level of the arch, the laparoscopist has usually reached the limits of the laparoscopic part of the dissection. The angles at which the laparoscopic instruments enter the mediastinum necessarily direct them posteriorly. This limits further proximal anterior dissection even in cases where longer instruments are used. Innovative semiflexible port and instrument design may alleviate this problem.

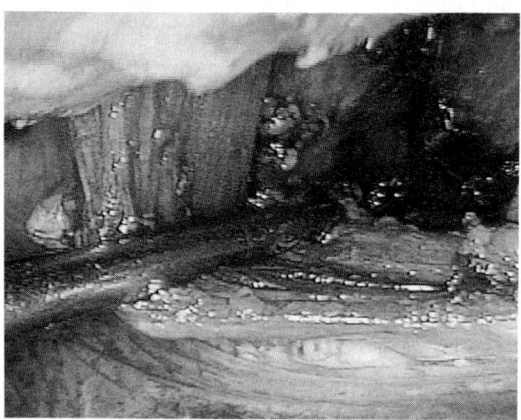

FIGURE 11.3. Mediastinal dissection: The esophageal hiatus, in the foreground, is rather easily dilated during the blunt dissection. It is usually not necessary to incise the diaphragm.

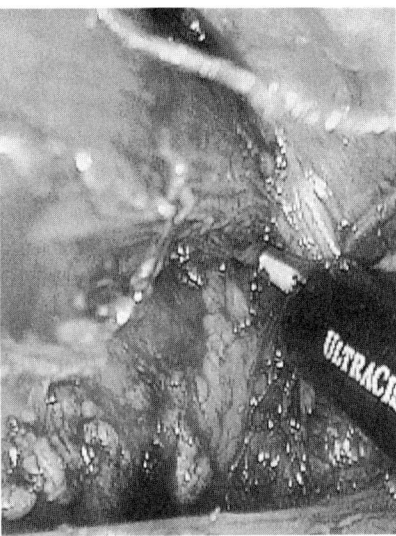

FIGURE 11.4. Mediastinal dissection: Here the dissection anterior to the esophagus is carried out with primarily blunt techniques. Harmonic scissors dissection is also useful in this area.

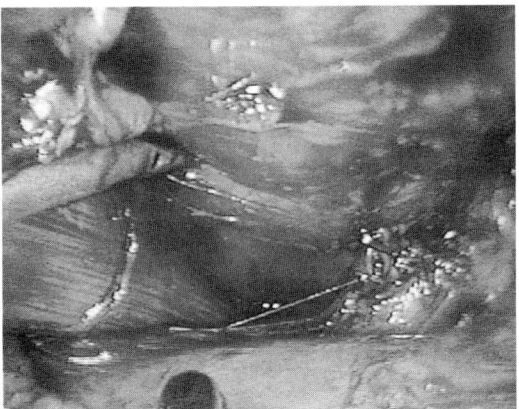

FIGURE 11.5. Mediastinal dissection: The proximal limit of the transhiatal dissection is reached. At the superior part of the picture, the transverse course of the pulmonary veins is noted. To the far left is the esophagus. Posteriorly, the aorta is easily identified.

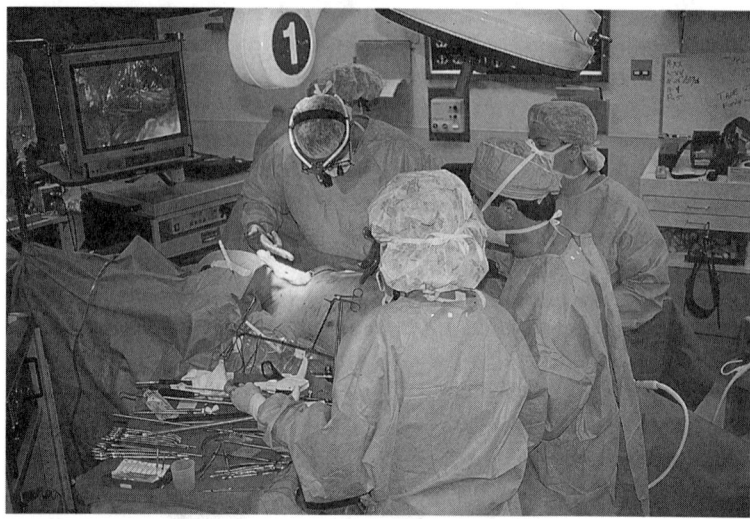

FIGURE 11.6. The second team pursues the cervical and upper mediastinal dissection from a left cervical approch. This team can usually work simultaneously with the laparoscopic team.

Cervical Dissection

During the laparoscopic mediastinal dissection, a second surgical team initiates cervical dissection (Fig. 11.6). An incision parallel to the anterior border of the sternocleidomastoid muscle is made. The cervical esophagus is carefully mobilized from the surrounding structures. Great care must be taken here to avoid injury to the recurrent laryngeal nerve. Blunt dissection around the esophagus in the superior mediastinum is carried down to meet the dissection below. It is usually wise and often helpful for the laparoscopic surgeon to observe the mediastinum and occasionally manipulate the esophagus during this part of the procedure.

Resection and Anastomosis

Upon completion of the proximal esophageal dissection, attention is then directed to transection of the proximal stomach. This is accomplished with an EndoGIA™ (United States Surgical Corporation, Norwalk, Connecticut) stapling and transection device. One or more firings of the device may be required to completely transect the stomach. Sutures are then placed between the stomach and distal esophagus to allow traction of the stomach

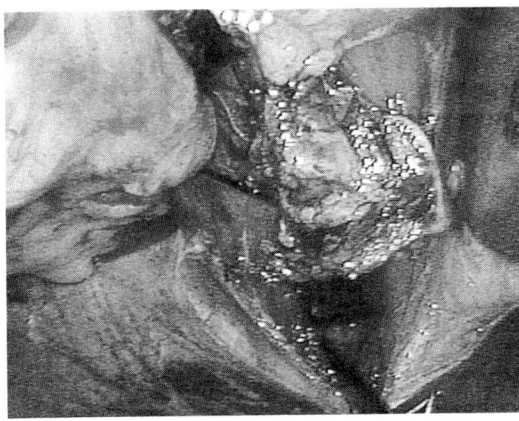

FIGURE 11.7. The distal line of resection has been created with endoscopic stapling/ cutting devices. A dark 0-silk suture is seen connecting the divided esophagus and stomach. This allows for retraction of the proximal stomach to the neck as the esophagus is withdrawn through the cervical incision.

proximally as the esophagus is then transected and the specimen removed from the field (Fig. 11.7). The esophagogastric anastomosis is hand sewn in a conventional manner.

As the cervical wound is closed, a final inspection of the abdomen is performed, the laparoscopic ports are removed, and the abdominal wounds are closed in routine manner. All port sites >10mm in diameter are closed at the fascial level as well as the skin.

Results of Laparoscopic Transhiatal Esophagectomy

DePaula has the largest series in the world and has performed more than 30 laparoscopic transhiatal esophagectomies at this time.[13] His current results are similar to his initial series. The procedure in his hands is successfully completed laparoscopically in nearly 100% of cases. Although this author has much less experience, all cases have been completed laparoscopically as well.

Operative times are long, but they decrease with experience. Mean operative time is approximately 4.5 hours. Mean postoperative length of stay is approximately 8 days. Complications include pneumothorax in approximately 10% of patients, transient dysphonia in up to 25% of patients, pleural effusion and/or atelectasis in approximately 25% of patients, anastomotic leak in approximately 3%, and dumping syndrome in approximately 3%. These are all early results and represent an aggressive learning curve by an accomplished laparoscopic surgeon.

These results compare quite favorably with those of other techniques, and in most cases they are significant improvements in patient outcomes.

Summary

Laparoscopic esophageal surgery is in its infancy. The technique of laparoscopic transhiatal esophagectomy has been shown to be feasible, and early results are encouraging. The operation, however, is not suited for the weak-hearted or the ill-prepared surgeon. Extensive laparoscopic experience in both general laparoscopy, especially in gastroesophageal laparoscopic procedures, is recommended before embarking on laparoscopic transhiatal esophagectomy. DePaula has shown us, however, that the potential patient benefits are worth the effort.

References

1. Turner GG, Durh MS. Excision of the thoracic esophagus for carcinoma with construction of an extrathoracic gullet. Lancet 1933;1:1315–1317.
2. Orringer MB, Sloan H. Esophagectomy without thoracotomy. J Thorac Cardiovasc Surg 1978;76:643–654.
3. Moreno-Gonzalez E, Pinto IG, Garcia I, et al. Esophageal resection through a translaparotomic-transcervical approach. Ann Ital Chir 1992;LXIII:1:33–37.
4. Bolton JS, Sardi A, Bowen JC, et al. Transhiatal and transthoracic esophagectomy: a comparative study. J Surg Oncol 1992;51:249–253.
5. Tialanus HW, Hop WCJ, Bernhard LAM, et al. Esophagectomy with or without thoracotomy: is there any difference? J Thorac Cardio Vasc Surg 1993;105(5):898–903.
6. Rahamim J, Cham CW. Oesophagogastrectomy for carcinoma of the oesophagus and cardia. Br J Surg 1993;80(10):1305–1309.
7. Krasna MJ, Flowers JL, Arrar S, et al. Combined throacoscopic/laparoscopic staging of esophageal cancer. J Thorac Cardiovasc Surg 1996;111(4):800–806.
8. Sadanaga N, Kuwano H, Watanabe M, et al. Laparoscopy-assisted surgery: a new technique for transhiatal esophageal dissection. Am J Surg 1994;168:355–357.
9. Cuschieri A. Thoracoscopic subtotal oesophagectomy. Endosc Surg Allied Technol 1994;2(1):21–25.
10. Coosemens W, Lerut TE, VanRaemdonck DE. Thoracoscopic surgery: the Belgian experience. Ann Thorac Surg 1993;56(3):721–730.
11. DePaula AL, Hashiba K, Ferreira E, et al. Laparoscopic transhiatal esophagectomy with esophagogastroplasty. Surg Laparosc Endosc 1995;5:1–5.

12. Yakoubian K, Bougeois B, Marty J, et al. Cardiovascular responses to manual dissection associated with transhiatal esophageal resection. J Cardiothoracic Anesth 1990;4(4):458–461.
13. DePaula AL. Personal Communication.

12
Laparoscopic Ulcer Surgery

Theodore Diamantis

The treatment of chronic peptic ulceration has changed considerably during the 1980s and 1990s. Elective operations for duodenal ulcer disease had previously dominated the clinical practice of a generation of abdominal surgeons. The incidence of the disease has changed and significant advances have been made in our understanding of its pathogenesis. Medical treatment and indications for surgery and surgical treatment have also changed. Elective operations have become very rare today.

There is a widely held misunderstanding that the introduction of cimetidine into clinical use, together with the other histamine H_2-receptor antagonists that followed, has been responsible for the decreasing incidence of duodenal ulcer.[1] In fact, there are no data to support this belief. On the contrary the incidence of duodenal ulceration has been declining in the Western world in the past four decades, which is long before the introduction of cimetidine. Studies from different sources support this observation. From 1970 to 1978, hospital admissions in U.S. hospitals for the treatment of duodenal ulcer were reduced by more than 40%. This reduction was mainly produced by the uncomplicated ulcer, not from the patients admitted with hemorrhage or perforation.[2] Unlike duodenal ulcer, hospitalization and mortality rates for gastric ulcer were not reduced.[3]

The introduction of histamine H_2—receptor antagonists and proton pump inhibitors in the medical therapy of peptic ulcer modified the clinical manifestation of the disease significantly, although its natural history remained unchanged. The recurrence rate without maintenance treatment was very high. There was no significant reduction in the number of patients operated on for complications, and the mortality rate from these complications was not reduced despite the fact that a healing rate of more than 90% could be achieved with antisecretory treatment.[4]

The identification of the importance of *Heliobacter pylori* infection in the ulcer diathesis, along with the dramatic reduction of the recurrence rate after its eradication, seems that it will change the natural history of the disease and that its complications will become less frequent.

Surgical treatment of peptic ulcer can be divided into two groups:

1. Treatment of uncomplicated ulcer
2. Treatment of the complications; namely bleeding, perforation, and obstruction

Laparoscopic Treatment of Uncomplicated Ulcer

Indications for elective surgical treatment of peptic ulcer have been restricted to:

1. Patients with intractable ulcer after an intensive medical treatment
2. *H. pylori* negative patients with relapsing duodenal ulcer

Although gastric ulcers and duodenal ulcers are often commonly felt to have common manifestations they have few pathophysiologic features in common. This fact, together with the possibility of cancer in cases of gastric ulcers that are unresponding to medical treatment, imposes different goals in the operative therapy.[2]

Duodenal Ulcer

The main goal of elective surgical treatment of duodenal ulcer should be alteration of the ulcer diathesis by reducing the acid secretion in a way that results in ulcer healing. Associated goals of the operation are the patient's safety, minimal ulcer recurrence rate, and freedom from chronic postoperative side effects. The ideal operation should be equally safe and effective, preventing recurrent ulceration and postoperative disability. As there is no such operation, the choice is based on the hierarchy of the various goals of the operation between:

- Truncal vagotomy with or without drainage
- Truncal vagotomy and antrectomy
- Proximal gastric vagotomy
- Posterior truncal vagotomy and anterior seromyotomy

Since its introduction by Dragstedt and Owens in 1943. Truncal vagotomy, combined with pyloroplasty, gastrojejunostomy, or antrectomy, has become and has remained the most popular surgical approach for duodenal ulcer therapy. As in the original series of patients, drainage procedure was advocated by Dragstedt because gastric outlet obstruction was observed in some cases. It has been proposed that this problem can be solved without a drainage procedure by pneumatic dilatation of the pylorus, resulting in rupture of the oblique and circular muscles, and giving a widely patent channel.[5] With this modification one can avoid the side effects of pyloroplasty or gastrojejunostomy. Recurrent ulcer rates following vagotomy and drainage are 5–15%, mortality is low (1%), and postoperative complications are between 11 and 26%.[13] (Table 12.1.)

The addition of antrectomy offers more intensive acid secretion reduction, which translates into lower recurrent ulcer rates. On the other hand, mortality and side effects are marginally increased.

In fact, the greatest contribution to duodenal ulcer surgery has been the application of proximal gastric vagotomy. The procedure consists of meticulous dissection and division of the multiple branches of the anterior and posterior nerves of Latarjet starting 5–7 cm proximal to the pylorus. The vagal trunks, their hepatic and celiac branches, and the nerves of Latarjet are left intact. All abdominal innervations except for the acid-secretory gastric mucosa are preserved, and near-normal gastric emptying and extragastric digestive tract functions are maintained. In addition, the operation requires a careful search for and division of all periesophageal vagal branches from anterior and posterior vagal trunks innervating the gastric fundus and the cardia. The procedure is technically demanding, and this can explain the fact that the reported recurrence rates range from as low as 5% to as high as 20%, which reflects different expertise with the procedure. Review of the literature in reports on more than 5,000 patients treated with proximal gastric vagotomy followed up to 18 years reveals a recurrent ulcer rate of 9.1%, a mortality rate of 0.2%, and side effects in 8% of cases.[6]

In 1980, Taylor introduced an interesting modification of proximal gastric vagotomy consisting of posterior truncal vagotomy combined with anterior lesser curvature seromyotomy of the corpus and fundus.[7] The devascularization of the entire lesser curvature of the stomach was avoided. Results were very encouraging, there was no significant alteration in gastric emptying, and safety and efficacy were comparable to those of proximal gastric vagotomy. The only disadvantage to this procedure is that the international experience is limited compared with proximal gastric vagotomy, and that it will remain so because the number of elective duodenal ulcer operations is diminishing every year.

The final decision about the operation to be performed is based on the personal philosophy of the surgeon, training, the general philosophy about what is more important to be avoided, and the possibility of recurrence or

TABLE 12.1. Results of operations used in the elective treatment of duodenal ulcer.

	Mortality rate (%)	Recurrent ulcer rate (%)	Side effects (%)
Truncal vagotomy/ antrectomy	1–2	1–2	13–29
Truncal vagotomy/ drainage	1	5–15	11–26
Proximal gastric vagotomy	0.1–0.3	9.1 (5–20)	8

the postoperative side effects. Proximal gastric vagotomy became popular in Europe long before it did in the United States, where medicolegal reasons influenced surgeons toward vagotomy and antrectomy, which is a more effective operation. More and more surgeons are now convinced that proximal gastric vagotomy or posterior truncal vagotomy and anterior seromyotomy are the operations of choice for the elective surgical treatment of duodenal ulcer because:

1. As no single operation for this disease has demonstrated uniform success in preventing ulcer recurrence, it appears reasonable to select the procedure that best minimizes morbidity.

2. In case of ulcer recurrence, its treatment is not necessarily surgical; however, even if this is the case, mortality and morbidity rates associated with operations for ulcer recurrence are less in patients who initially have undergone proximal gastric vagotomy than those who have undergone any other operation.

3. With laparoscopic surgery both proximal gastric vagotomy as well as posterior truncal vagotomy and anterior seromyotomy can be performed, which minimizes operative trauma and hospitalization.

Laparoscopic Proximal Gastric Vagotomy

It became evident very early that the laparoscopic approach could be used to successfully perform typical proximal gastric vagotomy.[8] The patient is placed in the so-called French position with the operating surgeon standing between the patient's legs.

The operation can usually be performed through two 10-mm and three 5-mm ports. As in most laparoscopic operations aiming at the gastroesophageal junction, the cannula to be used for the telescope should be placed 3–5 cm above the umbilicus, depending on the height of the patient (Fig. 12.1). The second port, which is placed on the right middle clavicular line under the costal margin, is used for retraction of the left hepatic lobe. The third port, which is low under the left costal margin, is used to retract the stomach laterally. Two other ports are placed in the epigastrium and are used by the surgeon for dissection and suturing.

After laparoscoic identification of the pylorus, the crowfoot of Latarjet nerve is identified and a distance of 6–7 cm from the pylorus is measured. Dissection and division of all vascular branches entering the lesser curvature is then begun. Some surgeons advocate that at least during initial operations both posterior and anterior vagal trunks must be identified, partially mobilized, and marked with an umbilical tape in order to reassure its preservation. The dissection can be made according to the surgeon's preference with dissecting scissors, hook, or ultrasonic scissors. The dissection should be meticulous. In obese patients it can occasionally be difficult; however we have found the ultrasonic scissors very helpful in these patients.

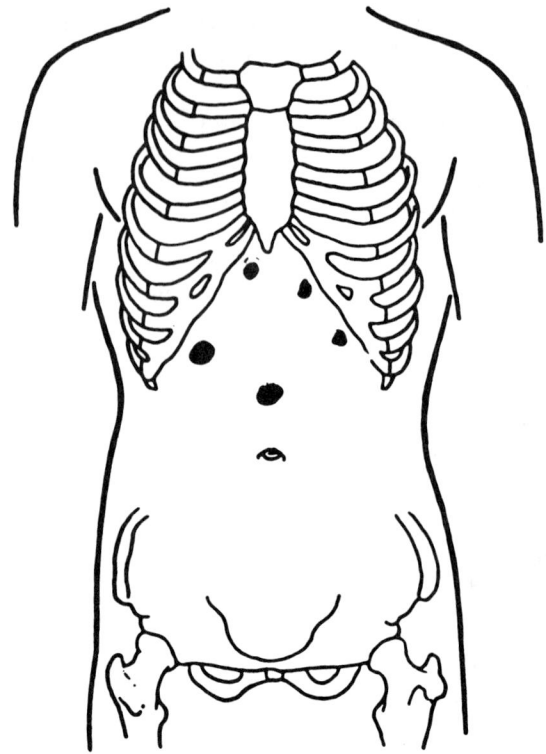

FIGURE 12.1. Usual sites of trocar placement for operations aiming at the gastroesphageal junction.

Some investigators advocate the use of intraoperative Congo red test in order to document the completeness of the vagotomy.[9]

Laparoscopic Posterior Truncal Vagotomy and Anterior Seromyotomy

Classic parietal-cell vagotomy was found by some surgeons to be an inordinately slow, laborious, and technically demanding operation requiring several hours. For this reason it is seen as a nonpractical proposition.[10] These surgeons have been advocating posterior truncal vagotomy and anterior seromyotomy as an alternative that is ideally suited to the laparoscopic approach. It has achieved the same acid-reducing effect and clinical results as in its open application.[5]

The access ports required for this procedure are the same with proximal gastric vagotomy. Dissection begins with the division of the peritoneum covering the right and superior margins of the hiatus. The first objective is to identify and expose the right crus of the diaphragm. The dissection is continued after that, between the right margin of the esophagus and the right crus toward its junction with the left crus. The posterior vagal trunk is found attached to the wall of the esophagus or lying over the left crus. It should be dissected free from the esophagus, clipped, and divided above the branches it gives to the cardioesophageal junction.[11]

Seromyotomy is carried out starting high on the fundus to the left of the esophagus to ensure complete parietal-cell denervation. It then follows the lesser curvature at a distance of about 1.5 cm from the edge to avoid vascular damage. The line of division of the seromuscular layer should be marked by superficial electrocautery with its lower end just proximal to the crowfoot of Latarjet's nerve. The close-up vision and the magnification of the laparoscopic approach facilitates division of the seromuscular layer down to the mucosa.

After completion, the myotomy wound is sutured with a continuous running absorbable 3-0 stitch.

Sharp dissection of the anterior seromuscular layer of the stomach may occasionally cause excessive blood loss and perforation of the mucosa. Several surgeons have reported that the use of carbon dioxide laser may reduce these problems. When used on the gastric serosal surface, the defocused carbon dioxide laser results in destruction of vagal fibers because its energy is preferentially absorbed by the neurons. Surgeons experienced with the use of carbon dioxide laser believe that it has other additional advantages over the scalpel in performing seromyotomy.[12,13] They report shorter operative time and do not consider the suture closure of the seromyotomy as necessary.

Laparoscopic Truncal Vagotomy and Pyloric Stretch

International experience with truncal vagotomy and pyloric stretch is limited,[14] long-term follow-up results are missing, and its principles are against what was for a long time considered as the gold standard for antiulcer surgery. It has not been confirmed that pyloric stretch is effective for long-term protection against delayed gastric emptying.

This procedure should be considered as experimental. Its simplicity cannot overcome the fact that it cannot be regarded as the endoscopic equivalent of any of the well-studied, well-established antiulcer procedures.

The final decision for the laparoscopic treatment of the uncomplicated duodenal ulcer using Taylor's operation should be made based on the surgeon's experience. It was reasonable for every individual surgeon to rely on personal experience before the era of laparoscopic surgery. The small number of these operations performed today will not allow any surgical team to collect adequate experience with any new procedure.

Gastric Ulcer

The important principles in the treatment of gastric ulcer are different from those of duodenal ulcer. Failure to complete healing after an intensive medical treatment of 4 weeks to a maximum of 8 weeks is an indication for surgical treatment. Size reduction is not a good indicator for continuation of medical treatment because gastric malignancies can show up to 50% reduction in diameter under antisecretory treatment. Conservative treatment longer than 8 weeks is suggested only for prepyloric ulcers with negative multiple biopsies.

The aims of surgical management are total excision of the ulcer, so that it can be examined histologically, and removal of the antrum to avoid recurrence. Billroth I gastrectomy is the operation of choice. When the ulcer is very high it may be excised separately.

Safety and efficacy of laparoscopic gastric resection and Billroth I or Billroth II anastomosis has been documented both experimentally and clinically, but operative experience to date is limited.[14,15]

For the time being the laparoscopic approach is not indicated for the surgical treatment of gastric ulcer. With the development of laparoscopic stapling technology, laparoscopic gastrectomy could be added to the armamentarium of the average laparoscopic surgeon in the future.

Laparoscopic Treatment of Complications of Peptic Ulcer Hemorrhage

Gastric or duodenal bleeding represents approximately 25% of upper gastrointestinal bleeding. Although there has been controversy about the value of diagnostic endoscopy in reducing mortality and mortality rates, the identification of the source of bleeding is mandatory for the selection of proper treatment. For this reason emergency endoscopy has been routinely performed for the last 15 years.

Since the late 1980s considerable progress has been made in endoscopic hemostasis.[16] Several methods are available for the endoscopic treatment of bleeding peptic ulcer, including some very simple ones such as epinephrine solution injection, as well as the sophisticated use of lasers. High success rates have similarly been reported with all methods. Hemostasis can be achieved in 80–95% of patients with active bleeding during endoscopy. The presence of bleeding stigmata (e.g., clot, black spot, or visible vessel) indicates that a repeat prophylactic session should be considered 24–48 hours after initial hemostasis. The choice between the various modalities is usually based on the availability in any different setting.

The wide use of endoscopic hemostatic techniques has decreased the mortality rates and the need for surgical intervention in patients with bleeding ulcers.

Although there has been an increasing number of preliminary reports of endoluminal laparoscopic surgery,[17] laparoscopic surgery for bleeding peptic ulcer should still be considered as experimental.

Obstruction

Gastric outlet obstruction complicates 10% of cases of duodenal ulcer disease in modern series. All patients that present with acute or chronic obstruction should initially be treated with medical therapy that consists of gastric decompression, intravenous hydration, and occasionally total parenteral nutrition. Surgical treatment for the obstruction is considered to be required if there is a positive gastric residual test after 4 or 5 days of medical treatment. It consists of 400 ml or more residual at 30 minutes after instillation of 750 ml of saline solution into the stomach. Upper gastrointestinal endoscopy should be performed in order to confirm the mechanical nature of obstruction and to exclude malignancy.

The operation performed should relieve both ulcer diathesis and treat obstruction. Three types of procedures are possible laparoscopically:

1. Laparoscopic total truncal vagotomy and pyloroplasty.
2. Laparoscopic total truncal vagotomy and gastrojejunostomy.
3. Laparoscopic total truncal vagotomy and antrectomy with a Billroth II reconstruction

The first operation is a simpler one, and is known to have a lower morbidity and mortality rate than open surgery. Extensive duodenal scarring makes a satisfactory pyloroplasty difficult.

Vagotomy and antrectomy is the most radical approach; however, it has a higher mortality and morbidity. All of the variables mentioned earlier apply in selecting the best operation for each individual patient.

Laparoscopic Total Truncal Vagotomy and Pyloroplasty

The patient is placed in a position as for all laparoscopic surgery. Placement of the trocars is as described earlier, except that the videolaparoscope should be entered at the level of the umbilicus to provide good access to both hiatus and pylorus.

Posterior truncal vagotomy is carried out as described for Taylor's operation. For the anterior vagus, the phrenoesophageal ligament is divided and the fat pad is removed enabling its identification. All small branches of both anterior and posterior vagus should be carefully divided. The esophagus should be cleaned of all nonelastic fibers using a monopolar hook as it is in open surgery.

Laparoscopic Heineke-Mikulicz pyloroplasty is performed exactly as it is in open surgery. A longitudinal incision of about 5 cm is made through all the pyloroduodenal segment. The wound is then sutured using continuous sutures of 3-0 Vicryl in two layers. We found that the magnification of the videoendoscope facilitates precise suture placement.

Laparoscopic Total Truncal Vagotomy and Gastrojejunostomy

There is often extensive scarring in the anterior surface of the duodenum that makes the construction of a pyloroplasty unsafe. A gastrojejuno-stomy can be performed, 8 cm proximal to the pylorus under these circumstances.[18]

Most surgeons are used to a posterior anastomosis, although others believe that an anterior gastrojejunostomy provides an equally sufficient drainage of the stomach. For retrocolic anastomosis, mobilization of the great curvature of the stomach should begin at the level of the entrance of the left gastroepiploic artery in the gastrocolic ligament. The dissection can be performed distal to the gastroepiploic arcade. The gastrocolic ligament is then opened, and retraction of the stomach upward allows exposure of the posterior aspect of the stomach. This dissection can be facilitated by the use of the harmonic scalpel. The best way to recognize the beginning of the jejunum is to follow it toward the ligament of Treitz. The operating surgeon should change position to the right side of the patient. Once the second jejunal loop is identified and mobilized it is approximated to the stomach with two endo-Babcock forceps. A gastrotomy and an enterotomy are performed and the linear cutter is then introduced. For an adequate stoma two firings of 35 mm or one with the 60-mm instrument are necessary. The suture line can be easily checked with the videolaparoscope for hemostasis, and one suture can be placed if necessary as in open surgery. The enterotomies are then closed with staplers or with a running suture in one or two layers. We have found that suture closure is much easier than staplers. A nasogastric tube should be placed in the efferent loop with some holes remaining in the stomach. It is usually removed the third day after reconfirmation of the integrity of anastomosis by gastrograffin swallow.

Laparoscopic Total Truncal Vagotomy and Antrectomy with a Billroth II Reconstruction

This procedure is more technically demanding, as well as more radical, than the other two. The first step is the opening of the gastrocolic ligament with the use of the harmonic scissors. Large vessels should be ligated with clips. The area of the posterior aspect of the first part of the duodenum must be dissected as in open surgery. The upper limit of the duodenum is dissected, and the right gastric artery is exposed, ligated with clips, and divided. The next step is transection and closure of the duodenum with an endoscopic cutter. With the distal part of the antrum retracted, the dissection along the lesser curvature can be completed with harmonic scissors and clips when needed. A posterior Billroth II gastrojejunostomy is then performed as described earlier, and the specimen is resected with several firings of the linear cutter.[19] The operation is completed with closure of the enterotomies with running sutures in two layers.

A laparoscopically assisted version of this technique is described by Katkhouda.[10] A 4-cm abdominal incision allows exteriorization of the stomach and the jejunum after its mobilization and duodenal division. The resection of the stomach and the anastomosis are completed extra-abdominally. This technique is probably quicker, easier, safer, and more suitable for most surgeons.

Truncal vagotomy and antrectomy is a difficult and long operation. Laparoscopic truncal vagotomy and pyloroplasty, whenever feasible, is the operation of choice for gastric outlet obstruction complicating duodenal ulcer disease. In cases with excessive scar tissue in the anterior aspect of the duodenum, we prefer to perform a gastrojejunostomy. Both operations can be performed safely by the average surgeon with experience in advanced laparoscopic surgery.

Perforation

The incidence of perforation of duodenal ulcer has not decreased proportionally to the overall decline of operations for peptic ulcer disease. The increased usage of nonsteroidal antiinflammatory drugs may be the cause of this phenomenon. Immediate simple closure of the perforation with or without an omental patch is the most common form of treatment for this emergency. Controversy remains over the indications, if any, of a definitive ulcer procedure at the time of closure of the perforation.

The two primary aims of the surgical procedure for perforated peptic ulcer are to close the perforation and to treat the peritonitis. Both aims can be accomplished through the laparoscopic approach.[9]

Four trocars are usually used. One is placed in the umbilicus for the laparoscope. Two other trocars are placed laterally on either side of the camera for each of the surgeon's hands. The forth trocar is placed under the right costal margin to be used as a retractor as well as for suction and irrigation.

After exploratory laparoscopy, the confirmation of peptic ulcer perforation is made by the presence of free fluid over the distal stomach and the duodenum, and the presence of false membranes in the area. The liver and/or the gallbladder usually cover the perforated ulcer with inflammatory adhesions. Dissection of these adhesions, starting from the edge of the liver, should be gentle, the liver and the gallbladder should be retracted superiorly, and the margin of perforation clearly seen.

Various techniques have been described for closure of the perforation[20-22]; however, one should use the same suture closure as in open surgery. The choice of needles, suture material, and needle holders is a mater of personal preference. We usually use 2-0 Vicryl sutures with a curved needle. Intracorporeal knot-tying technique is preferable because extracorporeal tying may result in excessive tension on the suture and tearing of the inflamed tissues around the perforation. Two or three sutures are usually used to bring the edges of the ulcer together. The anesthetist is asked to inflate the stomach with air through the nasogastric tube and air-tightness of the closure is tested. Whenever a part of the omentum is found free it is used as a patch.

In very rare cases the inflammatory tissue around the perforation does not permit a safe and air-tight closure of the perforation. In these cases excision of the ulcer, pyloroplasty, and truncal vagotomy may be indicated, depending on the patient's history and general condition.

The second aim of the operation is the treatment of peritonitis. This is probably the most important step of the procedure. The peritoneal cavity should be cleansed with at least 8 L of fluid. Suction/irrigation equipment can provide laparoscopic peritoneal lavage as effectively as it does in open surgery. Every quadrant of the peritoneal cavity should be treated with special care. Suction/irrigation should be considered complete only after elimination of all contaminated liquids and suction of clear irrigation fluid.

We routinely place a drain on the subhepatic space, as we do in open surgery. The drain is removed on the second postoperative day.

Prospective studies have demonstrated that laparoscopic closure of perforated ulcer is a relatively safe procedure.[6,7] In the hands of experienced laparoscopic surgeons, it is also a straightforward operation. Most procedures, unfortunately, are performed as an emergency during the night when the experienced laparoscopist is not always available. This is the reason that preliminary prospective studies failed to show the clear advantages of the laparoscopic approach over the open procedure. Since, then almost all surgeons under training have experience in laparoscopic surgery; therefore, the laparoscopic approach should be considered as the operation of choice for perforated duodenal ulcer.

The question of definitive ulcer procedure during the operation for perforation is under debate. We think that the indication for a definitive procedure is only for patients with recent perforation (less than 12 h) and a long history of ulcer disease, which had a successful *H. pylori* eradication treatment in the past, or those with local conditions necessitating excision of the ulcer and pyloroplasty. All other patients should have the chance to be treated postoperatively with antisecretory drugs and antibiotics, which promise a definitive treatment of ulcer disease in more than 95% of the cases.

Laparoscopic closure of the perforation and proximal gastric vagotomy or posterior truncal vagotomy and anterior seromyotomy are time-consuming operations. In case of an emergency operation for peritonitis we think that the open approach is more indicated, at least in centers with minimal experience in elective laparoscopic ulcer surgery.

Conclusions

Laparoscopic surgery is already playing an important role in both elective and emergency ulcer surgery. In the future, comparison of long-term results after *H. pylori* eradication and elective laparoscopic ulcer surgery will stimulate the interest of gastroenterologists and patients in favor of the minimally invasive approach for at least some forms of ulcer that are difficult to treat medically.

References

1. Kurata JH, Haile BM. Epidemiology of peptic ulcer disease. Clin Gastroenterol 1994;13:289–307.
2. Mulholland MW, Debas HT. Chronic duodenal and gastric ulcer. Surg Clin N Am 1987;67:489–507.
3. Elashoff JD, Grossman MI. Trends in hospital admissions and death rates for peptic ulcer in the United States from 1970 to 1980. Gastroenterology 1981;68:194–196.
4. Bardhan KD, Gust G, Hinchliffe RFC, et al. Changing patterns of admissions and operations for duodenal ulcer. Br J Surg 1989;76:230–236.
5. Pringle R, Irwing AD, Longrigg JN, et al. Randomized trial of truncal vagotomy with either pyloroplasty or pyloric dilatation in the surgical management of chronic duodenal ulcer. Br J Surg 1983;70:482–484.
6. Thompson JC, Wiener I. Evaluation of surgical treatment for duodenal ulcer: acute and long-term effects. Clin Gastroenterol 1984;13:569.
7. Taylor TV, Lythgoe JP, McFarland JB, et al. Anterior lesser curve seromyotomy and posterior truncal vagotomy versus truncal vagotomy and pyloroplasty in the treatment of chronic duodenal ulcer. Br J Surg 1990;77:1007–1009.
8. Frantzides CT, Ludwing KA, Quebbeman EJ, et al. Laparoscopic highly selective vagotomy: technique and case report. Surg Laparosc Endosc 1992;2:348–352.
9. Schneider TA, Andrus CH. The endoscopic Congo red test during proximal gastric vagotomy: an essential procedure. Surg Endosc 1992;6:16–17.
10. Mouiel J, Katkhouda N. Laparoscopic truncal and selective vagotomy. In: Zucker K (ed.). Surgical laparoscopy. Quality Medical Publishers, St. Louis, 1991, pp. 263–279.
11. McKernan JB, Wolfe BM, McFadyen BV, Jr. Laparoscopic repair of duodenal ulcer and gastroesophageal reflux. Surg Clin N Am 1992;72:1153–1167.
12. Qureshi A, Darzi A, Kay E, et al. Carbon dioxide laser vagotomy: early results. Min Inv Ther 1994;3:357–360.

13. Sakuramachi S, Kimura T, Harada Y. Experimental study of laparoscopic selective proximal vagotomy using a carbon dioxide laser. Surg Endosc 1994;8:857–861.
14. Anvari M, Park A. Laparoscopic-assisted vagotomy and distal gastrectomy. Surg Endosc 1994;8:1312–1315.
14. McDermott EWM, Murphy JJ. Laparoscopic truncal vagotomy without drainage. Br J Surg 1993;80:236–240.
15. Soper NJ, Brunt LM, Brewer JD, et al. Laparoscopic Billroth II gastrectomy in the canine model. Surg Endosc 1994;8:1395–1398.
16. Sugawa C. Endoscopic diagnosis and treatment of upper gastrointestinal bleeding. Surg Clin N Am 1989;69:1167–1183.
17. Potvin M, Gagner M, Pomp A. Laparoscopic transgastric suturing for bleeding peptic ulcer. Surg Endosc 1996;10:400–402.
18. Katkhouda N, Bremner R, Ortega A. Laparoscopic management of complications of peptic ulcer disease. Surg Techn Inter 1995;4:121–126.
19. Katkhouda N, Mouiel J. Laparoscopic treatment of peritonitis. In: Zucker K ed. Surgical laparoscopy update. Quality Medical Publishers, St. Louis 1993, p. 287.
20. Johansson B, Hallerback B, Glise H, et al. Laparoscopic suture closure of perforated peptic ulcer. Surg Endosc 1996;10:656–658.
21. So JBY, Kum CK, Fernandes ML, et al. Comparison between laparoscopic and conventional omental patch repair for perforated duodenal ulcer. Surg Endosc 1996;10:1060–1063.
22. Miserez M, Eypasch E, Spangenberger W, et al. Laparoscopic and conventional closure of perforated peptic ulcer; a comparison. Surg Endosc 1996;10:831–836.

13
Laparoscopic Band Plication for the Treatment of Morbid Obesity

Konstantinos Konstantinidis, Michael Vorias,
George Sambalis, and Michael Georgiou

Morbid obesity is considered a multifactorial disease that results from neurochemical, genetic, and psychological factors. It is considered to be a contemporary disease that inflicts all social classes. In the United States approximately 12 million people are morbidly obese, whereas 3–5% of the American population will develop serious and life-threatening complications related to their obesity.[1]

Is Obesity a Disease or a Condition?

In February 1985, it was considered necessary to convene a National Institutes of Health (NIH) Consensus to affirm that obesity is indeed a disease.[2] Public interest in controlling obesity sells the majority of books in the nonfiction category. The NIH's goal became the sensitization of the medical profession, especially the general surgeons, who were not willing to accept obesity as a disease, using proof demonstrating the increased morbidity and mortality related to this condition, which affects the cardiopulmonary system e.g., (coronary disease, hypertension, pulmonary insufficiency, sudden death, obesity–hypoventilation syndrome, sleep apnea, Pickwickian syndrome) and also leads to diabetes mellitus, thromboembolism, gallstones and liver disease, susceptibility to infection, esophagitis, increased operative risk, skin problems, pseudotumor cerebri, menstrual disorders, renal disease, osteoarthritis, varicose veins, infertility, urinary stress incontinence, psychosocial incapacity, depression, and cancer risk (e.g., endometrium, breast, prostate, kidney, colon, gallbladder).[3]

Studies have demonstrated that obese people have an altered social profile and that their social activities are meager.[4] The social–economic status mainly in females is inversely related with their degree of obesity,[5] which affects job employment. Sexual activity and behavior are also affected. The increase of body weight causes changes in external sexual characteristics. These individuals assume a generally asexual shape, which differs from the accepted body image, resulting in their social isolation and stigmatization, defined as the *obesity stereotype*.[6]

Definition

The ideal body weight (IBW) was defined by the Metropolitan Life Insurance Company in 1959.[7] Morbid obesity is usually defined as body weight exceeding the ideal by at least 100–110 lb, as being twice the ideal body weight, or as obesity that approaches those figures but is complicated by major weight-related complications.

The body mass index (BMI) is defined by Kilograms per square meter, and is a good clinical indicator for calculating weight with respect to height.[8]

A BMI < 25 is considered normal
A BMI 25–30 is considered overweight
A BMI > 30 is considered obese
A BMI > 40 is considered morbidly obese

Treatment

Nonsurgical Treatment

This mode of treatment focuses on reduced calorie intake (dieting) and/or increased energy expenditure (exercise). These modalities often are effective for weight reduction in the short term, but recidivism is nearly universal in the morbidly obese.

Surgical Treatment

Antiobesity surgery is used when all other conservative modalities have failed in order to avert potential and established complications.

Historical Aspect of Surgical Treatment

Approximately 50 years have passed from the initial surgical attempts to treat morbid obesity. There were three main types of operations performed:

1. those that produce a malabsorption state (bypasses)
2. those that restrict intake (gastric restrictive procedures)
3. combination of the two

Malabsorptive Procedures

In the early 1950s, Kremen, Linner, and Nelson[9] studied long-term consequences on the physiology of small bowel metabolism after removal or bypass of portions of the small bowel in canines. They concluded that these procedures could be adapted for the treatment of the morbidly obese patient. In 1954 they presented their 36–18 technique. Thirty-six inches of the jejunum is anastomosed end-to-end to 18 inches of the terminal ileum. In 1963 Payne and Dewind followed with their end-to-side jejunocolic shunt.[10] In 1969 they recommended their 14–4 technique,[11] which is an end-to-side jejunoileostomy that uses the first 14 inches of jejunum and the last 4 inches of the terminal ileum.

The years 1950–1970 were the "golden years" for the previously mentioned procedures, mainly due to their relative surgical safety and simplicity, even in the superobese patient. Long-term metabolic complications, however, outweighed the weight loss that was achieved, and surgeons slowly abandoned these techniques.

As interest for bypass procedures dropped, Billroth II reconstruction was gaining popularity for the treatment of duodenal ulceration. Once it was observed that weight-loss was one of the "complications," the stage was set for the so-called gastric restrictive procedures.

Gastric Restrictive Procedures

In 1966 Mason and Ito described the gastric bypass. They partitioned the upper one third of the stomach horizontally, and a loop gastrojejunostomy was created.[12] In 1971, in an attempt to simplify the procedure, Mason described the simple horizontal gastroplasty: partial gastric transection with a stoma on the greater curvature.[13] Although it is an easier operation, results were discouraging, and the procedure was discontinued.

Two modifications to Mason's gastric bypass were made in 1977.

1. The wide-spread use of surgical staplers led Alden to perform a partition using a linear stapler instead of gastric division.[14]
2. Griffen and Young suggest using a Roux-en-Y anastomosis instead of a loop, thus avoiding alkaline gastritis.[15]

Alden's idea to use a linear stapler led Pace in 1979 to use the stapler for a horizontal gastroplasty and to remove two to three staples from the center of linear stapler, thus forming a central stoma.[16] In 1980, Gomez, used the linear stapler, but left a channel on the greater curvature through which ingested food passed.[17]

The Achilles' heal of the previously mentioned procedures was the dilatation of the "stoma," which was related to two issues: pouch size and stoma stability. The problems were addressed by limiting the pouch to less than 50 ml and by supporting a 12-mm stoma with mesh.[17–19]

The initial enthusiasm for horizontal gastroplasty soon declined as a result of poor weight loss and late weight gain. Other problems included postoperative complications, such as staple-line break down, "stoma" obstruction from mesh erosion, failure of gastroscopic dilatation of the "stoma" in cases of stenosis, and alterations of gastric blood supply after horizontal partitioning. Problems contributed to a search for other gastric procedures.[20] Tretbar's gastric plication[21] and the formation of the "stoma" on the lesser curvature by Long in Australia in 1977[22,23] paved the road to vertical gastroplasty. Laws modified the procedure by placing a ring of silicone tubing around the outflow tract to avoid "stoma" dilatation.[24] Mason developed a breakthrough in 1980 with the presentation of the vertical banded gastroplasty.[25]

Biliopancreatic Diversion

The third type of procedure is the one combining the effects of intestinal bypass and gastric restrictive procedures. In 1976 Scopinaro in Italy described the technique of biliopancreatic diversion.[26]

Minimally Invasive Techniques

The morbidly obese constitute a subset of surgical patients in whom the avoidance of any type of postoperative complication is mandatory. These include anastomotic leaks, which are both difficult to diagnose and associate with a high mortality rate. Garren approached the avoidance of the "surgical risk" by endoscopic placement of gastric balloons.[27] Complications such as gastric ulceration, perforation, bleeding, intestinal obstruction, and balloon perforation made this treatment modality less popular.

In 1977 Wilkinson, who understood that the Achilles' heel is a volume-limiting pouch and a rate-limiting "stoma" in the gastric restrictive procedures, proposed the use of gastric banding[28] as a gastric "external" restrictive procedure, thus avoiding the feared, possible anastomotic, leaks. The Materials that were used initially, were Marlex and Dacron.[29-31] In 1983 Kuzmak[32] adopted gastric banding for the treatment of obesity, overcoming the disadvantages of the former materials by introducing the stoma adjustable silicone gastric band. The material is inert and the stoma is calibrated after operation.

The laparoscopic revolution and its adoption by the surgical community challenged those who deal with surgical obesity. Laparoscopy was less traumatic and offered the possibility for less-dangerous treatment of morbid obesity. Thus, the era of laparoscopic procedures for obesity has begun.

The advantage of laparoscopic procedures is mainly the avoidance of the surgical incision. This mainly eliminates the postoperative pain, and results in better respiratory function and faster patient ambulation. Wound-related complications were minimal, and they were never life threatening; however, the possible risk of an anastomotic leak still remains. The avoidance of the "risk" of complications, which are wound or pain related, is overcome by the laparoscopic approach. The "risk" of an anastomotic leak is overcome by the laparoscopic placement of an adjustable silicone gastric band. Belachew[33] and Cadiere[34] from Belgium and Favretti[35] from Italy were among the pioneers of this technique.

Surgical Technique of Laparoscopic Adjustable Silicone Gastric Band (LASGB)

1. *Patient positioning*—Supine with legs abducted and bent, and steep anti-Trendelenberg position, with the first assistant on the left and the second assistant on the right, and the surgeon located between the legs.

2. *Pneumoperitoneum*—Acquired with Hasson trocar (trocar #1) placement at the junction of the upper two thirds with the lower one third of the xiphoumbilical line; intraabdominal pressure is maintained at 15 mmHg.

3. *Trocar placement*—After establishment of the pneumoperitoneum and visualization of the abdominal cavity using a 30-degree laparoscope, four additional 10-mm trocars are introduced under laparoscopic vision. Trocar #2 is placed in the right hypochondrium through which grasping forceps, suction irrigation, and Lap-band closure tool are placed. Trocar #3 is placed in the subxyphoid region through which a fan liver retractor is inserted. Trocar #4 is placed in the left midclavicular line through which grasping forceps, cautery hook, bipolar dissector, and needle holder are inserted. Trocar #5 is placed in the left anterior axillary line below the costal margin. Trocars 2 and 4 are operative ports, whereas Trocars 3 and 5 are used for exposure instruments.

4. *Exposure*—A three- to five-digit liver retractor is introduced trough trocar #3 and the round ligament and the left lobe of the liver are retracted anteriorly for exposure of the gastroesophageal junction. A Babcock grasper is introduced through trocar #5 for later traction of the stomach fundus and thus lesser curvature exposure.

5. *Pouch calibration*—At this time the anesthetist introduces the calibration tube. When placement is verified in the stomach, a balloon is inflated with 15–20 ml of air. The tube is then withdrawn upward toward the gastroesophageal junction. This permits the surgeon to identify the areas of dissection as the inferior margins of the balloon.

6. *Initial dissection*—The lesser curvature dissection begins 2–3 cm from the GE junction, using a hook or a bipolar dissector staying close to the gastric wall, while preserving the vagus nerve. The greater curvature site is dissected with an opening made in the avascular phrenogastric ligament, close to the gastric wall. This is usually proximal to the first short gastric vessel.

7. *Retrorogastric tunnel*—With the balloon deflated the retrogastric dissection is begun using the bipolar dissecting instrument and the suction-irrigation probe. The dissection is made bluntly, as close as possible to the posterior gastric wall. The direction of the dissection is toward the opening made on the greater curvature. Once the retrogastric tunnel is created, a reticulating grasping forceps or the articulating dissector instrument (BioEnterics) is passed through and left in place.

8. *Band introduction and placement*—Replace trocar #5 with a 15- or 18-mm trocar, through which the lap-band is introduced into the abdominal cavity. It is placed around the stomach and the band-tubing end is inserted into the buckle and brought outside the abdomen at trocar #5. At this time the anesthetist again passes the calibration tube into the stomach and inflates the balloon with 15–20 ml of saline. The calibration tube is connected to the gastrostenometer electronic sensor and calibrated so that the first light is on. The lap-band closure instrument is then introduced from trocar site #2, and the band is locked. In order to achieve a stoma diameter of 12 mm, saline (<4 ml) is introduced from the external band tubing until the fourth light on the gastrostenometer turns on. Evidence supports leaving the band open in the postoperative period. All or part of the saline required to reach the fourth light is removed to avoid occlusions due to short-term edema.

9. *Stabilization of the lap band*—In order to avoid band slippage, four to six nonabsorbable retention sutures are placed above and below the band (stomach-to-pouch), beginning at the greater curvature. Placement of a posterior suture is mandatory and can be easily placed if the bursa omentalis was dissected.

10. *Access port placement*—After the fascia at trocar site #5 has been sutured, the lap-band external tubing is connected to the access port of the LAGBS system which is then secured with four nonabsorbable sutures to the musculoaponeurotic fascia at trocar #5.

Experience

Patients

We present our initial experience in placement of the laparoscopic adjustable silicone gastric band (LASGB). From January 1995 until May 1997 we attempted LASGB placement in 18 patients (7 males, 11 females) with a mean age of 39.8 years. Their average body weight was 143.2 kg (95–180 kg), average height was 1.65 m (1.52–1.88 m), and mean body mass index was 47.7 kg/m^2 (41.1–54.8 kg/m^2). All patients were morbidly obese with BMI over 41.1 kg/m^2.

Preoperative Assessment

Criterion for operation was a BMI > 40 kg/m^2. All patients were evaluated preoperatively by medical, psychiatric, and nutritional experts. A standard upper GI barium study, gastroscopy, and upper abdominal ultrasonography were performed on all patients.

Results

Three patients (all female) had gallstones, and laparoscopic cholecystectomy was performed concurrently. Operative time was 160 min (100–

270 min). In one patient, LASGB was not placed due to a hiatal hernia >3 cm discovered intraoperatively. There were no major intraoperative complications, and there were no conversions to open placement. Three minimal intraoperative complications were left lobe lacerations treated by coagulation. Postoperative complications were mainly four wound seromas (trocar #5) and two band slippage's, which resulted in band removal in one and band deflation in the other. Average postoperative hospital stay was 3 days (2–5 days). Patients had a close follow-up and a 3-month evaluation. The 3- and 6-month postoperative mean BMI was 38.9 kg/m^2 and 35.7 kg/m^2, respectively.

References

1. Griffen WO. Bariatric Surgery in the 1990's. Adv Surg 1992;25:99–117.
2. National Institutes of Health Consensus Development Statement. Health implications of obesity. National Institute of Health, Bethesda, 1985;(2):11–13.
3. Buchwald H, Rucker RD Jr. Rise and fall of jejunoileal bypass. In Nelson RL, Nyhus LM (eds.) Surgery of the small intestine. Appleton-Century Crofts, New York, 1987, pp. 529–541.
4. Kuskowska-Wolk A, Rossner S. Decreased social activity in obese adults. Diabetes Res Clin Pract 1990;10:65.
5. Sobal J, Stunkark AJ. Socioeconomic status and obesity: a review of the literature. Psychol Bull 1989;205:260.
6. Cowan G, Cowan K. Obesity stereotypes. Prob Gen Surg 1992;9(2).
7. Metropolitan Life Insurance Company. New weight standards for men and women. Stat Bull Metrop Insur Co 1959;40:1–4.
8. Frankel HM. Determination of body mass index JAMA 1968;255:12(Letter).
9. Kremen AJ, Linner JH, Nelson CH. An experimental evaluation of the nutritional importance of proximal & distal small intestine. Ann Surg 1954;140:439.
10. Payne JH, Dewind LT, Commons RP. Metabolic observations in patients with jejunocolic shunts. J Surg 1963;106:273.
11. Payne JH, Dewind LT. Surgical treatment of obesity. Am J Surg 1969;118:141.
12. Mason EE, Ito C. Gastric By-pass in obesity. Surg Clin North Am 1967;47:1345.
13. Mason EE, Printen KJ, Bloomers TJ, et al. Gastric bypass for obesity after ten years experience. J Obesity 1978;2:197.
14. Alden JF. Gastric and jejunoileal bypass. A comparison in the treatment of morbid obesity. Arch Surg 1977;112:799.
15. Griffen WO, Young UC, Stevenson CC. A prospective comparison of gastric and jejunoileal bypass procedures for morbid obesity. Ann Surg 1977;186:500.
16. Pace WG, Martin EW. Gastric partitioning for morbid obesity. Ann Surg 1979;190:392.
17. Gomez CA. Gastroplasty in the surgical treatment of morbid obesity. Am J Clin Nutr 1980;33:406.
18. Mason EE. Surgical treatment of obesity. W.B. Saunders, Philadelphia, 1981, pp. 408–419.

19. Freeman JB, Burchet HJ. A comparison of gastric bypass and gastroplasty for morbid obesity. Surgery 1980;88:433.
20. Grace DM. The demise of horizontal gastroplasty. Prob Gene Surg 1992;9(2).
21. Tretbar LL, Taylor TL, Sifers EC. Gastric plication for morbid obesity J Kans Med Soc 1976;77:488.
22. Long M, Collins VP. The technique and early results of high gastric reduction for obesity. Aust NZ J Surg 1980;50(2):146.
23. O'Leary JP. Partition of the lesser curvature of the stomach in morbid obesity. Surg Gyn Obstet 1982;154:85.
24. Laws H. Standardized gastroplasty orfice. Am J Surg 1981;141:393.
25. Mason EE, et al. Ten years of vertical banded gastroplasty for severe obesity. Prob Gene Surg 1992;9(2).
26. Scopinaro N, Gianetta E, Civalleri G, et al. Bilio-pancreatic bypass to obesity. II. Initial experience in man. Br J Surg 1979;55:518.
27. Garren L, Garren M. Gastric balloon implantation for weight loss in the morbidly obese. Am J Gastoenterol 1985;80;860.
28. Wilkinson LH, Pelosa OA, Milne RL. Gastric wrapping. In: Deitel Medical surgery for morbidly obese patients. Lea & Febiger, Philadelphia, 1989, p. 283.
29. Backman L, Granstorm L, Initial (1 year) weight loss after gastric banding, gastroplasty or gastric bypass. Acta Chir Scand 1987;153:215.
30. Molina M, Oria H. Gastric banding (abstract). Sixth annual bariatric surgery colloquium. Iowa City, iowa, 1983;15.
31. Lovig T, Haffer FW, Nygaard K, et al. Gastric banding for obesity: early results. Int J Obesity 1987;11:377.
32. Kuzmak LI. Stoma adjustable silicone gastric banding. Prob General Surg 1992;9(2)
33. Belachew M, Legrand M. Laparoscopic adjustable silicone gastric banding in the treatment of morbid obesity. Surg Endo 1994;1354–1356.
34. Cadiere GB. Laparoscopic gastroplasty for morbid obesity. Br J Surgery 1994;81:152.
35. Favretti F, et al. Laparoscopic placement of adjustable silicone gastric banding(ASGB): early experience. Abstact, 11th Annual Meeting of American Society for Bariatric Surgery, Minneapolis.

Part III
Other Abdominal Procedures

14
In Search of a Role for Laparoscopic Inguinal Hernia Repair

Rifat Latifi, Harold Brem, and James C. Rosser Jr.

Laparoscopic hernia repair is established as a safe and effective technique. Nevertheless, its indications are disputed, and the technique is not a matter of general agreement.

The requirement for general anesthesia, higher costs, and less-than-splendid results in the early experience led to skepticism for laparoscopic inguinal hernia repairs.[1] Furthermore, the results of open hernia repair are simply excellent, and they are accomplished with low cost under local anesthesia. The Lichtenstein hernia repair involves no tension, has little postoperative pain, makes early return to physical activities possible, and it has a low incidence of infection despite use of prosthetic material. This procedure is the technique of choice in the United States today despite the wide availability of laparoscopic surgery.[1]

Negligible pain and a rapid return to physical activities were originally the most promising elements of laparoscopic hernia repair. The safety and clinical efficacy of laparoscopic hernia repair was established years ago; for example, in an early report of 597 patients.[2] The technique was reported as safe and effective. Another study of 635 laparoscopic hernia repairs[3] reported a modest 8% complication rate and 1.7% recurrence rate in short term follow-up. Despite these studies, the uncertainty of the long-term outcome of laparoscopic hernia repair remains.[4]

Multiple laparoscopic techniques have been developed in an attempt to minimize complications and decrease recurrence rates. These techniques include transabdominal preperitoneal prosthetic repair (TAPP), intraperitoneal onlay mesh, and a total extraperitoneal approach (TEP).

In this chapter we will review the current results of clinical studies of laparoscopic repair of inguinal hernia. We will also describe details of TAPP, which is our preferred technique because of a lower rate of complication[5,6] (Table 14.1).

The advantages of using TAPP over TEP include:

1. Better visualization of anatomical structures in all types of inguinal hernia.

TABLE 14.1. Complications of TAPP versus TEP repairs.

	TAPP (%)	TEP (%)
Hematomas	2.3	3.6
Neuralgias	1.8	1.0
Urinary retention	1.0	0.9
SBO	0.2	0.0
Overall	8.2	10
Recurrence	1	0
	($N = 1,944$)	($N = 578$)

Source: Phillips et al. Surg Endosc 1995;9:16–21.
This table demonstrates the low recurrence and minimal morbidity of laparoscopic hernia repair, particularly with the TAPP procedure.[6]

2. Anatomical recognition follows a more logical order.

3. More widely applicable. Any previous lower abdominal or inguinal incision will obligate utilization of the TAPP. Furthermore, there is a high incidence of TEP failure in recurrent hernias because of scar retraction resulting in tearing of the peritoneum. This will result in conversion of the TEP to a TAPP repair.

4. In an indirect hernia the sac is not exposed by the balloon. The sac is dissected, ligated, and divided without having been able to identify its contents. This can lead to injury of critical structures.

Furthermore, the TAPP procedure must be familiar to all no what matter the surgeon's preference is because failure of the TEP approach mandates conversion to TAPP. The ability to perform a TAPP repair is fundamental to assure a minimally invasive alternative to open hernia repair.

Clinical Results

The laparoscopic TAPP hernia repair is an extension of the open preperitoneal Stoppa technique.[7] The TAPP is the most frequently performed type of laparoscopic hernia repair.[6] This technique has been associated with a low recurrence rate and minimal morbidity when compared with the open technique.[8] One hundred patients were randomized to undergo open hernia repair (Lichtenstein) or TAPP.[9] Patients after TAPP returned to work in an average 8.9 days, whereas those who had an open repair returned to work on an average of 17 days after the open procedure.

In a retrospective study, TEP[10,11] had a recurrence rate of 0.3%, whereas TAPP had a rate of 2.0%. In addition, the complication rate was 10.7% in the TAPP group versus 3.7% in the TEP. In another large study of 3,229 hernia repairs performed in 2,559 patients[6] the TAPP technique was the most commonly applied (60%). The TEP was performed in 18% of the patients while various other procedures were used in 22%. The overall complication rate in this study was 10%. The TAPP technique had 1.6% recurrence rate and 7% complications rate, most of which were hematomas, neuralgia, and urinary retention. There were 0.3% small bowel obstruction and two deaths. Critics of the TAPP suggest that this technique converts the extraperitoneal operation into a more invasive intraperitoneal one.[11]

A study of 733 patients undergoing the TAPP and 382 undergoing the TEP revealed that the TEP had no complications and one recurrence, whereas the TAPP had nine complications.[12] There were no differences in return to work. The extraperitoneal laparoscopic hernia repair was performed in 487 patients in a multicenter randomized study, and it compared with 507 patients undergoing conventional open approach.[13] Patients undergoing laparoscopic hernia repair had a lower incidence of wound infection, resumed physical activities earlier, and had fewer recurrences. Furthermore, although the operative time was slightly longer in laparoscopic group, and all underwent general anesthesia, these patients were discharged sooner than were open technique patients. Because hardly any patient is admitted after herniorrhaphy in current practice, the relevance of this observation is perhaps lost. Patients in the laparoscopic group returned to work much earlier than did those who underwent open hernia repair (a median of 7 days).

A prospective randomized controlled trial[4] assessed the interim benefits of laparoscopic hernia over the open technique repair and found no differences in length of the operation, hospital stay, or convalescence. Although the laparoscopic group had less pain and used less narcotic in the early days after operation, there was no differences in the amount of discomfort by 7 days. There were differences in perioperative quality of life at 7 days and at 1 month postoperatively. For these modest gains laparoscopic herniorrhaphy was 40% more expensive.[4]

Abdominal Preperitoneal TAPP Hernia Repair

This technique has been successfully employed by the authors in more than 250 patients.[14] We prefer the TAPP procedure because of the reduced cost as well as the decreased complication rate (Table 14.1). It must be emphasized that this procedure can be done equally well whether the surgeon is right handed or left handed; however, ambidexterity is an asset.

Before beginning the operation, 10 steps to anatomical recognition are recommended. These steps are divided into two phases.

Phase One

1. The medial umbilical ligament is identified upon entering the abdominal cavity.

2. In a male, follow the medial umbilical ligament posteriorly and you will encounter the vas deferens.

3. Turn your view laterally and you will observe a blue tubular structure coming to rendezvous with the vas deferens. These are the gonadal vessels.

4. The gonadal vessels join the vas at the internal inguinal ring and disappear into the canal.

5. This juncture forms a triangle that sits over the external iliac artery and vein, and the genitofemoral nerve. Because of the possibility of serious patient injury in this area it has been dubbed the "triangle of doom."

6. There is a peritoneal fold that covers the inferior epigastric vessels at the superior–medial aspect of the internal inguinal ring.

Phase Two

Reidentify the internal inguinal ring.

7. The inferior edge represents the iliopubic tract. Follow this structure medially until you encounter Cooper's ligament.

8. Reidentify the internal ring and identify the superior aspect, which is the folded edge of the transversus abdominus aponeurosis (i.e., "the arch"). All the fascia above this structure medially and laterally represent the transversus abdominus aponeurosis.

9. Reidentify the iliopubic tract above and lateral to the anterior superior iliac spine.

10. Identify the gonadal vessels. The area bounded by the iliopubic tract, the anterior superior iliac spine, and the gonadal vessels contains the femoral nerve and the lateral femoral cutaneous nerve. Use of the cautery in this area can lead to serious consequences; therefore, it is dubbed the "zone of electrical hazard."

Room and Patient Setup

The following procedure was designed to detail the procedure of unilateral right inguinal hernia (Figs. 14.1–14.3). As in all laparoscopic procedures optical correctness must be established. *Optical correctness* is defined as proper alignment of all of the optical equipment such that there is no "operative site/video monitor directional discrepancy." Optical correctness is established by having the surgeon, camera, operative site, and a monitor in a direct line (Figs. 14.1 and 14.2). In addition, the surgeon must never operate with the monitor over the shoulder. Nothing is more frustrating or potentially harmful than moving the tip of an instrument to the right and seeing it move to the left on the monitor.

Trocar Placement

After general anesthesia is induced, a nasogastric tube and a bladder catheter are inserted. For a left inguinal hernia, 12- and 5-mm ports are placed

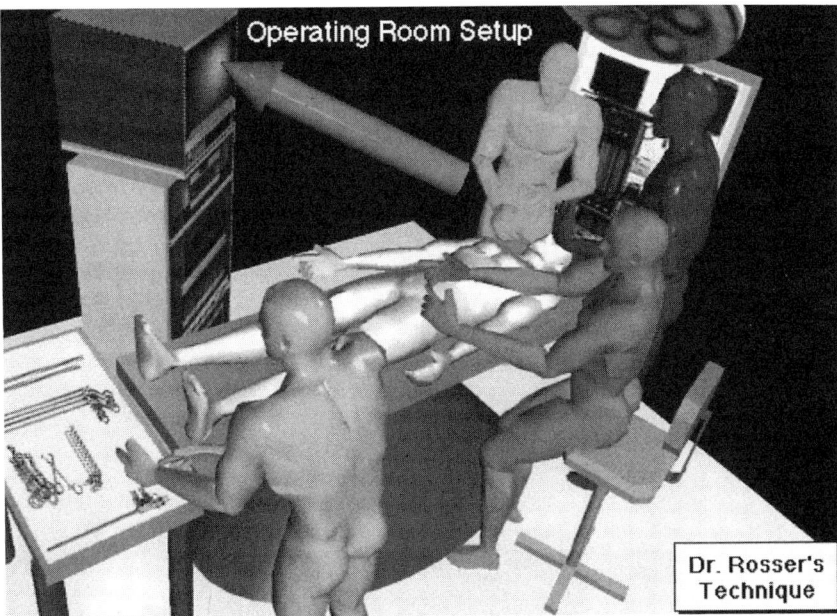

FIGURE 14.1. Schematic illustration of optical correctness in a patient undergoing a right inguinal hernia repair. Note that the surgeon is sitting down. As in all laparoscopic procedures when a surgeon moves to the right, the image should move to the right on the television monitor; similarly, when the surgeon moves to the left, the image on the television screen should move to the left.

on the right side. A 12-mm trocar is placed just below the umbilicus. Pneumoperitoneum is accomplished through this trocar. The 30-degree scope is then inserted, and the second and third trocar are placed under direct visualization. The second port (12 mm) is placed contralateral to the hernia at the level of the umbilicus, immediately lateral to the rectus abdominus muscle. The third trocar (5-mm) is placed two to three fingerbreadths below the second trocar (Fig. 14.3).

Initial Incision and Aquadissection

The Rosser-Cabot aquadissection probe is inserted immediately lateral to the medial umbilical ligament. When the probe is inserted, saline is infused under pressure, which effectively separates the peritoneum from underlying structures.

Advancement and Maturation of Peritoneal Flap

A vertical incision is made in the peritoneum extending down to the vas deferens. This is followed by a transverse incision extending 2 cm lateral to

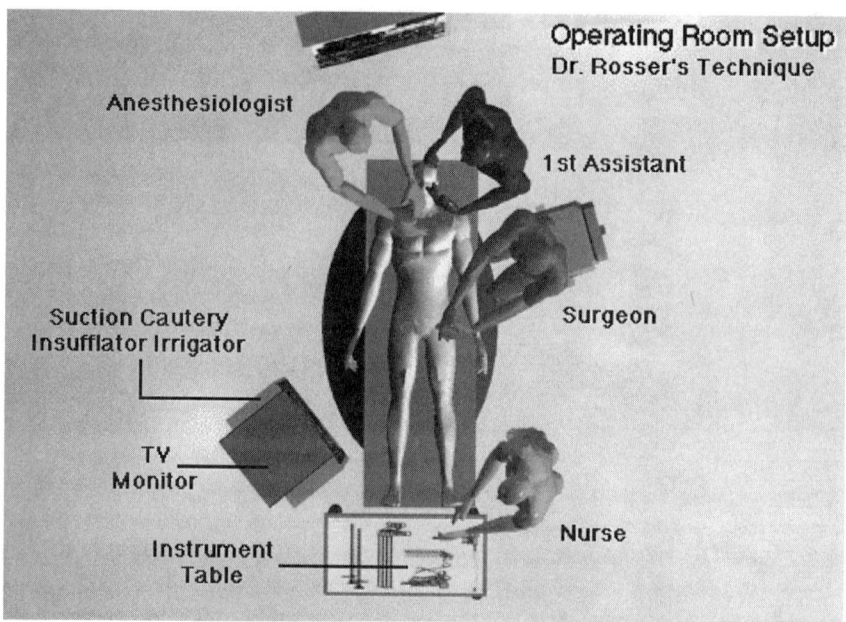

FIGURE 14.2. Correct positioning of the surgeon and assistants prior to repair of an inguinal hernia.

the hernia defect. It is important to mature the peritoneal flap by blunt dissection and not by cautery. The peritoneal flap is matured by fully separating the peritoneum from the underlying structures, which include the transversus abdominus aponeurosis, the vas deferens, and gonadal vessels. A large pocket is created to allow the mesh to lie flat against the abdominal wall and cover all of the sites of potential herniation through the myopectinal orifice. The advancement flap technique is advantageous because it allows excellent visualization of the anatomical structures while allowing for additional peritoneum to cover the mesh.

Placement of the Mesh

The placement of the mesh requires application of several steps. First, by using palpation, then traction and countertraction, one must identify the white ligaments medial to Cooper's ligament. The lateral iliopubic tract is subsequently identified. Cooper's ligament and iliopubic tract represent the inferior points of fixation for the mesh. The superior, medial, and lateral surface for fixation of the mesh is the aponeurosis of the transversus abdominus muscle. Second, the nonabsorbabale mesh is spread and grasped at its center with a dissector, pushed through the 12-mm port, and placed over the dissected preperitoneal area. Third, staple the mesh inferi-

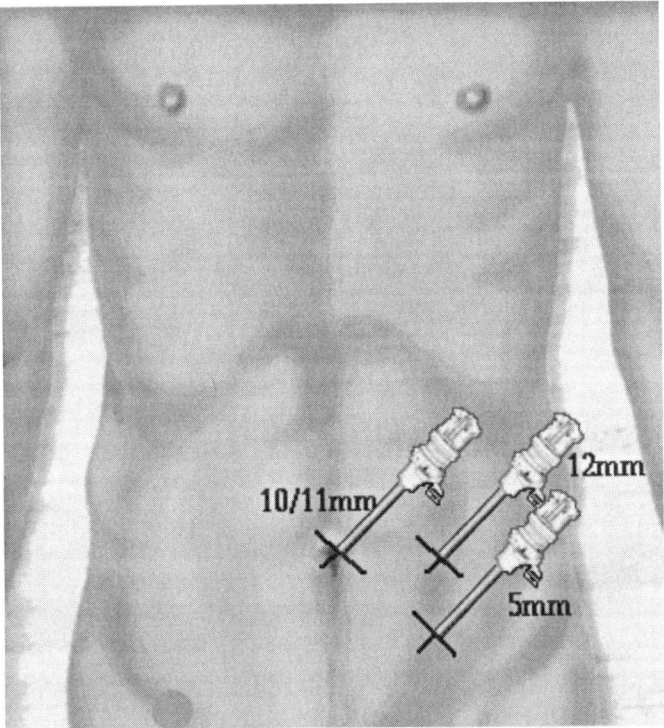

FIGURE 14.3. Schematic diagram of placement of all three ports. These areas should be marked on the patient prior to port placement.

orly, first to the iliopubic tract, and then to the Cooper's ligament. The mesh is then stapled superiorly and laterally to the aponeurosis of the transversus abdominus. Caution is exercised to avoid injury to the inferior epigastric vessels. In order to prevent a medial recurrence of the hernia the medial border between Cooper's ligament and the transversus fascia must be sealed.

Last, the superior edge of the mesh is lifted and stapled to the transversus abdominus aponeurosis. Note that medial to the internal inguinal ring the transversus abdominus layer is almost entirely aponeurotic, while lateral to the internal inguinal ring the transversus abdominus layer is less aponeurotic.

Reapproximation of the Peritoneum

The intraabdominal pressure is reduced to 8–10mmHg. Begin staple approximation of the peritoneum at the lateral corner, which becomes an anchor point. Always maintain excellent visualization of both sides of the peritoneum before actually firing the stapler. It is important to have a very short distance between the staples to prevent adhesive fixation or herniation of abdominal content into the area of repair.

Closure

Irrigation and inspection are meticulously completed. The fascia of both of the 10–12-mm ports is closed. The skin is approximated with 5-0 absorbable suture. The nasogastric tube and bladder catheter are removed while the patient is anesthetized. The patient is usually discharged to home on the day of surgery following short-term recovery in the postanesthesia care unit.

Total Extraperitoneal (TEP) Hernia Repair

The technical details of TEP procedure are as follows.[5,9] This procedure can be performed under local or regional anesthesia. The procedure advocated by John Payne is described here.[5,9]

Port Placement

A 10-mm port is placed below the umbilicus and the balloon is placed here and directed through towards the symphysis pubis. The second trocar with a 5-mm port is placed two to three fingerbreadths above the symphysis pubis. If location is critical to subsequent mesh placement, then the third trocar is either a 5- or 10- or 12-mm port depending, on the mesh fixation device that will be used. This third port is placed between the first two ports. This trocar allows for two-handed dissection, mesh placement, and fixation. The last two ports are placed under direct vision to avoid entering the peritoneal cavity. If the peritoneal cavity is entered the subsequent pneumoperitoneum can significantly limit the extraperitoneal space. A countermeasure to this can be accomplished anytime during the operation by placing a Veress needle, lateral to the rectus abdominus muscle, into the peritoneal cavity to vent the excess gas and thereby restore the extraperitoneal space for dissection and hernia repair.

Exposure

Make the first incision immediately lateral to the midline in the inferior fold of the umbilicus, on the side of the hernia. Either side can be used for a bilateral repair. Use blunt dissection with hemostats and small S-shaped retractors to expose the anterior rectus sheath clearly. Incise the anterior rectus sheath and then initially use a hemostat to separate the rectus abdominus muscle from the posterior rectus sheath. Continue to utilize blunt dissection to visualize the posterior rectus sheath clearly.

Insertion of Balloon Trocar

A Young or army–navy retractor is used to elevate the rectus abdominus muscle for insertion of the balloon trocar. Minimal or no resistance should be encountered as the balloon trocar is inserted gently in the plane parallel to the rectus in the direction of the symphysis pubis. The tip of the trocar should be palpable at the level of the symphysis pubis. Remove the cover and inflate the balloon with either saline or air. (Some balloons accept the laparoscope for direct observation of the inflation.) The initial balloon dissection is then completed. Suction may be used to evacuate the saline from the balloon. Withdraw the balloon from the extraperitoneal space. The trocar is then passed down the guidewire, and an airtight seal is secured.

Insufflation and Trocar Insertion

Insufflate with 10–12 mmHg and insert a 30- or 45-degree laparoscope. The space being visualized is behind the posterior aspect of the rectus abdominus muscle that was developed by the previously placed balloon. Insert trocars # 2 and #3 under direct visualization.

Dissection

1. Start the dissection in the midline and identify the symphysis pubis. Course along inferiorly and laterally to expose Cooper's ligament. The inferior epigastric vessels are then identified as they course along the ceiling of the extraperitoneal space. Search for an aberrant obturator artery, which originates from the inferior epigastric artery and crosses Cooper's ligament to the obturator foramen. This aberrant obturator artery may occur in 30% of patients and could result in dramatic bleeding as a result of overaggressive dissection or misplacement of a staple.

2. Dissect lateral to the symphysis and above Cooper's ligament to expose the iliopubic tract. (*Note*: Femoral hernias will be found in the space between these structures.) The transversus abdominus aponeurotic arch forms the remainder of the medial pelvic floor. It is the weakness in the transversalis fascia in this area that allows a direct hernia to form. Note that all lipomas should be completely reduced; however, the excess "pseudosac" does not necessitate excision. At this point the medial dissection is complete and the lateral aspect is dissected.

3. The lateral myopectineal orifice is identified. The peritoneal envelope is dissected off the anterior abdominal wall. This is an area where particular caution must be used to avoid injury to the peritoneal envelope, particularly in patients with recurrent and/or large indirect hernias.

Continue the dissection cephalad and lateral to the anterior superior iliac crest. It is imperative that you do not use cautery in this area because sensory nerves to the thigh run in this area, particularly in the iliacus fascia.

4. Reidentify the spermatic cord and reduce any indirect sac. Use careful blunt dissection to reduce the indirect sac and adjacent lipomas completely into the extraperitoneal space.

5. Transect the sac in a patient with a particularly large indirect sac (only if you are certain that all the viscera have been reduced). Then ligate the proximal sac while leaving the distal sac open. Note as the cord is mobilized caution not to use electrosurgery or excessive dissection in the triangle of doom (see the previous text in TAPP procedure) in order to avoid testicular atrophy and genito-femoral nerve injury.

Preparation of the Mesh

The mesh graft must be large enough to cover the myopectineal orifice completely. A slit is placed in the middle of the mesh, followed by a small keyhole to place around the spermatic cord. In order to facilitate passage of the mesh into the extraperitoneal space, suture the two tails of the mesh.

Placement of the Mesh

The mesh may be folded or directed toward the symphysis. The shorter segment may be passed under the cord and oriented for further deployment. Once the mesh is properly positioned beneath the cord, the suture securing the two ends of the tail is cut. The mesh is then completely positioned over the pelvic floor. Patience and persistence are the most important factors in mesh placement, although a small right angle clamp may be helpful in positioning the mesh. The mesh must lie across the midline and completely cover all sites of potential herniation site. The mesh must overlap beyond the border of any direct hernia by 1 cm, even if a second piece of mesh becomes necessary.

Mesh Fixation

The first and perhaps most important suture or staple for mesh fixation is between the mesh and Copper's ligament. In the lateral aspect of Cooper's ligament caution should be directed so as not to staple or suture the iliac or obturator vessels. All staples are placed above the iliopubic tract to avoid structures in the triangle of doom. Additional staples are then used to secure the mesh well across the midline and the undersurface of the rectus and transversus abduminus muscles. Note that staples placed along the margins of a large direct defect may prevent the mesh from being pushed out of the direct defect. All lateral staples are placed above the iliopubic tract and medial to the anterior superior iliac crest. This will prevent injury to the sensory nerves of the thigh, which run in the iliacus fascia. If the head of the stapler can be palpated from the anterior abdominal wall, then one can be sure that the staples will be placed in the correct area. If too much pressure is used in a very slender patient, however, then it is possible for these staples to penetrate the muscle and injure either the ilioinguinal or iliohypogastric nerves. Check that the tails of the mesh are: (1) covering all spaces of potential herniation, (2) not creating tension on the spermatic cord, and (3) if a slit has been made in the mesh, check that the tails are overlapped and secured without injuring the epigastric vessels.

Closure

Make sure all of the gas is released. Remove the trocars under direct vision. No fascial sutures are needed.

Completion of Operation

The urinary catheter is removed and after recovery, the patient is discharged home after they have demonstrated that they can spontaneously void.

Complications of Laparoscopic Hernia Repair

In general the most common complications of laparoscopic hernioplasty are hematomas, neuralgia, urinary retention, and testicular pain.[8] Other complications, such as chronic pain, small bowel obstruction, trocar site infection and hernia, and vascular and visceral injuries, are less common.

Although 9% of patients undergoing laparoscopic hernia repair have some form of complications only 1% of them are significant.[6] While no major differences in complication rates were found among different techniques in this study,[6] simple closure of the internal ring without mesh had a 3% recurrence rate. Other complications, such as bladder injury or colon injury, were also documented.

Paresthesia and nerve injuries have not been commonly reported; however, they do occur in the laparoscopic technique.[5] The recurrence of a hernia after a laparoscopic repair is almost always a consequence of a technical error such as failure to properly stabilize the mesh or to adequately cover the hernia defect. Many of these complications can be easily avoided by a thorough understanding of the inguinal anatomy as visualized through the laparoscope[5] (Fig. 14.4).

Summary

Although the laparoscopic herniorrhaphy has become part of the general surgeon's armamentarium, its role in hernia treatment is uncertain and the choice of the technique is evolving; however, there has been no outcry from

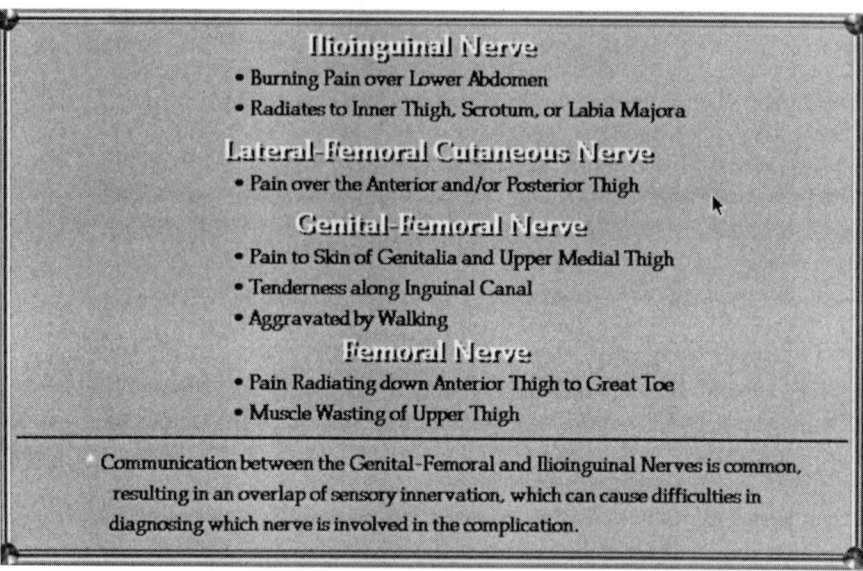

Ilioinguinal Nerve
- Burning Pain over Lower Abdomen
- Radiates to Inner Thigh, Scrotum, or Labia Majora

Lateral-Femoral Cutaneous Nerve
- Pain over the Anterior and/or Posterior Thigh

Genital-Femoral Nerve
- Pain to Skin of Genitalia and Upper Medial Thigh
- Tenderness along Inguinal Canal
- Aggravated by Walking

Femoral Nerve
- Pain Radiating down Anterior Thigh to Great Toe
- Muscle Wasting of Upper Thigh

Communication between the Genital-Femoral and Ilioinguinal Nerves is common, resulting in an overlap of sensory innervation, which can cause difficulties in diagnosing which nerve is involved in the complication.

FIGURE 14.4. Nerve injury following an inguinal hernia repair can be avoided by a detailed understanding of the anatomy of the nerves of this region.

patients to perform laparoscopic repairs. There has been ample opportunity for patients to discuss this procedure in detail in the past years, and there may not be such a quantum difference between the options as there was with open versus laparoscopic cholecystectomy. With laparoscopic cholecystectomy there was no question in the mind of patients, in a matter of months of introduction, that the previous procedure was no longer desirable. We currently recommend laparoscopic hernia repair for patients with bilateral hernias, working patients who need to return to regular physical activity promptly, and those with large inguinal hernias requiring mesh and those with recurrent hernias. Specific complications of laparoscopic hernia repair are well recognized.[5]

As with all surgical procedures, proper selection of patients is of utmost importance. Similar to other laparoscopic procedures long-term outcomes and complications will not be known for decades.

References

1. Memon MA, Rice D, Donohue JH. Laparoscopic herniorrhaphy. J Am Coll Surg 1997;184:325–335.
2. Fitzgibbons R, Anibali R, Litke B, et al. A multicentered clinical trial on laparoscopic inguinal hernia repair: preliminary results. SAGES Annual Meeting, Phoenix, Arizona, April 1993.

3. MacFayden BV, Arregui M, Corbitt J, et al. Complications of laparoscopic herniorrhaphy. Surg Endosc 1993;7:155–158.
4. Barkun JS, Wexler MJ, Hinchey EJ, et al. Laparoscopic versus open inguinal herniorrhaphy: preliminary results of a controlled trial. Surgery 1995;118:703–710.
5. Rosser JC. CD-ROM: Laparoscopic hernia repair. Surgical procedure. Springer-Verlag, New York, 1997.
6. Phillips EH, Arregui M, Carroll BJ, et al. Incidence of complications following laparoscopic hernioplasty. Surg Endosc 1995;9:16–21.
7. Stoppa RE. The treatment of complicated groin and incisional hernias. World J Surg 1989;13:545–554.
8. Newman L, Eubanks S, Mason E, et al. Is laparoscopic herniorrhaphy an effective alternative to open hernia repair? J Lap Surg 1993;3:121–127.
9. Payne JH, Griniger LM, Izawa MT, et al. Laparoscopic or open herniorrhaphy? Arch Surg 1994;129:973–979.
10. Ramshaw BJ, Tucker JG, Conner T, et al. A comparison of the approaches to laparoscopic herniorrhaphy. Surg Endosc 1996;10:29–32.
11. Ramshaw BJ, Tucker JG, Masson EM, et al. The comparison of transabdominal preperitoneal (TAPP) and total extra peritoneal approach (TEPA) laparoscopic herniorrhaphies. Am Surg 1995;61:279–283.
12. Felix EL, Michas CA, Gonzalez MH. Laparoscopic hernioplasty. TAPP vs TEP. Surg Endosc 1995;9:984–989.
13. Niem MSL, van der Graff Y, van Steersel CJ, et al. Comparison of conventional anterior surgery and laparoscopic surgery for inguinal hernia repair. N Engl J Med 1997;336:1541–1547.
14. Rosser JC. Unpublished data.

15
Laparoscopic Colectomy for Benign and Malignant Disease

Joseph B. Petelin

Laparoscopic methods for the treatment of colonic pathology have been the subject of intense interest, surgical innovation, and controversy since the first reports of these techniques surfaced in 1991.[1-5] The well-known benefits of laparoscopic treatment of biliary tract problems, including greater patient comfort, less surgical insult to the body wall, shorter hospitalization, and a more rapid return to normal activity, are among the reasons for the pursuit of similar methods in colonic surgery.[6]

In the United States alone, approximately 300,000 colectomies are performed yearly. The application of minimally invasive techniques to this population certainly has far-reaching physical, social, and economic implications. More important, the surgical, medical, and potential oncologic issues associated with the new technology have stimulated a lively and ongoing discussion of the role of laparoscopic colectomy in the surgical armamentarium.

This chapter reviews the progress that has been made in this field, as well as technical accomplishments and methods of resection, contentious issues, and future directions of research and practice.

Indications for Laparoscopic Colectomy

Most authors agree that any benign colonic pathology is potentially amenable to laparoscopic surgery. Indications include, but are not necessarily limited to, polyps, diverticular disease, bleeding, colitis, endometriosis, arteriovenous malformations, volvulus, rectal prolapse, and revision of a Hartman procedure.[1-9] Certain prerequisites must be satisfied, however, before embarking on such a surgical venture. These include proper patient selection, surgeon preparation, surgical team preparation, and facility preparation. In this regard, patients selected should be able to withstand a prolonged general anesthetic, and they should be aware of the difference between open and laparoscopic approaches.

The laparoscopic treatment of colonic malignancies is much more controversial. The topic generates vigorous and sometimes heated debate among general and colorectal surgeons alike. There are many reasons for this controversy: some scientific, some social, some financial, and some almost irrational. The most important of these concerns relates to whether or not the laparoscopic approach provides an equivalent, or better, treatment of curable colon and rectal cancer as compared with surgery via laparotomy. There are numerous authors who strongly believe that laparoscopic resection of colon and rectal cancer is not only equivalent to open resection in this regard, but is, in fact, superior to it as a treatment modality.[6,10–18] There are an equal number of surgeons strongly opposed to this viewpoint.[19]

As surgical history has demonstrated in the past, emotion rather than fact too often influences these initial responses to new technology and/or new techniques. Both the innovators of the new method and those upholding the tenets of the "open" standard have important points to make. Laparoscopic surgeons have provided evidence that the minimally invasive techniques of colon resection produce equivalent margins of resection, less postoperative pain, less postoperative narcotic analgesic use, less prolonged postoperative ileus, less immunosuppression,[20,21] shorter hospitalization, more rapid return to prehospitalization activity, and greater patient satisfaction than open colectomy. Surgeons concerned about this viewpoint have raised questions about the adequacy of the margins of resection, the adequacy of the lymph node harvest, the ability to survey the abdomen completely for synchronous or metastatic disease, and the incidence of port and/or extraction site recurrence of cancer in patients undergoing laparoscopic resection of colorectal malignancies.[22–28]

The literature regarding this relatively new topic abounds with volleys of support and/or criticism for each viewpoint. Each individual surgeon must carefully analyze the literature, and objectively assess his or her own capabilities, as well as those of the team and facility where the proposed operation is scheduled, in order to make an informed decision about the preferred approach to the patient with colorectal cancer. He or she must then be able to convey this information to the patient for the final decision as to which approach will be employed.

Contraindications to Laparoscopic Colectomy

Contraindications to laparoscopic colectomy include inability of the patient to tolerate general anesthesia, patient unwillingness to undergo laparoscopic colectomy, uncorrectable coagulopathy, facility and/or team inability to provide adequate support for such a procedure, and surgeon inability to perform laparoscopic colectomy in an effective and efficient manner. Relative contraindications, such as obesity, inflammation, and history of previous abdominal surgery, are usually dependent on the expertise and experience of the surgeon. Laparoscopic surgery for colorectal malignancy is still a controversial issue, and it may be contraindicated if the surgeon does not agree to study his or her own results and that of the published literature.

Techniques of Laparoscopic Colectomy

The approach to laparoscopic colectomy varies depending on both the location of the lesion as well as the personal preference of the surgeon. Totally laparoscopic and laparoscopic-assisted techniques have been described, although the latter are much more commonly practiced than the former. When reviewing the literature, the reader should be cognizant of the various names given to the approach, and should carefully analyze the description of the named approach in each report. Some authors refer to a laparoscopic-assisted approach wherein four or five ports are placed, the lateral attachments to the colon are divided, and the remainder of the procedure is then performed through a larger incision. Others believe that a true laparoscopic-assisted approach requires that at least some, if not all, mesenteric dissection is done laparoscopically, and that the extraction and anastomosis may be performed through a larger incision. It is this author's opinion that the latter description is more appropriately designated laparoscopic-assisted, and that the results of the procedure, especially duration of ileus, analgesic requirements, length of stay, and return to activity, are directly related to this distinction. The reader, therefore, should pay particular attention to the description of the procedure in a series reported in the literature.

The following descriptions of procedures represent the general steps employed by the majority of surgeons performing laparoscopic colectomy. Whereas port number and placement may vary from surgeon to surgeon, the basic steps are essentially equivalent. The author's preferences will be described here. It will be noted where some surgeons prefer a significant deviation or alternate approach to a given part of the procedure.

Right Colectomy

The operating theater is arranged so that one monitor is located superior to the patient on the right and one monitor is located inferior to the patient on the left. Some authors may prefer to have both monitors located at the head of the table. The Mayo stand is usually located at the foot of the table. The patient is usually placed in the supine position without abduction of the lower extremities.

Pneumoperitoneum is usually initiated at the umbilicus using either a Veress needle or an open laparoscopic technique. The port size and placement preferences of the author are demonstrated in (Fig. 15.1). The 12-mm diameter port is placed at the umbilicus to allow access for the scope and possible stapling devices later. A 10-mm port is placed in the suprapubic region; the scope is later transferred to this port. A 5-mm port is placed directly over the cecum, and another 5-mm port is placed in the epigastrium, usually just to right of the midline. All of these secondary ports are placed under direct vision.

After placement of the secondary ports, a thorough exploration of the abdominal cavity is performed; the laparoscope is then transferred to the suprapubic port, and scissors are introduced through the umbilical port. The lateral attachments of the cecum and ascending colon are divided. The attachments of the terminal ileum are also divided at this time. The hepatic flexure of the colon is freed from its superolateral attachments and the omentum. This allows full mobility of the right colon. The base of the mesentery of the right colon is then incised and the right colic artery and vein are ligated or clipped and divided. The remainder of the mesenteric dissection is then performed, usually laparoscopically. Some authors prefer to use clips or automatic staplers to divide the mesentery, while others use bipolar cautery or harmonic scissors. The potential advantage of the latter is that both vascular control of small vessels and division of the mesentery may be accomplished with the same instrument.

The mobilized segment of the ascending colon, terminal ileum, and transverse colon is then grasped through the umbilical port. The incision at the umbilicus is then extended, usually inferiorly if possible, and the specimen is delivered onto the abdominal wall without contaminating the incision.

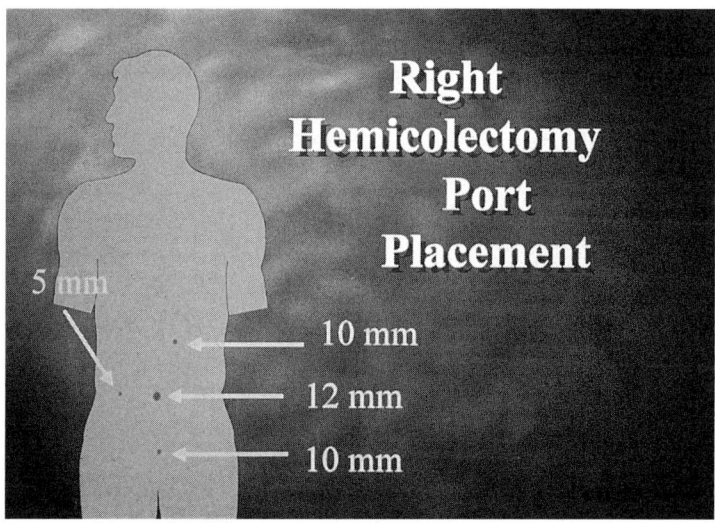

FIGURE 15.1. Right colectomy port sites.

The proximal and distal resection margin is then created either with conventional techniques or with automatic stapling and cutting devices. The specimen is removed from the operative site. The anastomosis is then created at the surface, using either automatic devices or employing conventional suturing techniques. The colon and small bowel is reduced into the peritoneal cavity, and the umbilical site is closed at the fascial level, allowing enough room for replacement of the 12-mm port.

The abdomen is reinsufflated. The mesenteric defect is then closed with either continuous or interrupted suture. The abdomen is inspected for hemostasis. The various ports are then removed and each port site ≥10mm in diameter is closed with zero or number 1 polyglycolic acid suture. Skin incisions are closed with absorbable suture.

Left/Sigmoid/Low Anterior Colectomy

The operating theater is arranged so that one monitor is located superior to the patient on the right and one monitor is located inferior to the patient on the left. The Mayo stand is usually located at the foot of the table. The patient is usually placed in the supine position with both lower extremities placed in a low lithotomy position. This allows access to the anus for intraluminal inspection and placement of instruments.

Flexible or rigid sigmoidoscopy or flexible colonoscopy is performed prior to final sterile preparation in order to identify the location of the lesion and the adequacy of the preoperative mechanical colonic preparation.

After sterile preparation and draping, pneumoperitoneum is usually initiated at the umbilicus using either a Veress needle or an open laparoscopic technique. The port size and placement preferences of the author are demonstrated in (Fig. 15.2). The Veress needle is replaced with a 10-mm port through which the laparoscope is inserted. A 12-mm port is placed in the right lower quadrant. A 5-mm port is placed in the left lower quadrant, and another 5-mm port is placed in the left upper quadrant. All of these secondary ports are placed under direct vision.

After thorough exploration of the abdominal cavity and pelvis, the patient is placed in Trendelenburg position. Occasionally, rotation of the table to the right allows displacement of the viscera away from the base of the left/sigmoid mesentery, thereby enhancing exposure. The location of the lesion is identified without manipulating it. If adequate exposure is not available, then another 5-mm port may be placed under direct vision in the appropriate position to provide access for a retractor.

The lateral attachments of the descending and sigmoid colon are divided and the left ureter is identified. The right ureter is also identified, if it has not been located prior to this time. Attention is then directed to the base of the mesentery. The inferior mesenteric artery and vein are identified, and

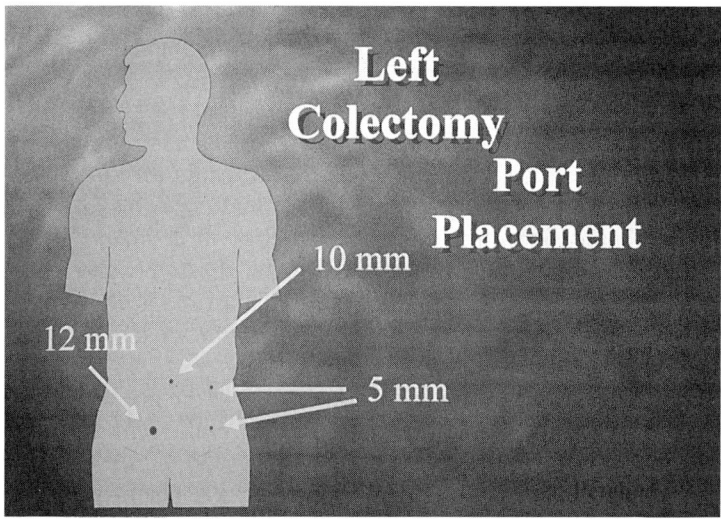

FIGURE 15.2. Left/sigmoid colectomy port sites.

the appropriate level of transection is identified. The mesentery is incised, and these vessels are secured with clips or ligatures. It is wise at this time to identify the proposed mesenteric path of dissection by scoring the perito-neum with the hook cautery device. The remainder of the mesenteric dissection is then performed using both scissors and hemoclips or bipolar cautery or harmonic oscillating scissors. The distal margin of resection is then secured and defined with an automatic stapling/cutting device, such as the Endo-GIA™ (USSC, Norwalk, Connecticut).

The distal aspect of the specimen may then be brought to the left lower quadrant site for final definition of the proximal line of transection, or the proximal line of transection may be defined with another series of applica-tions of the Endo-GIA™ device laparoscopically. If the latter method is selected, as is the case in patients with cancerous lesions, then the specimen is placed in an impermeable bag, which is inserted through the 12-mm right lower quadrant port. The specimen is then brought to the left lower quad-rant port site, where the abdominal wall incision is extended to allow delivery of the specimen without contamination. The anvil of the EEA Stapler™ is then placed in the proximal colon, which is secured around the anvil with a purse string suture. This is then reduced into the abdominal cavity, and the left lower quadrant wound is closed with zero or number 1 absorbable polyglycolic acid suture. If necessary, the left lower quadrant 5-mm port may be replaced to facilitate closure of the mesentery.

Pneumoperitoneum is then reestablished, and exposure of the pelvis once again established. The EEA™ handle is the advanced through the anus, and the spike driven through the distal staple line, or adjacent to it.

The spike is removed from the handle and withdrawn through the right lower quadrant port. The anvil is then docked to the handle and the handle is closed. As this closure is performed, the descending colon is observed to insure that the colon is not rotated at the anastomosis. After this is confirmed, the handle is closed and fired. The handle is then removed from the anus and the tissue rings from the anvil are inspected for integrity.

The surgeon then moves to the perineum and performs an endoscopic evaluation of the anastomosis to insure that it is intact, hemostatic, and without abnormality. If the integrity of the anastomosis is questioned, then the pelvis may be filled with liquid laparoscopically while air is insufflated through the sigmoidoscope. Bubbles indicate insufficiency of the anastomosis.

The surgeon changes gown and gloves, returns to the operating table, and inspects the anastomosis once again. If suture reinforcement is required, then it is accomplished at this time using interrupted 3-0 silk suture. Knots are secured with intracorporeal knotting techniques. The mesentery is then usually closed with either interrupted or continuous absorbable suture.

One final pelvic and abdominal inspection is completed. A closed system drain may be placed in the pelvis if necessary. It is usually brought out of the abdomen through the left lower quadrant. The ports are then removed and all port sites ≥10 mm are closed with suture at the fascial level.

Abdominal Perineal Resection

The operating room arrangement, patient position, and abdominal and pelvic dissection are essentially identical to that used for left or sigmoid colectomy. Further laparoscopic dissection of the rectum is carried down to the level of the levator muscles. After this is complete, the surgeon moves to the perineum for excision of the anus in the conventional manner. The specimen is usually delivered through the perineal wound. This obviously requires proximal transection of the rectosigmoid colon prior to the perineal dissection. The perineum is closed in the usual manner.

The construction of the colostomy is usually accomplished while the laparoscope is still in place, although the pneumoperitoneum is intermittently reduced to facilitate fascial fixation of the colon. The ports are then removed and all ports sites ≥10 mm are closed with suture at the fascial level. After the port site wounds are closed, the colostomy is matured to the skin in the conventional manner.

Transverse Colectomy

The operating theater is arranged so that both monitors are located superior to the patient on the right and the left. The Mayo stand is usually located at the foot of the table. The patient is usually placed in the supine low lithotomy position.

Pneumoperitoneum is usually initiated at the umbilicus using either a Veress needle or an open laparoscopic technique. Location of ports is quite variable for transverse colectomy. The 12-mm diameter port is placed at the umbilicus to allow access for the scope and possible stapling devices later. A 10-mm port is placed in the suprapubic region, usually either to the right or left of the midline; the scope is later transferred to this port. A 5-mm port is placed directly over the cecum, and another 5-mm port is placed in the left upper quadrant. All of these secondary ports are placed under direct vision.

The lateral attachments of the ascending and descending colon are divided as previously described. The surgeon may wish to stand in the perineal position for this and remaining parts of the procedure. The omentum is then incised to further mobilize the transverse colon. This is most easily accomplished with the harmonic oscillating scissors, which provide vascular control and division almost simultaneously.

The base of the mesentery is then incised and major vascular branches are secured with ligatures or clips and then divided. The remainder of the mesentery may be controlled and divided with the harmonic scissors or with scissors and clips. The specimen is delivered through the umbilical port site after the abdominal wall is opened sufficiently there. Proximal and distal transection, as well as the anastomosis, are performed at the surface. A portion of the entire mesenteric defect may be closed at this time, or it may be closed laparoscopically after the remaining colon is reduced into the peritoneal cavity. Each port site is closed as described previously.

Total Colectomy

The operating room is arranged so that the surgeon and the monitors may move as necessary to accomplish resection of the entire colon. The patient is placed in the low lithotomy position. Total laparoscopic colectomy is essentially a combination of all of the procedures described earlier. It is admittedly a major undertaking and considerable planning and preparation of the surgeon, the team, and the patient should be accomplished beforehand.

Results of Laparoscopic Colectomy

In general, the results of laparoscopic colorectal surgery have been encouraging in recent years. Improvements in equipment and technique have resulted in shorter operating times, fewer conversions, and fewer complications than were noted in the reports of the early 1990s. Surgical judgment in regard to patient selection, preparation, and intraoperative assessment has also matured. The anecdotal reports of initial experience with various laparoscopic techniques of colon resection in small numbers of patients have been replaced with critical evaluations of a relatively large series of patients. Even though the issues regarding the place of laparoscopic colon resection for malignancy are not yet resolved, the utility of laparoscopic colectomy for treatment of benign disease in unquestionable.

Operative Time

The site of resection, the nature of the disease process, and the experience of the surgeon all affect the operative time. In experienced hands, operative times range from 1.5 to 4.5 hours. Right-sided resections are usually associated with shorter operative times, whereas abdominal–perineal resections, transverse colectomies, and total colectomies have been reported to take as long as 6 hours. Nearly all reported series indicate that operative time decreases significantly as experience is gained. Nevertheless, it appears that an average operating time for a segmental resection will continue to be approximately 2 hours for most experienced laparoscopic colonic surgeons.[6,10,15,29]

Conversion Rate

Initial reports indicated conversion to open colectomy rates greater than 40%.[28] It is fortunate that with experience and better patient selection, mean conversion rates of 4–10% are common. The most common reasons for conversion include "difficult anatomy," severe inflammation, visceral or vascular injury, "frozen pelvis," or dense colonic fixation to adjacent structures.[11–16,29,30]

Duration of Ileus

Nearly all authors indicate that the perceived duration of ileus is significantly less in laparoscopic patients as compared with patients undergoing open colectomy. Most authors do not use nasogastric tubes in the postoperative period unless the patient experiences severe nausea and vomiting. Most patients are allowed to consume liquids within 24 hours, and many authors indicate that solid food consumption is begun within 48 hours of the operation. The reasons for this apparent benefit remain unproven, but most authors believe that it is secondary to less tissue manipulation, less exposure of the intestine to dessication, less need for narcotic analgesia postoperatively, and earlier ambulation of these patients. The success of this protocol for early oral intake following laparoscopic colonic surgery has stimulated new interest in applying similar protocols to patients undergoing open colectomy. Nevertheless, most laparoscopic surgeons would argue that there is still a subjective significant difference in the ability of these patients to tolerate enteral feeding in the early postoperative period.[6,10–16,30]

Length of Stay

Patients have been discharged from the hospital, without complication, as early as 24 hours following laparoscopic colectomy, although this is not the norm. It is more common that the length of stay averages 4.5 days. In the author's experience over the 2 years (after prior experience with >100 cases), most (of the subsequent 80) patients were discharged on the morning of the third postoperative day without any incidence of readmission.

This practice has been facilitated because of greater patient mobility, less dependence on parenteral narcotics and fluids, shorter duration of ileus, and improved patient comfort following laparoscopic colectomy.[6,10–16,29,30]

Complications

Complications occur in approximately 10–16% of patients and include atelectasis, urinary retention, urinary tract infection, colitis, anastomotic bleeding, parastomal hernia, enterotomy, small intestinal obstruction, and major vascular injury. Mortality rates in most series are zero to 1%.[6,10–16,29,30] Anecdotal reports of tumor seeding of the peritoneal cavity port sites and extraction sites have stimulated much discussion. In most large series, however, where the surgeon has performed more than 100 laparoscopic colectomies, and where extensive training and experience in laparoscopic surgery predated the authors' experience with laparoscopic colectomy, no port site tumor implantation has been noted to date. This topic is still under intense study, and it will probably require more time before the actual cause of these reported incidents is elucidated.

Summary

Laparoscopic colectomy is certainly feasible for the treatment of most colorectal disorders. In selected centers and in selected patients, the results of a laparoscopic approach to colorectal surgery compare quite favorably with open techniques; however, this field is still in its infancy. Laparoscopic colectomy, therefore, should only be considered by surgeons who are expertly trained in colon and rectal surgery and laparoscopic surgery, and who are willing to study both their own outcomes as well as those reported in the literature.

References

1. Fowler DL, White SA. Laparoscopy-assisted sigmoid resection. Surg Lap Endosc 1991;1(3):183–188.
2. Lange V, Meyer G, Schardey HM, et al. Laparoscopic creation of a loop colostomy. J Laparo Endosc Surg 1991;1(5):307–312.
3. Redwine DB, Sharpe DR. Laparoscopic segmental resection of the sigmoid colon for endometriosis. J Laparo Endosc Surg 1991;1(4):217–220.
4. Monson JRT, Darzi A, Carey PD, et al. Prospective evaluation of laparoscopic assisted colectomy in an unselected group of patients. Lancet 1992;340:831–833.
5. Peters WR. Laparoscopic total protocolectomy with creation of ileostomy for ulcerative colitis: report of two cases. J Laparo Endosc Surg 1992;2(3):175–178.
6. Phillips EH, Franklin ME, Carroll BJ, et al. Laparoscopic colectomy. Ann Surg 1992;216:703–707.
7. Romero CA, James KM, Cooperstone LM, et al. Laparoscopic sigmoid colostomy for perianal Crohn's disease. Surg Lap Endosc 1992;2(2):148–151.
8. Ballantyne GH. Laparoscopically assisted anterior resection for rectal prolapse. Surg Lap Endosc 1992;2(3):230–236.
9. Milson JW, Lavery IC, Bohm B, et al. Laparoscopically assisted ileocolectomy in Crohn's disease. Surg Lap Endosc 1992;3(2):77–80.
10. Franklin ME, Ramos R, Rosenthal D, et al. Laparoscopic colonic procedures. World J Surg 1993;17(1):51–56.
11. Lord SA, Larach SW, Ferrara A, et al. Laparoscopic resections for colorectal carcinoma: a three-year experience. Dis Colon Rectum 1996;39:148–154.
12. Franklin ME, Rosenthal D, Norem RF. Prospective evaluation of laparoscopic colonic resection versus open colon resection for adenocarcinoma: a multicenter study. Surg Endosc 1995;9(7):811–816.
13. Lumley JW, Fielding GA, Rhodes M, et al. Laparoscopicassisted colorectal surgery: lesson learned from 240 consecutive patients. Dis Colon Rectum 1996;39:155–159.
14. Plasencia G, Jacobs M, Verdeja JC. Laparoscopic-assisted sigmoid colecotmy and low anterior resection. Dis Colon Rectum 1994;37(8):829–833.
15. Zucker KA, Pitcher DE, Martin DT, et al. Laparoscopic-assisted colon resection. Surg Endosc 1994;8:12–18.
16. Dean PA, Beart RW, Nelson H, et al. Laparoscopic-assisted segmental colectomy: early Mayo Clinic experience. Mayo Clin Proc 1994;69:834–840.
17. Musser DJ, Boorse RC, Madera F, et al. Laparoscopic colectomy: at what cost? Surg Lap Endosc 1994;4(1):1–5.
18. Jacobs M, Verdeja G, Goldstein D. Minimally invasive colon resection. Surg Laparosc Endosc 1991;1:144–150.
19. Beart R, Peracchia A, Croce S, et al. Laparoscopic surgery panel. Dis Colon Rectum 1994;37(2):S144–S150.
20. Allendorf JPF, Bessler M, Whelan RL, et al. Better preservation of immune function after laparoscopic assisted vs. open bowel resection in rats. Accepted for publication, Dis Colon Rectum, 1996;39(10 suppl):S67–S72.
21. Harmon GD, Senagore AJ, Kilbride MJ, et al. Interleukin-6 response to laparoscopic and open colectomy. Dis Colon Rectum 1994;37(8):754–759.
22. Wexner SD, Cohen SM. Port site metastases after laparoscopic colorectal surgery for cure of malignancy. Br J Surg 1995;82:295–298.

23. Hewitt P. Intraperitoneal cell movement during abdominal CO_2 insufflation and laparoscopy—an in vivo model. Accepted for publication, Dis Colon Rectum, 1996;39(10 suppl):562–566.
24. McDermott JP, Devereaux DA, Caushaj PF. Pitfall of laparoscopic colectomy: an unrecognized synchronous cancer. Dis Colon Rectum 1994;37(6):602–603.
25. Ramos JM, Gupta S, Anthone GJ, et al. Laparoscopy and colon cancer: is the port site at risk? A preliminary report. Arch Surg 1994;129:897–899.
26. Walsh DCA, Wattchow DA, Wilson TG. Subcutaneous metastases after laparoscopic resection of malignancy. Aust NZ J Surg 1993;63:563–565.
27. Fusco MA, Paluzzi MW. Abdominal wall recurrence after laparoscopic-assisted colectomy for adenocarcinoma of the colon. Dis Colon Rectum 1993;36(9):858–861.
28. Falk PM, Beart RW, Wexner SD, et al. Laparoscopic colectomy: a critical appraisal. Dis Colon Rectum 1993;36:28–34.
29. Beart RW. Laparoscopic colecotmy: status of the art. Dis Col Rectum 1994;37(2):S47–S49.
30. Franklin ME, Rosenthal D, Dorman JP, et al. Prospective comparison of open versus laparoscopic colon surgery for carcinoma: five year results. Paper read at the meeting of the American Society of Colon and Rectal Surgeons, Seattle, 1996;(6):9–14.

16
Laparoscopic Splenectomy

Periclis J. Tzardis and Vasillis Laopodis

Since the first cautious steps in laparoscopic surgery after its advent at the late 1980s, minimal access surgical techniques are now well established and applicable in the management of various surgical pathology. In the course of time, the experience and dexterity of surgeons in laparoscopic surgery have widened considerably. On the other hand, technology in the field of imaging and image transportation, as well as the functional design and construction of advanced laparoscopic instruments, are rapidly progressing. Combined with the enthusiastic acceptance by the public of laparoscopic procedures, these facts resulted in a tremendous increase of the number of classical surgical operations that are now performed laparoscopically.

Laparoscopic splenectomy, although described by Cushieri[1] since the early 1990s, was not often performed until the last half of the decade. It was only then, therefore, that this procedure was undertaken in a series of patients large enough to permit objective evaluation of the method and produce rather reliable conclusions.[1,2,3]

Indications/Contraindications

The indications for laparoscopic splenectomy remain more or less the same as they are for the open procedure; however, there are several additional contraindications imposed by the peculiarities and limitations of laparoscopic techniques. Idiopathic thrombocytopenic purpura (ITP) is the most common indication for laparoscopic splenectomy, followed by familial spherocytosis and Hodgkin's disease. Laparoscopic splenectomy has also been performed in hemodynamically stable patients with traumatic rupture of the organ. Hematological disorders causing enlargement of the spleen and hypersplenism are relatively common and could be managed laparoscopically[4-10] (Table 16.1). B-homozygous Mediterranean hemolytic anemia (Cooley's disease) is quite common in Mediterranean countries; therefore, such patients, who have developed hypersplenism, could benefit from laparoscopic removal of their spleen. Prospective controlled studies

192

TABLE 16.1. Indications for splenectomy.

A. Cure of underlying disease
- Hereditary spherocytosis
- Immune thrombocytopenic purpura (ITP)
- Autoimmune hemolytic disease
- Thrombotic thrombocytopenic purpura
- Splenic trauma
- Splenic cyst
- Splenic abscess
- Splenic tumor

B. Treatment of hypersplenism
- Hairy cell leukemia
- Chronic lymphatic leukemia
- Myelofibrosis
- Thalassemia major
- Felty's syndrome
- A.I.D.S.
- Splenic vein thrombosis

C. Staging
- Hodgkin's disease

D. Diagnostic
- Splenomegaly of unknown etiology

evaluating the efficacy and safety of the procedure in this particular high-risk group of patients are on their way.

On the other hand, the major restraining factor for laparoscopic splenectomy is considered to be the large size of the spleen. Attempts to laparoscopically remove very large spleens are usually followed by increased conversion rates. Certain authors consider a longitudinal axis of the organ longer than 20 or 30 cm, as estimated by ultrasonography, as an absolute contraindication for laparoscopic splenectomy.[3,7] Others have advocated preoperative embolization of the splenic artery under these circumstances.[2] Relative contraindications for laparoscopic splenectomy are disorders of the clotting mechanism, which are not so rare in patients suffering from hematologic disease, multiple previous operations in the upper abdomen, portal hypertension, obesity, and enlargement of portal splenic lymph nodes.[7]

Preoperative Work-Up

Standard preoperative work-up should be carried out in all patients. Furthermore, the underlying disease leading to splenectomy must be carefully evaluated because it may cause coagulation disorders and/or hematological sequela. Whole blood or platelet transfusions may be warranted in order to maintain hemoglobin levels above 9.5 g% and platelet numbers higher than 90,000/ml. Platelet transfusion should ideally take place immediately following the ligation of the splenic vessels. It should be kept in mind that patients with ITP, or other hematological pathology, may be under treatment with corticosteroids and should be managed accordingly.

Preoperative ultrasound is imperative in order to determine the exact size of the spleen, which is a very important factor in planning laparoscopic splenectomy. Some authors advocate preoperative splenic artery embolization in cases of extreme splenic enlargement (e.g., patients suffering from β-thalassemia major). Embolization may produce dramatic reduction in splenic size, but there have been reports of several complications, such as pulmonary embolism, or infarcts in other organs. Pain may also be quite disturbing; therefore, embolization should only be attempted a few hours prior to the operation.[2,8–11] Apart from determining splenic size, ultrasound helps in locating ectopic spleneculi, whose removal is imperative, particularly in patients undergoing splenectomy for hematological disease.

The incidence of overwhelmingly postsplenectomy infection, although relatively small in the general population, is rather alarming in a patient harboring some kind of immunodeficiency or hematological disorders, as are most of the patients who undergo elective splenectomy. For this reason, polyvalent antipneumonococcal vaccine should be administered 2–4 weeks preoperatively. Likewise, preoperative antibiotic prophylaxis is mandatory for infectious complications in these susceptible patients.

Operative Technique

Positioning of Patient and Operating Team/Creation of Pneumonoperitineum

The operation is conducted under general anesthesia with endotracheal intubation. The patient is lying in the lithotomy position and the video monitor is placed over his/her left shoulder. A urinary bladder catheter and a nasogastric tube are inserted in order to empty the bladder and deflate the stomach, thus facilitating the safe placement of the trocars. Hourly urinary output is also monitored, especially in lengthy operations. The surgeon stands either between the patient's abducted legs, or to the right side of the operating table. The first assistant stands on the left, and the second assistant is on the right side of the patient. The scrub nurse stands on the right side of the patient, too (Fig. 16.1). Pneumoperitoneum is induced with the use of a Verress needle through an umbilical skin incision. Particular care should be taken in patients with marked enlargement of the spleen, where the lower pole of the organ may cross the midline near the umbilicus. The deep Trendelenburg position helps the cephalad shift of the organ and the insertion of the needle. Hasson's open technique can also be utilized in such

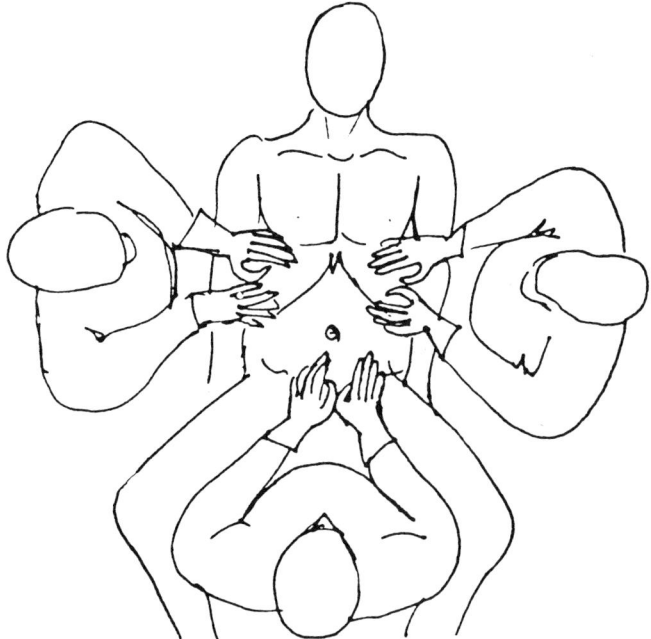

FIGURE 16.1. Positioning of surgical team.

cases or in cases of previous abdominal operations. After the insertion of the laparoscope, the peritoneal cavity is explored and the spleen is inspected. The other cannulae are then placed as follows: one 12-mm port is inserted in the midline between the umbilicus and the xiphoid, one 15-mm port in the midline halfway between the umbilicus and the pubic tubercle, another 15-mm port in the left flank along the anterior axillary line, and a 12-mm port by the left anterior superior iliac spine (Fig. 16.2). The use of five or six large 12–15-mm canulae facilitates the alternation of the instrument's positions and surgical manipulations in the course of the operation. The precise trocar positions are not constant, depending on the splenic size and the patient's physique. Thus, the definite cannulae placement should be decided after the insertion of the laparoscope and during the procedure.

Splenic dissection is facilitated by placing the patient in a reverse Trendelenburg position and by tilting the operating table 15–20 degrees to the right (Fig. 16.3). With this maneuver the spleen drops away from the diaphragm and the greater omentum and the stomach move to the right of the midline. The short gastric vessels are thus placed under tension and are easily dissected. In the same manner the hilum of the spleen and the tail of the pancreas are exposed.

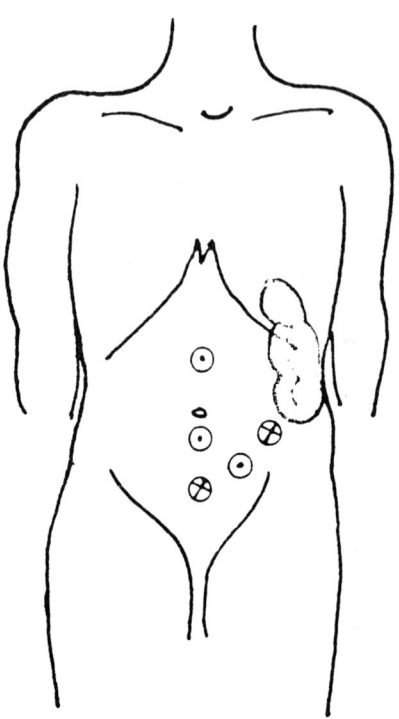

FIGURE 16.2. Trocar sites.

Search for Accessory Spleens

Following adequate insuflation and proper trocar placement, the stomach is grasped with an endobabcock clamp halfway along the greater curvature and retracted to the right. Division of splenococlic ligament and the spleen is commenced, and the spleen is manipulated using a blunt instrument, such as the suction-irrigation instrument, in order to reveal accessory spleens in the area of the splenic hilum, the tail of the pancreas, and the gastrocolic ligament. Spleneculi can also be found along the mesentery of the small bowel, the presacral space, and adjacent to the ovaries (Fig. 16.4). The search for ectopic splenic tissue should be done as an initial step of the operation in order to avoid difficulties in detecting the spleneculi due to

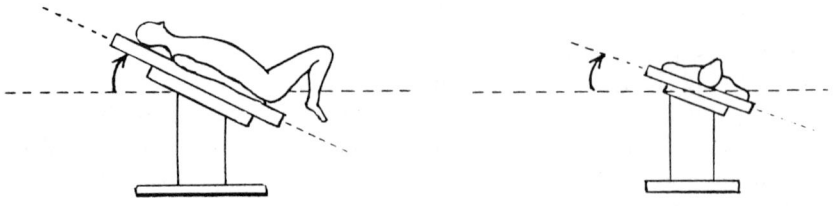

FIGURE 16.3. Operating table positioning.

FIGURE 16.4. Sites of ectopic splenic tissue. a. splenic hilum; b. pancreatic tail; c. splenocolic ligament; d. gastrocolic ligament; e. mesentery; f. presacral space; g. adnexa; h. scrotum.

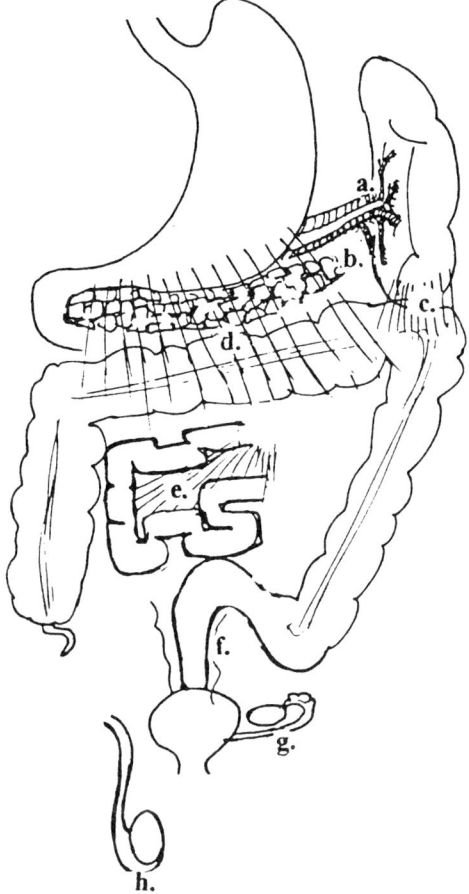

possible hemorrhage and blood infiltration of tissues. After removal of the spleen an additional search is necessary, because the organ itself may obscure the operating field. Complete removal of all ectopic splenic tissue is mandatory, especially when splenectomy is undertaken for hematological disease.

To this respect laparoscopy offers the advantage of magnification and close-up search of all of the sites possibly harboring spleneculi, but lacks the ability of digital investigation. Ectopic spleens are reported to be found in 30% of splenectomies performed laparoscopically.[2,9–11] Laparoscopic detection and removal of an accessory spleen overlooked during an open splenectomy has been reported.[7]

Mobilization and Devascularization of the Spleen

After the meticulous search for spleneculi, the division of the splenocolic ligament is completed with the use of diathermy and/or clips. The left colic flexure is pushed downward along the corresponding paracolic gutter (Fig. 16.5). All adhesions between the lower pole and the posterior abdominal wall are then divided. The stomach is retracted to the right by one of the assistants and the spleen is elevated upward and to the left with the use of the suction-irrigation instrument. These last maneuvers are necessary in order to identify and dissect the main vessels at the hilum of the spleen. These vessels are best ligated with the endoGIA loaded with the vascular-clip cartilages. The instrument may be fired once or twice, while smaller vessels may be controlled with simple clips. Some authors prefer to dissect the principal branches of the splenic artery and vein and ligate them separately, but this may cause bleeding, which can prove difficult to control and may require conversion of the operation. Clear visualization of the tail of the pancreas is mandatory during this part of the procedure. The remaining adhesions with the posterior abdominal wall and the diaphragm are then transected (Fig. 16.6). The short gastric vessels are then ligated and divided between clips, and the spleen is completely freed from its bed. In some instances division of the short gastrics are taken prior to the main splenic artery and vein. Some authors advocate ligation of the splenic artery at the superior border of the pancreas, as an initial step of the procedure in order to reduce the size of the spleen. We have found this to be quite difficult and

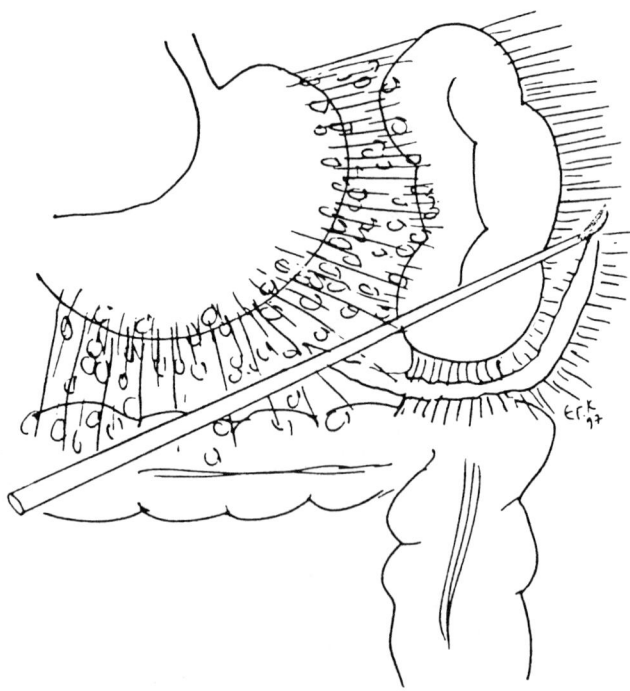

FIGURE 16.5. Division of splenocolic ligament.

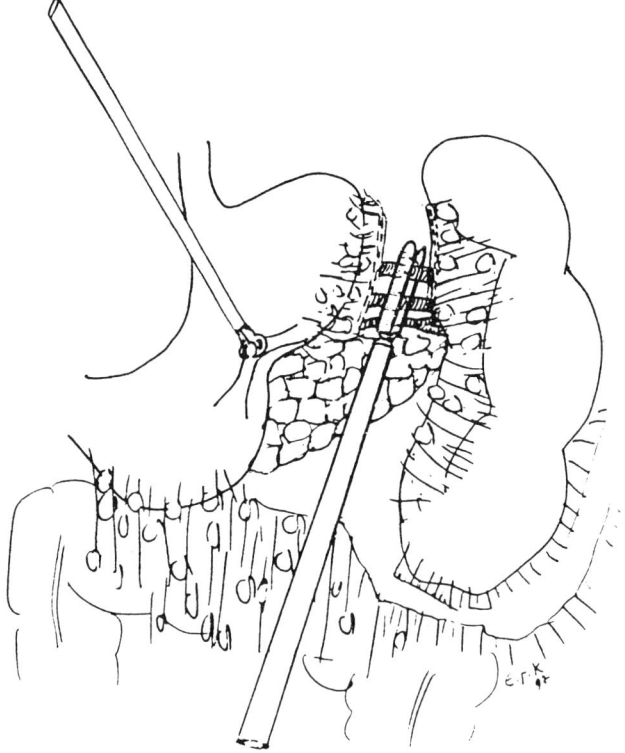

FIGURE 16.6. Splenic vessel division with endoGIA.

time consuming, and it produced troublesome bleeding in two cases. As already mentioned preoperative splenic artery embolization can produce splenic size reduction, although not without complications.

Removal of the Spleen from the Abdomen

The standard procedure for removing the spleen from the abdominal cavity entails placement of the organ in large endobag, morcellation in small pieces, and removal of the bag with its contents. Morcellation may be carried out either with a pair of ordinary forceps or with the use of a specially designed morcellator. The placement of a very large spleen (i.e., cases of hypersplenism) in a retrieving bag, however, can be quite difficult. In such cases retrieval of the spleen through a Pfannenstiel incision or through an incision in the posterior wall of the vulva have also been reported[9,11] (Fig. 16.7). Our practice is to create a 5-cm incision by joining the two trocar sites in the left flank and recover the specimen through it. Any of these alternative small incisions do not cause serious discomfort to the

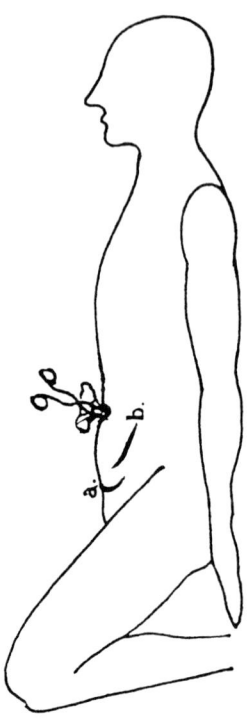

FIGURE 16.7. Removal of the spleen from the peritoneal cavity. a. pfannenstiel incision; b. trocar site joining incision; c. specimen morcelation.

patients, and they do not interfere with their early ambulation. Following the removal of the organ the abdominal cavity is irrigated with normal saline and meticulous hemostasis is maintained. A search for ectopic spleneculi is performed last, and a drain is placed in the left subcostal space.

Postoperative Care

The nasogastric tube and the bladder catheter are removed the day following surgery. On the second postoperative day the subcostal drain is either removed or shortened. Patients should be ambulated on the day of surgery or on the first postoperative day and are allowed a liquid diet. Antibiotics are administered during the first 24 hours, as are opioid analgesics. Oral or rectal analgesia with acetaminophen is then sufficient. Mean postoperative stay following laparoscopic splenectomy is reported between 3 and 5 days.[2,7,9] The most common complications encountered are atelectasis of the left lung, left subcostal collection, or abscess, prolonged serosanguineous drainage, and trocar site inflammation.

Experience

We present a series consisting of 17 patients, 12 of which had hypersplenism secondary to β-thalassemia major, three familial spherocytosis, and two ITP. Patients with β-thalassemia major underwent cholecystectomy and appendectomy simultaneously with the splenectomy. This group of patients will be addressed separately due to the complexity of this procedure and the excessive size of the spleen.

Our initial experience was acquired from five patients: three with spherocytosis and two with ITP. The patients had small or moderately enlarged spleens. Although the procedure was quite novel, we concluded the operations laparoscopically in four cases. One patient was converted due to hemorrhage complications from the short gastric vessels. Patients received 1–2 units of washed red blood cells on average. The specimens were extracted from the abdominal cavity rather easily with the use of a laparo-bag. Postoperative complications were limited to one case of left lung atelectasis. All patients were discharged by the fourth postoperative day.

As a consequence to this encouraging results we decided to apply the method to β-thalassemia major patients. The concept for this decision was based on the high incidence of the disease in Greece and therefore on the large number of patients who develop hypersplenism requiring splenectomy. These patients would probably benefit from the advantages offered by a laparoscopic approach. All 12 of our patients had a longitudinal axis of the spleen, measured by ultrasound, that exceeded 25 cm (range 25–44 cm, mean 32 cm). They had severe hypersplenism with increased transfusion requirements and thrombocytopenia, whereas the huge spleen produced discomfort and abdominal fullness. Nine out of the 12 patients also had cholelithiasis, which was symptomatic in seven. These nine patients underwent laparoscopic cholecystectomy along with the splenectomy. All patients were submitted to prophylactic appendectomy as well. This additional procedure is indicated because of the related immunodefeciency and the associated dangers of a nonelective operation in the patient population. Finally, liver biopsy was taken for the assessment of the degree of hemosidirosis.

The operation was conducted laparoscopically in 10 patients, while in the second and fourth case it was converted because of severe hemorrhage from branches of the splenic vein. Control of the hemorrhage was not feasible laparoscopically. Preliminary ligation of the splenic artery was attempted in two cases and was successful in one. Spleneculi were found in one patient located in the hilum of the spleen and were removed laparoscopically. Operation time ranged from 4.5 hours in the first case to 2.5 hours in the last three patients, including cholecystectomy and appendectomy. All patients received up to 3 U of washed red blood cells, whereas the need for further transfusions was one of the criteria for conversion. The patients tolerated the procedure very well, especially when compared with our experience with open procedures.[12] The postoperative hospitalization ranged between 3 and 6 days. The analgesia requirements were confined to the first 48 hours, and pain was easily controlled. Four patients presented with low-grade postoperative fever, caused by left lung atelectasis and were treated conservatively. Two patients exhibited excessive serous discharge from the splenic bed drain, which stopped 2 days later. A limited suppuration of a trocar site was noted in one patient. Aesthetic results were considered to be most satisfactory by all patients.

Conclusions and Perspectives

The main advantages of laparoscopic surgery over conventional open techniques is remarkably decreased postoperative pain, decreased hospitalization, and relatively rapid rehabilitation and return to full activity. Before laparoscopic splenectomy is established as a procedure of choice, it should entail all these advantages. Above all, this operation must be proved to be effective and safe as well. It seems that these criteria are met quite satisfactory, as long as the disease for which splenectomy is indicated is not complicated with extreme splenomegaly.[2,7,9,11] The two major taxing points in this position are the difficult surgical manipulations in cases of extreme splenomegaly and the rich vascularity of the organ. Most authors are troubled by the increased possibility of hemorrhage complications during laparoscopic splenectomy; hemorrhage is referred as the principal cause of conversion.[1,11] Accumulated experience and standardization of the operating steps on one hand and familiarity with the use of the endoGIA instrument loaded with vascular clips on the other contribute to keep hemorrhagic events to a minimum while at the same time lowering the operating time significantly. We consider, however, that time limits must not be a principal goal when such a potentially hemorrhagic procedure is undertaken. The cost of laparoscopic splenectomy is quite high compared with the open, but shorter hospitalization and earlier return to full activities must be taken into account. Patient acceptance of this method is impressive, due to the minor postoperative pain and the excellent aesthetic result.

Laparoscopic removal of the spleen can be established as the method of choice in patients requiring elective splenectomy. It must be stressed, however, that this procedure is still in evolution and further experience is needed in order to achieve better results and to come to safer conclusions.

References

1. Cushieri A, Shimi S, Banting S, et al. Technical aspects of laparoscopic splenectomy. J R Coll Surg Edinb 1992;37:414–416.

2. Poulin EC, Thibault C, Mamazza J. Laparoscopic splenectomy. Surg Endosc 1995;9:172–177.
3. Cushieri A. Laparoscopic splenectomy. In: Cushieri A, Buess G, Perissat J (eds.). Operative manual of endoscopic surgery. Springer-Verlag, New York, 1992; Vol. 2, Chap. 11, pp. 208–219.
4. Gigot JF, Healy ML, Ferrant A. Laparoscopic splenectomy for idiopathic thrombcytopenic purpura. Br J Surg 1994;81:1171–1172.
5. Hashizume M, Sugimachi K, Kitano S. Laparoscopic splenectomy. Am J Surg 1994;167:611–614.
6. Philips EH, Carrol BJ, Fallas MJ. Laparoscopic splenectomy. Surg Endosc 1994;8:931–933.
7. Emmermann A, Zornig C, Peiper M, et al. Laparoscopic splenectomy. Technique and results in a series of 27 cases. Surg Endosc 1995;9:924–927.
8. Rege RV, Merriam LT, Joehl RJ. Laparoscopic splenectomy. Surg C.I.N. Am 1996;76(3):459–469.
9. Thibault C, Mamazza J, Letournau R, et al. Laparoscopic splenectomy: operative technique and preliminary report. Surg Laparosc Endosc 1992;2(3):257–261.
10. Yoshida K, Yamazaki Y, Mizuno R, et al. Laparoscopic splenectomy in children. Preliminary results and comparisons with the open technique. Surg Endosc 1995;9:1279–1282.
11. Ferzli G, Fiorillo M. A Posterior gastric approach to laparoscopic splenectomy. Surg Endosc 1995;9:1017–1019.
12. Golematis B, Tzardis P, Legakis N, et al. Overwhelming postsplenectomy infection in patients with thalassemia major. Mount Sinai J Med 1989;56:97–99.

17
Evaluation and Technique of Laparoscopic Adrenalectomy

FRANK G. SCHOLL and BARBARA K. KINDER

Historical Perspective

A. M. Shipley performed the resection of the first preoperatively diagnosed pheochromocytoma in 1927 using an open anterior approach. Since then, a number of techniques for accessing the adrenal glands have been proposed. The introduction of the posterior retroperitoneal approach by Young in 1936 allowed surgeons the ability to operate on adrenal pathology without opening the abdomen. With the advent of high-quality optics and improved laparoscopic instrumentation in the late 1980s, a laparoscopic approach to the adrenals became feasible. Gagner and Higashihara both reported successful laparoscopic adrenalectomy in 1992.[1,2] Since that time, there have been several reports of safe and effective laparoscopic treatment of functional and nonfunctional adrenal disease.[3-9]

Several approaches for laparoscopic adrenalectomy have been developed. In general, these can be divided into two main groups: the retroperitoneal posterior approach and the transperitoneal anterior and lateral approaches.[10,11] The major advantage of the transperitoneal approach is perhaps that it provides the surgeon with a large clear operative field with excellent visualization of the retroperitoneum. It also allows the surgeon to perform a laparoscopic abdominal exploration.[6] The retroperitoneal posterior approach has been advocated by some authors who feel the visualization of the vasculature of the gland is better, especially on the right where the right adrenal vein drains into the posterior aspect of the inferior vena cava.[12] This technique has also been advocated for tumors less than 6 cm and for bilateral disease.[10]

Indications for Laparoscopic Adrenalectomy

Based on our experience and that of others, we found that laparoscopic adrenalectomy is the procedure of choice for functional and nonfunctional adrenal tumors that are benign and less than 8–10 cm in size.[9,13] The preoperative assessment takes one of two general directions, and is based on the method of presentation of the patient.

Asymptomatic patients, identified because of an incidental finding of an adrenal mass (incidentaloma), need to be evaluated for evidence of secretory function of the tumor and assessment of the likelihood of malignancy. Clinical and familial history will alert the clinician to the possibility of familial syndromes such as the multiple endocrine neoplasias, Von Hippel-Lindau, and other neuroectodermal dysplasias, which include adrenal tumors (usually pheochromocytomas) as part of their disease complex. Metastases to the adrenal should be considered in asymptomatic patients with a prior history of malignancy.

Hypertensive patients must be screened for pheochromocytoma, Cushing's syndrome, and hyperaldosteronism. The prevalence of adrenal masses in essential hypertension in one series was quoted as being as high as 12%.[6] Twenty-four–hour urinary screen for catecholamines and metabolites (as well as epinephrine/norepinephrine fractions in the MEN 2 patients) is a simple and reliable method of ruling out pheochromocytoma.

Loss of diurnal variation of serum cortisol levels suggests a cortisol-secreting adenoma in the presence of a unilateral adrenal mass and a patient with the stigmata of Cushing's syndrome. Confirmation of the diagnosis can be achieved by demonstrating elevated urinary cortisol metabolites, lack of suppression of serum cortisol by the low dose dexamethasone suppression test, and a low adronocorticotrophic hormone (ACTH) level. It is important to identify patients with subclinical cortisol production preoperatively as they may develop adrenal insufficiency after resection of an adrenal "incidentaloma."[14]

Diagnosis of primary hyperaldosteronism is made in the hypertensive patient by the presence of spontaneous hypokalemia and a plasma aldosterone (ng/100 ml) to plasma renin (ng/ml) ratio greater than 15. Existence of an adenoma (aldosteronoma) must be confirmed because the treatment of bilateral adrenal nodular hyperplasia causing hyperaldosteronism is primarily medical. Random plasma levels of testosterone, dehydroepiandrosterone (DHEA sulfate), androstenedione, or estradiol associated with suppressed luteinizing hormone, and follicle-stimulating hormone suggest the presence of excess sex hormone production. Absence of biochemical abnormalities does not mean that the adrenal mass is nonfunctional; rather, it indicates that no secretory hyperfunction can be identified systemically.

Contraindications

Absolute contraindications for the laparoscopic approach to the adrenals include those for other laparoscopic procedures; severe cardiac disease, portal hypertension, shock, coagulopathy, and a definite diagnosis of adrenal malignancy. Some authors have advocated laparoscopic intervention for metastatic disease located in the adrenal.[13] The list of relative contraindications is decreasing as more experience is gained with the laparoscopic approach. These include morbid obesity, severe pulmonary disease, and extensive upper quadrant surgery (particularly hepatic resection in the case of a right-sided adrenal tumor or diaphragmatic hernia repair in the case of a left-sided tumor). In general, prior abdominal surgery is not as problematic in adrenal cases due to the more posterolateral location of the adrenal gland.

Surgical Technique

We have used the transperitoneal lateral approach pioneered by Gagner et al.[15] The main advantage of this approach is that it provides a larger operative field (compared with the retroperitoneal balloon approach). In addition, lateral positioning of the patient allows gravity to retract the spleen, in the case of the left adrenal, and the liver, in the case of the right adrenal, once a peritoneal flap has been developed. Dependent drainage also helps to keep blood and irrigation fluid out of the operative field. Both of these are advantages over the anterior approach.

Using this technique the patient is positioned on the table in the lateral decubitus position, after placement of an orogastric tube, Foley catheter, and application of sequential compression boots. The table is fully flexed and the kidney rest extended, thus opening the space between the costal margin and iliac crest. A beanbag is used to maintain position.

The operating suite is set up for optical correctness, with both the surgeon and assistant placed on the same side of the table, on the side opposite the adrenal pathology. All monitors and insufflation equipment should be on the opposite side of the patient from the operative team to allow an unobstructed view of these items throughout the case. Establishment of the pneumoperitoneum is achieved via the Veress needle using alternative sites in the right or left subcostal region at the lateral border of the rectus muscle. In very thin patients the open Hassan technique is used. Carbon dioxide insufflation to 15mmHg is performed and once adequate pneumoperitoneum is achieved, and assessed by percussion of the abdomen, a 10-mm trocar is inserted, and the abdominal exploration is carried out. Two other 10-mm trocars are inserted under direct vision laterally along the costal margin, with care taken to stay well away from the iliac crest, which may limit mobility of the most lateral trocar. On the right, a fourth trocar may occasionally be needed more medially to permit insertion of a fan retractor for retraction of the liver. The 30-degree laparoscope is required for the laparoscopic adrenalectomy. The renal promontory is the initial anatomic landmark. A peritoneal flap is developed from the renal promontory extending superiorly to the diaphragm. On the left, this permits the spleen and tail of the pancreas to fall away by gravity, facilitating the rest of the dissection. On the right, the dissection of the peritoneal flap culminates in division of the triangular ligament of the liver and mobilization of that organ. The splenic and/or hepatic flexure usually does not need to be mobilized. At this point, an adrenal tumor mass of 2 cm or greater can readily be appreciated. In the case of small aldosteronomas, the characteristic yellow color of the normal adrenal cortex can be seen within the periadrenal fat and the gland identified for dissection; thereafter, the medial edge of the peritoneal flap is grasped and dissection of the anterior and superior surface of the adrenal gland can be carried out. Division of the many small vessels supplying the adrenal gland can be expedited by using the harmonic scalpel.[9] We have used this instrument extensively in both adrenalectomy and other laparoscopic operations and found that with judicious use it can safely replace small vascular clips, thus helping to reduce operative time. After dissection of the superior pole, the lateral aspect of the gland is dissected and elevated anteriorly and medially, allowing dissection of the posterior aspect of the gland. Finally, the inferior (renal) and medial aspects can be approached.

Major vascular structures are identified and divided between clips. The main right adrenal vein is often short and wide and is quite delicate. Caution must used to avoid avulsion of the vein from the posterolateral aspect of the vena cava. The superior optical detail afforded by the laparoscopic approach shows the multiple major adrenal veins which are common and should be anticipated. The gland is then placed in a 10-cm plastic bag and removed through the lateral port site. Extension of both the skin and fascial incision may be necessary to facilitate removal of large tumors. Fascial closure is performed either laparoscopically or externally under direct vision at all port sites greater than 5 mm. The skin is closed and sterile dressings are applied.

Results

Between 1986 and January 1997 we performed 17 open and 15 laparoscopic adrenalectomies for unilateral benign disease at Yale-New Haven Hospital. There were 6 males and 11 females in the open group. Mean operative time was 162 minutes, with a median time of 168 minutes and a range of 105 to 225 minutes. The mean hospital stay was 7.2 days, a median stay of 6.5 days and a range of 2 to 14 days. The group undergoing laparoscopic adrenalectomy had seven males and seven females (one male patient with Von Hippel–Lindau disease underwent two unilateral operations, at separate times.) The mean operative time was 239 minutes, with a median time of 240 minutes and a range of 160 to 360 minutes. The mean length of hospital stay was 2.3 days with a median stay of 2.0 days and a range of 1 to 4 days. These results are compared in Table 17.1.

A variety of benign adrenal tumors were encountered. The breakdown of diagnoses for the laparoscopically removed tumors is shown in Table 17.2.

TABLE 17.1. Comparison of open and laparoscopic adrenalectomy performed at Yale since 1986.

	Open adrenalectomy N = 17	Laparoscopic adrenalectomy N = 15
Operative time in minutes		
Mean	162	239
Median	168	240
Range	105–225	130–360
Hospital stay in days		
Mean	7.4	2.3
Median	6.5	2.0
Range	2–14	1–4

The largest tumor removed laparoscopically was an 8-cm pheochromocytoma. Consistent with other reports, hemodynamic changes in well-blocked patients with pheochromocytoma were not significantly different using the laparoscopic approach.

The open adrenalectomy group had one significant postoperative complication in a patient who needed reoperation and splenectomy for postoperative bleeding. There were no mortalities in this group. To date there have been no mortalities and no significant morbidity related to the use of the laparoscopic technique at our institution.

Discussion

The laparoscopic age is upon us. Operations that require a large incision to remove a relatively small volume of pathologic tissue are ideally suited to laparoscopic surgery, as evidenced by the tremendous success of laparoscopic cholecystectomy. The removal of adrenal tumors is another area where the laparoscopic approach is clearly associated with less morbidity.

TABLE 17.2. Types of laparoscopically removed adrenal tumors.

Diagnosis	Number
Aldosteronoma	5
Pheochromocytoma	4
Cortisol-secreting adenoma	3
Nonfunctional	2
Testosterone-secreting adenoma	1
Total	**15**

TABLE 17.3. Results of laparoscopic adrenalectomy in comparative retrospective studies of laparoscopic versus open adrenalectomy, including current Yale series and recent literature.

Author	Year	#Patients	Mean operative time	Mean length of stay	Major complications	Mortality
Brunt[16]	1996	24	183	3.2	2	0
Guazzoni[21]	1995	20	170	3.4	1	0
Jacobs[17]	1997	19	164	2.3	1	0
Korman[18]	1997	10	164	4.1	2	0
Prinz[22]	1995	10	212	2.1	N/A	N/A
Yale	1997	15	239	2.3	0	0

Successful laparoscopic adrenalectomy was first described in 1992 by Gagner and Higashihara.[1,2] More than a dozen series have reported results of laparoscopic adrenalectomy since then, mainly at university teaching hospitals and tertiary care centers.[9,13,16–20] In fact, at the time of this writing there are 118 citations under combined textword *laparoscopic* and *adrenalectomy* in the medline database. These reports have shown that in experienced hands laparoscopic adrenalectomy is the procedure of choice for removing many adrenal neoplasms. There have been a number of large series that have shown that laparoscopic adrenalectomy can be performed safely and with decreased hospital stay and morbidity over the open technique. Some of these, as well as the results of the current series, are summarized in Tables 17.3 and 17.4.

Gagner has reported on a series of 100 adrenal exploration/resections, with no mortalities and a 12% complication rate. No patients have had hormonal recurrences, although two have renovascular hypertension of unknown etiology, and of eight patients treated for what ultimately ended

TABLE 17.4. Results of open anterior adrenalectomy in comparative retrospective studies of laparoscopic versus open adrenalectomy, including current Yale series and recent literature.

Author	Year	#Patients	Mean operative time	Mean length of stay	Major complications	Mortality
Brunt[16]	1996	24*	142	8.7	9	1
Guazzoni[21]	1995	20**	145	9	4	0
Jacobs[17]	1997	19	151	5.1	6	0
Korman[18]	1997	10	124	5.9	2	0
Prinz[22]	1995	11*	174	6.4	N/A	N/A
Yale	1997	17	162	7.4	1	0

* includes only those patients who underwent open anterior adrenalectomy out of a larger group.
** includes patients who underwent both open anterior and retroperitoneal adrenalectomy.

up as malignant disease, none have recurred locally. Follow-up in this series ranged from 1 to 44 months.[13] This is by far the largest experience in the literature, and with this tremendous operative experience has come proficiency as mean operative times are reported to be 123 minutes, with bilateral procedures averaging only 45 minutes more.

Laparoscopic adrenalectomy for benign functional and nonfunctional adrenal tumors less than 8–10 cm can be done safely and effectively with less morbidity and shorter hospital stay than the open approach. Although not included in this series, we have found it to be ideal for the performance of bilateral adrenalectomy in patients' with Cushing's disease who have failed other therapies. Some advantages of the modified transperitoneal lateral technique we describe are optical correctness, "gravity" retraction, a clear, large operative field, use of a peritoneal retraction flap, and the judicious use of the harmonic scalpel. The learning curve for laparoscopic adrenalectomy is steep; however, it is likely that as experience and familiarity with this technique grow, operative times will continue to decrease, and this will surely become the gold standard of care for patients with benign adrenal neoplasms. The necessity for a high level of dedication to the refinement of the application of laparoscopic techniques to endocrine surgery remains clear if we are to continue to improve the quality of patient care into the next millenium.

References

1. Gagner M, Lacroix A, Bolte E. Laparoscopic adrenalectomy in Cushing's syndrome and pheochromocytoma [letter]. N Engl J Med 1992;327:1033.
2. Higashihara E, Tanaka Y, Horie S, et al. [A case report of laparoscopic adrenalectomy]. Nippon Hinyokika Gakkai Zasshi 1992;83:1130–1133.
3. Guazzoni G, Montorsi F, Bergamaschi F, et al. Effectiveness and safety of laparoscopic adrenalectomy. J Urol 1994;152:1375–1378.
4. Go H, Takeda M, Takahashi H, et al. Laparoscopic adrenalectomy for primary aldosteronism: a new operative method. J Laparoendosc Surg 1993;3:455–459.
5. Go H, Takeda M, Imai T, et al. Laparoscopic adrenalectomy for Cushing's syndrome: comparison with primary aldosteronism. Surgery 1995;117:11–17.
6. Gagner M, Breton G, Pharand D, et al. Is laparoscopic adrenalectomy indicated for pheochromocytomas? Surgery 1996;120:1076–1079; discussion 1079–1080.
7. Takeda M, Go H, Imai T, et al. Laparoscopic adrenalectomy for primary aldosteronism: report of initial ten cases. Surgery 1994;115:621–625.
8. Fletcher DR, Beiles CB, Hardy KJ. Laparoscopic adrenalectomy. Aust N Z J Surg 1994;64:427–430.
9. Hansen P, Bax T, Swanstrom L. Laparoscopic adrenalectomy: history, indications, and current techniques for a minimally invasive approach to adrenal pathology. Endoscopy 1997;29:309–314.
10. Duh QY, Siperstein AE, Clark OH, et al. Laparoscopic adrenalectomy. Comparison of the lateral and posterior approaches. Arch Surg 1996;131:870–875; discussion 875–876.

11. Gagner M, Lacroix A, Prinz RA, et al. Early experience with laparoscopic approach for adrenalectomy. Surgery 1993;114:1120–1124; discussion 1124–1125.
12. McDougall EM, Clayman RV. Advances in laparoscopic urology. Part I. History and development of procedures. Urology 1994;43:420–426.
13. Gagner M, Pomp A, Heniford BT, et al. Laparoscopic adrenalectomy—lessons learned from 100 consecutive procedures. Ann Surg 1997;226:238–246.
14. Caplan RH, Strutt PJ, Wickus GG. Subclinical hormone secretion by incidentally discovered adrenal masses. Arch Surg 1994;129:291–296.
15. Gagner M, Lacroix A, Bolte E, et al. Laparoscopic adrenalectomy. The importance of a flank approach in the lateral decubitus position. Surg Endosc 1994;8:135–138.
16. Brunt LM, Doherty GM, Norton JA, et al. Laparoscopic adrenalectomy compared to open adrenalectomy for benign adrenal neoplasms [see comments]. J Am Coll Surg 1996;183:1–10.
17. Jacobs JK, Goldstein RE, Geer RJ. Laparoscopic adrenalectomy. A new standard of care. Ann Surg 1997;225:495–501; discussion 501–502.
18. Korman JE, Ho T, Hiatt JR, et al. Comparison of laparoscopic and open adrenalectomy. Am Surg 1997;63:908–912.
19. Ishikawa T, Sowa M, Nagayama M, et al. Laparoscopic adrenalectomy: comparison with the conventional approach. Surg Laparosc Endosc 1997;7:275–280.
20. Horgan S, Sinanan M, Helton WS, et al. Use of laparoscopic techniques improves outcome from adrenalectomy. Am J Surg 1997;173:371–374.
21. Guazzoni G, Montorsi F, Bocciardi A, et al. Transperitoneal laparoscopic versus open adrenalectomy for benign hyperfunctioning adrenal tumors: a comparative study [see comments]. J Urol 1995;153:1597–1600.
22. Prinz RA. A comparison of laparoscopic and open adrenalectomies. Arch Surg 1995;130:489–489; discussion 492–494.

18
Laparoscopic Placement of Feeding Tubes

Robert Bell and James C. Rosser Jr.

Under normal circumstances, oral intake of carbohydrates, proteins, and fats is sufficient to meet daily caloric requirements. Upper gastrointestinal cancer, mental obtundation or retardation, multiple trauma, and sepsis are special conditions that make it impossible to obtain an adequate amount of nutrients by mouth. Short-term parenteral nutrition is necessary in instances such as enterocutaneous fistulas and short bowel syndrome; however, patients with functional gastrointestinal tracts should be fed enterally. Enteral feeding locally stimulates enterocyte growth and enhances intestinal immune function. Most enteral formulas provide glutamine, which is the principle enterocyte nutrient. Standard total parenteral nutrition (TPN) solutions do not contain glutamine as it is unstable in solution. Even with optimal parenteral nutrition, enterocyte atrophy is well documented. Animal studies demonstrate impaired mucosal immunity when TPN is compared with enteral feeding.[1] The combination of mucosal atrophy and decreased local immunity may predispose for bacterial translocation and sepsis. In a study of trauma patients, septic complications were decreased when enteral nutrition was compared with parenteral nutrition.[2]

Short-term enteral feeding can be accomplished with nasogastric or nasointestinal feeding tubes. They are the initial mode of nutrition in patients unable to tolerate oral feedings. Nasointestinal feedings can be used in patients without paralytic ileus or high nasogastric outputs (>600ml/ day), as long as there is a reasonable length of bowel available for nutrient absorption. Enteric feeding should be avoided in patients with gastrointestinal hemorrhage, bowel obstruction, or severe pancreatitis. Although they can provide an optimal delivery of nutrients, nasoenteric tubes are uncomfortable and increase the risk of aspiration pneumonia. When long-term enteric feeding is anticipated, patients are best served with operative feeding tube placement.

The surgical placement of feeding tubes has long been a role of the general surgeon. In 1875, a London surgeon, Sidney Jones, performed the first successful feeding gastrostomy.[3] He fashioned a cone of gastric tissue, which he brought out to the skin. In 1891, Witzel was the first to employ a rubber catheter for gastrostomy. Over the years, these basic procedures were modified, most notably by Stamm in 1894 and Janeway in 1913. The first feeding jejunostomy was performed in 1879 by Surmay of Harve.[4] Stamm, Mayo and Witzel refined the procedure over the ensuing years. Laparotomy was the only method to provide long-term enteral feeding until 1979. At that time, Ponsky and Gauderer developed an endoscopic percutaneous technique for placing feeding tubes.[5] Percutaneous endoscopic gastrostomy (PEG) has become the first-line procedure of choice for feeding tube placement. Percutaneous gastrostomy has several limitations, however, and open gastrostomy or jejunostomy had previously provided the only alternative to PEG. If PEG must be avoided, then a minimally invasive means for providing enteral nutrition should be sought. With the emerging role of laparoscopy, so has its application to various general surgical procedures. Several laparoscopic techniques have been developed for the placement of long-term feeding tubes. The indications for feeding tube placement, laparoscopic or percutaneous, are listed in Table 18.1.

The majority of laparoscopic procedures are a variation of the PEG technique; therefore, a brief description of the percutaneous procedure and its limitations will now be given.

TABLE 18.1. The indications for feeding tube placement.

Intracranial disease
Traumatic head injury
Cerebrovascular accident
Brain tumor

Progressive organic brain disease
Parkinson's Disease
Multiple Sclerosis
Dementia
Cerebral Palsy
Mental retardation
Status post brain surgery

Local disease
Oral cavity tumor
Pharyngeal tumor
Esophageal carcinoma

Laryngeal carcinoma
Facial fractures

Other
Pancreatic carcinoma (preop neoadjuvant therapy)
Enteral medications
Inflammatory Bowel Disease
Ventilator Dependency

Percutaneous Endoscopic Gastrostomy (PEG)

Endoscopic feeding tube placement has proven to be effective in most patients in need of nutritional support. Several methods have been described. With all techniques, the patient should have oral intake stopped 8 hours prior to the procedure. A first-generation cephalosporin is given "on call" to the endoscopy suite. Local anesthesia is injected subcutaneously in the left upper quadrant at the catheter exit site.

The "pull" technique was described by Ponsky with the initial description of the procedure.[5,6] After the endoscope is passed into the stomach, the area of maximal transillumination is observed in the left upper quadrant. A small incision is made in the skin at this site, and a 16-gauge needle is inserted into the stomach under endoscopic visualization. A suture is then passed through the needle and grasped with a polypectomy snare. The suture is brought out the patient's mouth and secured to the tapered end of a gastrostomy catheter. The catheter is then pulled through the stomach and exits the abdominal wall where it is secured. The "push" technique is comparable to the pull technique except that a guide wire is passed through the needle and brought out the patient's mouth. The gastrostomy tube is then passed over the guide wire via Seldinger technique until it advances through the stomach and exits the abdominal wall. These technical variations allow some degree of operator flexibility, but neither technique has proven to be superior to the other.

The Russell modification, which is probably the most commonly used method for PEG placement, utilizes a "peel away" introducer.[7] A 16-gauge needle punctures the gastric lumen under endoscopic surveillance and a guidewire is passed through the needle. The needle is removed and an introducer with sheath is then passed over the guide wire using the Seldinger technique. The introducer is removed and a Foley catheter (14-Fr) is inserted through the sheath. The balloon is inflated and the sheath is then peeled away from the catheter. The catheter is then secured externally.

All three procedures are safe and easy to perform by a skilled endoscopist. The procedure is performed with local anesthesia and intravenous sedation. Operative time is usually less than 30 minutes and postprocedural discomfort is minimal. A randomized, prospective trial, however, demonstrated that PEG was not more efficacious than traditional Stamm open gastrostomy (OG).[8] Both groups experienced a 25% postoperative complication rate. The 30-day mortality rate was 12.5% for PEG and 8.8% for open gastrostomy. Finally, whereas the initial costs of PEG are less than OG, a repeat endoscopy for a tube change equalizes the difference.

PEG has a complication rate of 5–32% and a 30-day mortality of up to 17%.[9] The morbidity and mortality of PEG is similar to open gastrostomy and jejunostomy and reflects the seriousness of underlying patient disease. Death is rarely attributable to the procedure alone. It is ironic that patients may be referred for PEG or gastrostomy because of repeated aspiration; however, neither open gastrostomy nor PEG protects against aspiration. In patients prone to aspiration, pressurization of the stomach as a feeding reservoir probably contributes to aspiration. Jarnigan et al.[9] reviewed complications of PEG in 60 patients. They found an overall rate of aspiration pneumonia of 15% of patients. Of those who aspirated, 77% had a history of aspiration prior to operation. Furthermore, aspiration pneumonia after PEG was responsible for over 50% of deaths in their series. Patients at risk for aspiration should be treated with jejunostomy. Placement of a jejunal tube through the PEG catheter (JET-PEG); however, fails to reduce aspiration risk. Instead, two thirds of patients who had JET-PEGs placed to reduce the risk of aspiration continued to aspirate.[10] Furthermore, nearly half of those patients died as a consequence of aspiration pneumonia. When open jejunostomy is performed as an isolated procedure, feeding-related aspiration can be completely eliminated.[11] For aspiration risk patients, PEG should be abandoned in favor of jejunostomy, as long as jejunostomy can be accomplished by minimally invasive means.

While PEG is widely applied in many patients who require long term nutritional support, there are other limitations and contraindications. PEG is also contraindicated in patients with ascites, bleeding disorders, large hiatal hernias, facial trauma and in patients with pharyngeal or esophageal tumors for whom endoscopy would be dangerous or difficult. Furthermore, the failure rate of PEG is about 5%.[8] Technical failures usually result from inability to transilluminate through the abdominal wall. Laparotomy in these cases generally reveals the left lobe of the liver covering the anterior wall of the stomach. When PEG is contraindicated or unsuccessful, direct intubation is necessary. Laparoscopy is a minimally invasive variant of direct intubation.

Laparoscopic Gastrostomy

Edelman presented the first description of laparoscopic gastrostomy in 1991.[12] Most techniques are modifications of Russell's endoscopic technique. Laparoscopic gastrostomies are usually performed under general anesthesia. However, for patients with a contraindication to general anesthesia, laparoscopic gastrostomy may be performed with local anesthesia and intravenous sedation.[13]

Technique

A first-generation cephalosporin is give intravenously just prior to the procedure and the abdomen is prepped and draped in a sterile fashion. Several techniques have been described.[12-15] With the surgeon and camera operator on the patient's right and the first assistant on the patient's left, a pneumoperitoneum is created using a Veress needle. Carbon dioxide is insufflated to a pressure of 10–15 mmHg. For procedures done under local anesthesia, insufflation pressure should be less than 10 mmHg. The first trocar is placed in the infraumbilical fold. A second 10-mm trocar is placed under direct visualization into the left upper quadrant. An atraumatic grasper is inserted through the second trocar site. At this point in time, stay sutures may be placed[14] directly followed by percutaneous insertion of a 16-gauge needle. A guidewire is placed through the needle and the needle is removed. An introducer and a "peel-away" sheath are exchanged via Seldinger technique. A Foley catheter is placed through the sheath as described earlier.

As an alternative, a transverse incision is initially made in the upper quadrant about 2–3 cm below the left costal margin lateral to the left rectus muscle. Using a hemostat, the underlying fascia is cleared. Four stay sutures are then placed laparoscopically using an Endostitch™ device; the sutures can be brought out of the abdominal wall through the incision using an Endoclose™ instrument. Needle puncture of the stomach can then be achieved using the sutures for retraction. After the gastrostomy tube is inserted, the sutures are secured externally and the transverse incision closed.

Other techniques obtain needle puncture of the anterior wall of the stomach without stay sutures[12] or by using T-bars for counter-retraction.[16] Tubes secured to the posterior fascia, however, are more easily replaced should the tube become inadvertently dislodged. This is especially important within the first week after the procedure, before adhesions have had time to develop between the anterior wall of the stomach and the posterior rectus fascia. The Foley catheter used for gastrostomy may range from #14Fr to #24Fr, with care to ensure that the introducer used is 2Fr sizes larger than the gastrostomy tube. Enteral feeding can begin from 12 to 24 hours after the operation.

Results

Most reports of laparoscopic gastrostomy consist of a small series of patients with emphasis on technique. Two series have included more than 20 patients,[13,17] and one series contained more than 40 patients.[14] All procedures in these series proved technically successful with an operating time less than 30 minutes. The catheter proved usable for an average of more than 10 months.[14] Relatively few deaths were reported in all series of laparoscopic gastrostomy. In a retrospective review,[18] the 30-day mortality rate was 7%. Complications after laparoscopic gastrostomy are difficult to assess because the current studies[13,14,16–18] were limited to inpatient records. The postoperative stay was short, however, and the majority of complications occurred after the patient left the hospital. No series to date has adequately addressed the problem of postoperative aspiration after laparoscopic gastrostomy. Long-term follow up of nursing–home patients after open gastrostomy revealed a 19% incidence of postoperative aspiration.[19] Aspiration pneumonia in these patients was lethal in 29%. Until the aspiration risks are adequately documented, jejunostomy is indicated in patients prone to aspiration. These include patients with a history of aspiration and those without faculties necessary for airway protection.

When PEG is not technically feasible, laparoscopic gastrostomy should be the alternative, provided the patients are mentally alert and not prone to aspiration. The advantages of gastrostomy over laparoscopic jejunostomy are related to a larger catheter size with gastrostomy. Laparoscopic gastrostomy catheters are typically 24Fr, as opposed to 14Fr with LJ catheters. Larger catheters allow for bolus feeding and the use of mashed home-made food. In the long run, the use of home-made preparations is less costly. Finally, gastric feedings may be hyperosmolar, which may be necessary in patients who need a large amount of calories but require fluid restriction. Patients with renal failure or congestive heart failure may benefit from hyperosmolar feeding.

Laparoscopic Jejunostomy

Laparoscopic placement of jejunal feeding tubes was first described in 1992.[20] Like gastrostomy, most series of laparoscopic jejunostomies are limited and emphasize technique rather than long-term results. Laparoscopic jejunostomy may be performed under general anesthesia or with local anesthesia and intravenous sedation.[21] Unless contraindicated, general anesthesia is preferred. For long-term nutrition, laparoscopic jejunostomy is the procedure of choice for patients with resectable esophageal cancer (future gastric pull-up procedure) and those at risk for aspiration. Aspiration risk patients include those with gastroparesis, gastric outlet obstruction, and those with a history of aspiration. It is the responsibility of the attending endoscopist or surgeon to obtain a thorough history to assess the patient's aspiration risk prior to operative placement of feeding tubes.

Technique[15]

A first generation cephalosporin is given immediately prior to anesthesia. The abdomen is prepped and draped in a sterile fashion and the bed is placed in slight reverse Trendelenberg. This table position allows the small intestine to fall into the pelvis and facilitates location of the ligament of Trietz. The surgeon is placed on the right side of the patient along with the camera operator, and the first assistant is placed on the left. The jejunostomy exit site is located in the patient's left upper quadrant. The position is at least 2cm lateral to the left rectus muscle and 2–3cm inferior to the left costal margin. Once this site is identified, a 3–4-cm transverse incision is made. Hemostats are then used to clear the subcutaneous tissue until the fascia is identified. A 2.5 × 2.5-cm area of fascia must be exposed. The first trocar is placed in the right upper quadrant about 2 cm lateral to the right rectus muscle and about 2 cm inferior to the right costal margin. Pneumoperitoneum is established through this site. The second trocar is placed just lateral to the left rectus muscle about halfway between the umbilicus and anterior superior iliac spine. The third trocar is about 15 cm directly inferior to the first trocar (Fig. 18.1). All three trocars are usually 10 mm in size, but a 5-mm trocar can be used with a smaller laparoscope. The laparoscope is inserted through the second trocar site and instruments are inserted into the first and third sites. The greater omentum is gently retracted cephalad and the small bowel is gently displaced inferiorly until the ligament of Trietz is identified. The jejunostomy tube will be placed about 40 centimeters distal to the ligament of Trietz. Four sutures, in a diamond fashion, will ultimately fix the bowel to the posterior fascia. A corresponding diamond grid is identified on the exposed anterior fascia and an Endoclose™ instrument is inserted through the fascia at the apex of the diamond into the abdominal cavity. About 30 cm of suture is brought into the abdominal cavity with an Endostitch™ instrument. The first stitch is placed through the jejunum at the apex of the diamond grid. Using the Endoclose™ device both limbs of the suture are brought out of the anterior abdominal wall through separate stab wounds where both limbs are secured

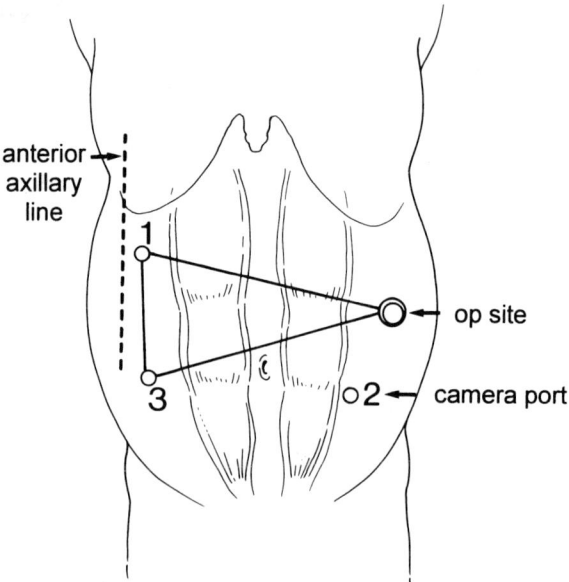

FIGURE 18.1. Port placement.

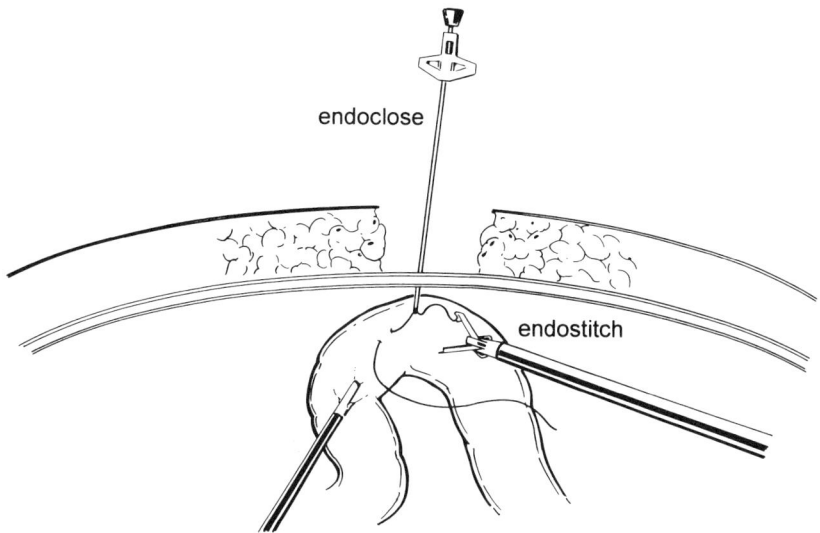

endoclose

endostitch

FIGURE 18.2. Initial suture placement.

with a hemostat (Fig. 18.2). The preceding steps are repeated for the three remaining sutures. When finished, the suture pattern will be about 2.5 cm long and about 2.5 cm wide (Fig. 18.3). A 16-gauge needle is then place through the center of the four fixation points and a guidewire is passed through the needle (Fig. 18.4). The needle is exchanged for an introducer and "peel-away" sheath via the Seldinger technique (Fig. 18.5). The introducer is removed. The sutures are then secured externally beneath the skin (Fig. 18.6) and infusion of water-soluble contrast verifies adequate tube position.

As an alternative, four T-fasteners may be used to draw the jejunum against the posterior rectus sheath and secured externally. The jejunostomy catheter is placed in the center of the four T-fasteners, and the fasteners are secured externally. This technique is similar to that described above for laparoscopic gastrostomy. After 2 weeks, to allow adhesions to form between the posterior rectus sheath and the jejunal serosa, the fasteners are severed externally and the T- fasteners subsequently pass into the feces. A prospective study of 36 laparoscopic jejunostomies[22] using this technique revealed a 14% incidence of postoperative tube dislodgment. Furthermore, 8% of cases were converted to open jejunostomy due to inadvertent enterotomies.

In a review of 32 laparoscopic jejunostomies,[23] Hotokezaka and colleagues revealed a 30-day mortality rate of 10.7%, again reflective of underlying patient disease. They observed a 6% risk for aspiration pneumonia; however, they failed to mention if aspiration was truly feeding related. In a Weltz's review of open jejunostomies,[11] 37% of aspirations occurred before

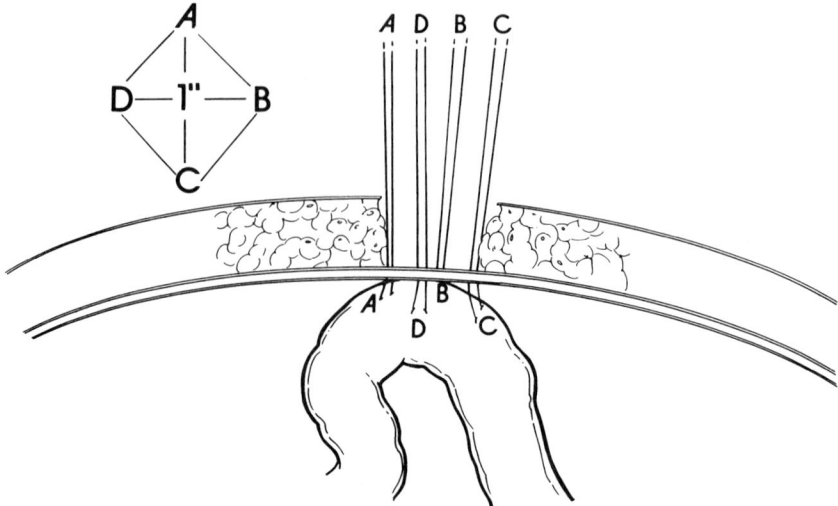

FIGURE 18.3. Facial suture pattern.

feeding was initiated. Furthermore, with Hotokezaka's described technique the jejunostomy catheter was placed between 25 and 30 cm beyond the ligament of Trietz. Placement of feeding tubes 40 cm beyond the ligament of Trietz may further reduce the risk of aspiration, as described in the technique earlier.

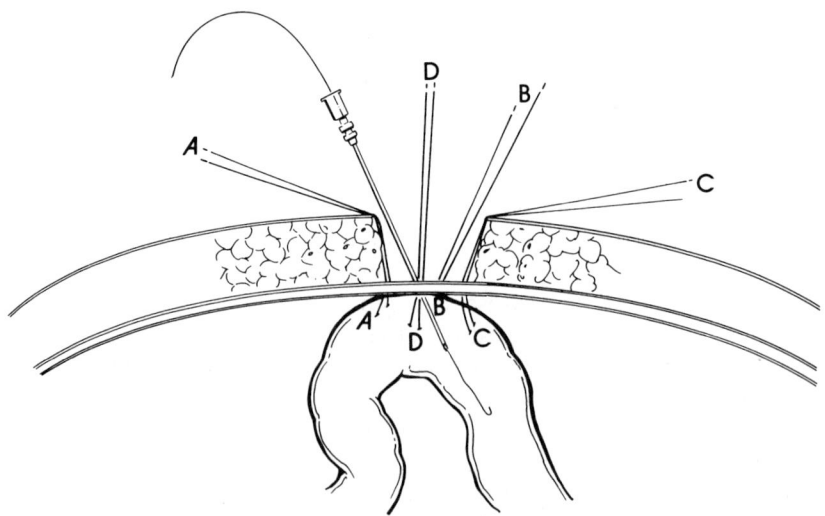

FIGURE 18.4. Needle and guidewire placement.

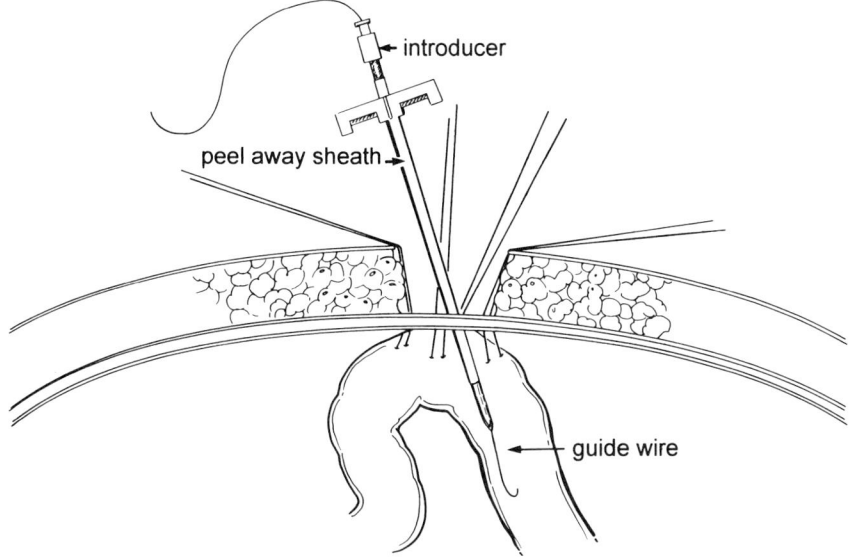

FIGURE 18.5. Introducer and peel away sheath.

The smaller catheter size of jejunostomy tubes renders them more applicable to continuous feeding rather than to bolus feedings. This also reduces the utility of using home-made preparations. Furthermore, jejunal feedings require iso-osmolar formulas as hyperosmolar feeding into the jejunum may lead to osmotic diarrhea. This is only problematic in fluid-restricted

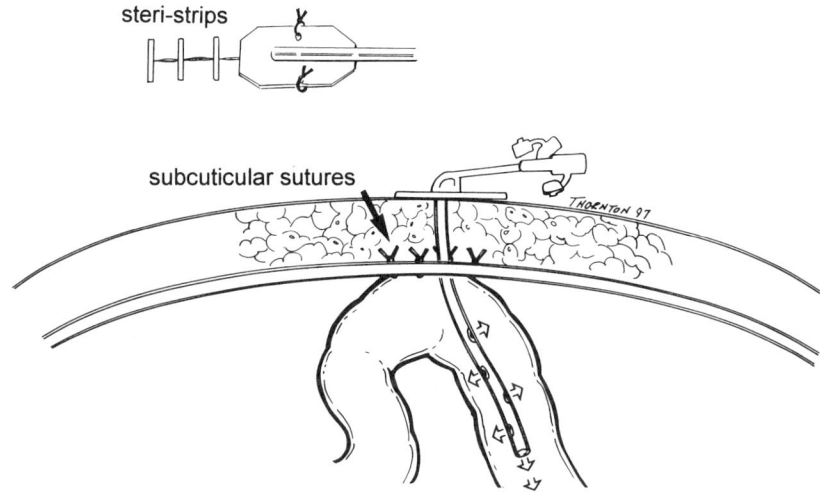

FIGURE 18.6. Jejunostomy tube in place.

patients. Fluid-restricted, jejunally fed patients cannot increase the formula concentration to meet nutritional goals. Fluid-restricted patients, therefore, will also be calorically restricted. Patients with congestive heart failure and renal insufficiency have relative contraindication to laparoscopic jejunostomy.

Conclusion

Over the past 20 years great strides have been made to meet the nutritional goals of critically ill patients. Due to medical, surgical, or psychological illness, patients may be unable to tolerate long-term oral feedings. While TPN is useful for providing immediate nourishment, patients should be fed enterally when possible. Enteral feeding tubes should be placed by a minimally invasive means. Percutaneous and laparoscopic procedures have proven to be a safe, effective, and durable means of providing enteral nutrition. PEG remains the standard method for obtaining enteral access. When PEG is contraindicated or unsuccessful, laparoscopic methods provide a minimally invasive alternative to open feeding tube placement. Laparoscopically placed tubes are amenable to day surgery, which facilitates rapid placement to rehabilitation or nursing home facilities. There is little postoperative discomfort, and enteral feeding may begin within 24 hours of surgery. As surgeons become more facile with laparoscopic techniques, an increasing number of gastrostomies and jejunostomies will be performed laparoscopically. In the upcoming years, after laparoscopic techniques become refined and patients are carefully followed long-term, laparoscopic placement of feeding tubes may become the procedure of choice for providing enteral nutrition.

References

1. Alverdy J, Hoon SC, Sheldon GF. The effect of parenteral nturition on gastrointestinal immunity: the importance of enteral stimulation. Ann Surg 1985;203:681–684.
2. Moore F, Moore E, Jones T, et al. TEN versus TPN following major abdominal trauma reduced septic morbidity. J Trauma 1989;29:916–923.
3. Harkins HN, Nyhus LM. Surgery of the stomach and duodenum, 1st ed. Little, Brown and Company, Boston, 1962, p. 5.
4. Shackelford RT. Surgery of the alimentary tract, 1st ed. WB Saunders, Philadelphia, 1955, p. 1041.
5. Gauderer MWL, Ponsky JL, Izant RJ. Gastrostomy without laparotomy: a percutaneous technique. J Pediatr Surg 1980;15:872–875.
6. Ponsky JL, Gauderer MWL, Stellato TA. Percutaneous endoscopic gastrostomy. Arch Surg 1983;118:913–914.
7. Russell TR, Brotman M, Norris F. Percutaneous gastrostomy: a new simplified technique. Am J Surg 1984;148:132–137.

8. Stiegmann GV, Goff JS, Silas D, et al. Endoscopic versus operative gastrostomy: final results of a prospective randomized trial. Gastrointest Endosc 1990;36:1–5.
9. Jarnagin W, Duh QY, Mulvihill SJ, et al. The efficacy and limitations of percutaneous endoscopic gastrostomy. Arch Surg 1992;127:261–264.
10. DiSario JA, Foutch PG, Sanowski RA. Poor results with percutaneous endoscopic jejunostomy. Gastrointest Endosc 1990;36:257–260.
11. Weltz CW. Morris JB, Mullen JL. Surgical jejunostomy in aspiration risk patients. Ann Surg 1992;215:140–145.
12. Edelman DS, Unger SW. Laparoscopic gastrostomy. Surg Gynacol Obstet 1991;173:401.
13. Ng PCH. Laparoscopic-assisted gastrostomy in 26 patients: indications and outcome at 2 years. J Laparoendosc Surg 1996;6:25–28.
14. Peitgen K, Walz MK, Krause U, et al. First results of laparoscopic gastrostomy. Surg Endosc 1997;11:658–662.
15. Rosser JC, Salem RR, Rodas EB, et al. A simplified technique for laparoscopic jejunostomy and gastrostomy. Am J Surg 1998; in press.
16. Duh QY, Way LW. Laparoscopic gastrostomy using T-fasteners at retractors and anchors. Surg Endosc 1993;7:60–63.
17. Edelman DS, Unger SW. Laparoscopic gastrostomy and jejunostomy: review of 22 cases. Surg Laparosc Endosc 1994;4:297–300.
18. Edelman DS, Arroyo PJ, Unger SW. Laparoscopic gastrostomy versus percutaneous endoscopic gastrostomy: a comparison. Surg Endosc 1194;8:47–49.
19. Cogen R, Weinryb J. Aspiration pneumonia in nursing home patietns fed via gastrostomy tubes. Am Gastroenterol 1989;84:1509–1512.
20. Albrink MH, Foster J, Rosemurgy AS, et al. Laparoscopic feeding jejunostomy: also a simple technique. Surg Endosc 1992;6:259–260.
21. Duh QY, Way LW. Laparoscopic jejunostomy using t-fasteners as retractors and anchors. Arch Surg 1993;128:105–108.
22. Duh QY, Senokozlieff-Englehart AL, Siperstein AE, et al. Prospective evaluation of the safety and efficacy of laparoscopic jejunostomy. West J Med 1995;162:117–122.
23. Hotokezaka M, Adams RB, Miller AD, et al. Laparoscopic percutaneous jejunostomy for long-term enteral access. Surg Endosc 1996;10:1008–1011.

19
Live Donor Nephrectomy

JOHN L. FLOWERS

The gap between the number of patients listed for renal transplantation and the number of kidney transplants continues to grow. In March 1997, the United Network for Organ Sharing (UNOS) national patient waiting list contained 35,121 registrations for kidney transplantation; however, only 10,892 kidney transplants were performed during 1995, the latest year for which data are available.

One method of addressing the growing shortage of organs for kidney transplantation is the increased use of living kidney donors. Potential advantages of living donation include superior graft function and survival when compared with cadaveric donors,[1,2] the ability to time the transplant when the recipient is in optimal condition and limit waiting time on dialysis, and a limit to the possibility of HLA sensitization during blood transfusions often necessary during dialysis. Nearly all of the 250 transplant centers in the United States perform live donor kidney transplants. Live donors accounted for 3,209 of 10,892 kidney transplants (29%) reported to UNOS in 1995.[1,2]

Nephrectomy using an extraperitoneal flank approach is the most common method of live donor renal allograft procurement. The procedure is safe and produces a kidney in optimal condition with minimal warm ischemia. Mortality is approximately 0.003%, but long-term morbidity may be substantial, ranging from 15 to 20% or higher.[3,4] Wound complications including infection and hernia formation occur in approximately 9% of patients with a flank approach.[1] Pneumothorax requiring pleural space drainage occurs in approximately 8% of cases. Chronic wound "diastases" or bulging and chronic incisional pain has been reported in up to 25% of patients. Return to normal activity may not occur for as long as 6–9 weeks, and "full recovery" of up to 9.5 months after surgery.[3,5] The rationale for the development of minimally invasive donor nephrectomy comes from a combination of the realization of the limitations of extraperitoneal flank nephrectomy, and the demonstration of the technical feasibility and efficacy of other similar laparoscopic procedures such as splenectomy and adrenalectomy.[6,7]

Potential benefits of a laparoscopic approach to live donor nephrectomy include less postoperative pain, shorter hospitalization, less incisional morbidity, more rapid return to normal activity, and improved cosmesis. The biggest potential advantage of the laparoscopic approach, however, that the sum of these improvements in patient recovery may result in increased acceptance of the donor operation and expand the pool of potential kidney donors. This is especially true in areas where cadaveric kidneys are not widely available or political policy considers the use of live donors unacceptable.[8]

Laparoscopic live donor nephrectomy has been performed in more than 80 patients at the University of Maryland Medical System (UMMS) since March 1996. This chapter details our initial experience with laparoscopic live donor nephrectomy. The laparoscopic donors are compared with a cohort of age-matched controls undergoing traditional donor nephrectomy with a flank incision, in order to determine whether early graft survival, intraoperative variables, and postoperative recovery are similar between open and laparoscopic donor nephrectomy.

Patients and Methods

Patient Selection

Seventy patients underwent laparoscopic live donor nephrectomy at the UMMS from March 1996 through March 1997. Laparoscopic donors were compared with a cohort of 65 patients undergoing open donor nephrectomy at UMMS from January 1994 through March 1997. The two groups were matched for age, sex, race, and comorbidity. Patient data were obtained from a combination of a prospective longitudinal database, medical record review, and personal and telephone interviews. Graft function and survival and patient recovery data were compared using analysis of covariance and multiple logistic regression. P values of less than 0.05 were considered statistically significant.

Absolute contraindications to either open or laparoscopic donor nephrectomy included absence of two functional kidneys, ABO incompatibility, pregnancy, certain infectious diseases (hepatitis B or C, human immunodeficiency virus), significant renal arterial occlusive disease, renal parenchymal diseases (e.g., malignancy or polycystic kidney disease), uncorrectable coagulopathy, and horseshoe kidney. Relative contraindications to laparoscopic donor nephrectomy include underlying medical conditions (e.g., extremes of age, hypertension, diabetes mellitus, nephrolithiasis) inability to tolerate general anesthesia or pneumoperitoneum, prior left colonic or splenic surgery, retroperitoneal inflammatory processes (e.g., diverticulitis, retroperitoneal fibrosis), morbid obesity, and ascites. Laparoscopic donor nephrectomy was performed on the left kidney in all cases in this patient cohort to maximize the length of renal vein available to the transplant surgeon. We have successfully performed right laparoscopic live donor nephrectomy in three cases recently.

Operative Technique

Laparoscopic live donor left nephrectomy is performed under general endotracheal anesthesia with the patient in the right decubitus position. The patient is draped to allow access for both a standard left flank incision if necessary and extraction of the kidney through a 6–7-cm midline incision.

A total of five operating ports are used. Four ports (three 12 mm and one 5 mm) are arranged parallel to the left costal margin and are used for the initial dissection. A 15-mm operating port is placed later during the procedure through a 6–7-cm midline incision to aid in extraction of the kidney. The camera is placed in the uppermost subcostal port and two dissection ports are located along the left costal margin. A 5-mm-retraction port is located in the posterior axillary line near the tip of the eleventh or twelfth rib; this port can occasionally be omitted.

The operative procedure begins with mobilization of the left colon and spleen. This step is followed by dissection of the renal vein and artery, dissection of the ureter, mobilization of the kidney (i.e., opening the renal fascia and division of perinephric fat), creation of the extraction incision and deployment of the extraction bag, and renal extraction. Renal extraction is accomplished by systemic anticoagulation followed by division of the ureter, renal artery, and renal vein, in that order. A 3-cm Endo-GIA stapler with a vascular cartridge is used for division of the renal vessels (United States Surgical Corporation, Norwalk, CT).

The extraction process begins with a 6-cm midline umbilical incision through the abdominal wall fascia without violating the peritoneum. A 15-mm operating port is placed through the extraction incision and a large plastic extraction sac is inserted and deployed over the liver, in preparation to receive the kidney. The patient is anticoagulated with 100 U/kg intravenous heparin sodium. The distal ureter is clipped and divided. After division of the renal artery and vein, the kidney is placed into the extraction sac and delivered through the midline wound. The kidney is immediately placed in iced saline solution and transferred to an adjoining operating suite where it is perfused and prepared for transplantation. Anticoagulation is reversed with 100 mg protamine sulfate and the midline extraction incision is closed. The abdomen is reinsufflated and inspected for hemostasis prior to conclusion of the procedure.

Results

Laparoscopic live donor nephrectomy was attempted in 70 patients and successfully completed in 66 cases (94%) (Table 19.1). A successful laparoscopic harvest was performed in one case, but the kidney was not

TABLE 19.1. Patient demographics and operative data.

Number of patients	70
Sex	
Male	26 (37%)
Female	44 (63%)
Age	37.9 years (range, 19–67 y)
Weight	78.1 kg (range, 51–127 kg)
Conversion to laparotomy	4 (5.7%)
Warm ischemia time	3.0 minutes (range, 1.9–6.9)
Reoperation	1 (1.4%)

transplanted due to discovery of an incidental 1 cm renal cell carcinoma. A total of 65 patients eventually received kidneys from laparoscopic donors. Conversion to laparotomy was necessary in 6% of cases (four patients: three for vascular injury and one for a combination of morbid obesity and inability to sustain pneumoperitoneum). Vascular injuries included hemorrhage during renal artery transection, external iliac artery injury during division of the ureter, and avulsion of a small posterior renal vein branch. All four patients experienced uneventful recovery after laparotomy. An additional patient (1.4%) required laparotomy and splenorrhaphy for postoperative hemorrhage from a splenic capsular tear.

Graft survival in laparoscopic allografts is 97% (67 of 69 patients) with a mean follow up of 7 months (range, 2–12 months). Reasons for graft failure include severe rejection in one patient and gangrenous cholecystitis with septicemia in another. No evidence of acute tubular necrosis was present on duplex flow scan or renal biopsy in either case. Delayed graft function occurred in 3% of patients in the laparoscopic group (2 of 69). Spontaneous recovery of function occurred within 10 days of surgery in both cases (Table 19.2).

Perioperative variables and early recovery data are listed in Table 19.3. Intraoperative blood loss, return of gastrointestinal function, postoperative parenteral narcotic use, and length of stay were all significantly shorter in the laparoscopic group. Return to normal activity is compared with open donor nephrectomy in Table 19.4. Laparoscopic donors returned to housework in 33% of the time necessary for the open group. In the laparoscopic group, ability to drive an automobile occurred in 35% of the time and

TABLE 19.2. Graft function and survival.

Function	# Patients	Graft survival (%)	Delayed graft
Laparoscopic	69	67 (97)	2 (3)
Open	65	64 (98)	1 (2)
P-value		0.6191	0.4961

TABLE 19.3. Intraoperative data and early post-operative recovery.

	Laparoscopic	Open	P-value
OR Time (min)	226.3	212.8	0.1658
Estimated blood loss (ml)	122.3	408.0	0.0001
Diet (h)			
Liquids	16.3	51.0	0.0001
Solids	40.0	77.7	0.0001
Parenteral narcotic use (h)	28.6	60.1	0.0001
Length of stay (d)	2.2	4.5	0.0001

Table legend: min = minutes; ml = milliliters; h = hours; d = days.

return to employment in 31% of the time necessary for the open nephrectomy group.

Morbidity occurred in 14% of patients (10 of 69) undergoing laparoscopic donor nephrectomy (Table 19.5). Four patients required blood transfusion (5.8%). Postoperative hypoxia occurred in 2 cases (2.9%). Congestive heart failure, renal artery injury, external iliac artery injury, and urinary retention all occurred in one patient each. There were no statistically significant differences in complication rates after open laparoscopic donor nephrectomy [Tables, 19.5 and 19.6, (odds ratio, 4:1)]. There was no mortality in either the laparoscopic or open donor group.

Discussion

Live donor nephrectomy is truly a surgical procedure where there is zero tolerance for error. This operation is unique among major surgical procedures in that an otherwise healthy patient is subjected to the risks of major surgery solely for the benefit of another person. In order to justify the laparoscopic approach for live donor nephrectomy, several conditions must be met. First (and most importantly), the laparoscopic donor should be subject to no unique or excessive morbidity when compared with the open donor. Second, kidneys procured using laparoscopic techniques must have graft survival and function rates equivalent to those obtained using open

TABLE 19.4. Postoperative recovery: Return to normal activity.

	Laparoscopic	Open	P-value
Housework (days)	8.8	26.9	0.0001
Driving (days)	11.1	31.6	0.0001
Employment (days)	15.9	51.5	0.0001

TABLE 19.5. Perioperative morbidity: Laparoscopic donor nephrectomy.

	Number of patients (%)
Hemorrhage	4 (6)
Hypoxia	2 (3)
Renal artery injury	1 (1)
External iliac artery injury	1 (1)
Urinary retention	1 (1)
Congestive heart failure	1 (1)
Total	**10 (14)**

nephrectomy with an extraperitoneal flank approach. Finally, the laparoscopic approach should result in some patient advantage such as less pain, shorter hospital stay, and earlier return to normal activity.

Preliminary graft survival rates (97%) after laparoscopic procurement compare favorably with both recent historical controls at our institution as well as the latest data reported by UNOS. There was no difference in graft survival between the laparoscopic cohort and open donors at UMMS during the time of study. Through October 1995, one year UNOS graft survival rates after living donor renal transplants ranged from 89 to 95%, depending on the histocompatability of the donor and recipient.[3] Graft failures after laparoscopic donor nephrectomy in this series occurred as a result of overwhelming sepsis and severe rejection. In both cases the transplanted kidneys functioned immediately, and there is no evidence to suggest laparoscopic procurement as a factor leading to graft failure. Longer follow-up is necessary, however, to determine the true incidence of graft survival after laparoscopic donor nephrectomy.

Two instances of delayed graft function (3%) occurred in this series. The incidence of acute tubular necrosis (ATN) after traditional living related kidney donation ranges from 1 to 6%, depending on the series.[2,3,9] Delayed

TABLE 19.6. Perioperative morbidity: Open donor nephrectomy.

	Number of patients (%)
Pneumothorax	14 (22)
Hemorrhage	7 (11)
Fever	6 (9)
Persistent incisional pain	5 (8)
Ileus/vomiting	4 (6)
Wound hernia/seroma	4 (6)
Urinary retention	4 (6)
Dyspnea	2 (3)

Note: Several patients had more than a single complication.

graft function/ATN after renal transplantation is presumed to be an ischemic event. Though neither allograft experienced prolonged warm ischemia, one obese donor had a long, technically difficult procedure that may have resulted in excessive manipulation and vasospasm. The recipient in the second case of ATN experienced significant hypotension in the immediate postoperative period that may have contributed to delayed graft function. Both kidneys recovered spontaneously and continue to function well.

Patient outcome after laparoscopic donor nephrectomy was impressive when compared with that seen with open donor nephrectomy. Operative times were similar between the two groups, which is a finding not seen in other comparisons of open and laparoscopic nephrectomy.[10,11] Return of gastrointestinal function, narcotic use, and hospital stay averaged less than half of the corresponding times for open donor nephrectomy. The benefits of the laparoscopic approach were even more impressive in the convalescent phase of postoperative recovery. Laparoscopic donors returned to housework, drove an automobile, and returned to work in 34–38% of the time necessary for their open counterparts. Hospital stay ranges from 5 to 17.6 days after open donor nephrectomy, with the most typical stay being 5.6–7.9 days.[2,4,5,9,12–15] There is little current data regarding long-term recovery after flank donor nephrectomy. One series of 29 cases reported "return to usual activities" at 2.25 months and "time to full recovery" of 9.46 months.[10] The improvements in inhospital and postoperative recovery associated with laparoscopic donor nephrectomy have been verified by two other series comparing laparoscopic nephrectomy for benign disease to transperitoneal and extraperitoneal flank nephrectomy.[10,11]

Initial data from our experience at UMMS suggests that these improvements in patient recovery may indeed be accomplishing our ultimate goal of increasing willingness to donate kidneys. Since the beginning of the laparoscopic donor program in March 1996, the number of patients evaluated for the kidney transplant waiting list has increased by 40%, and the number of screening cross-matches performed for potential live donors has increased by 37%. The number of actual living donor harvests increased by 85% from the year preceding the study period (from 41 cases in 1995 to 76 cases in 1996).

Despite our enthusiasm and the initial success of laparoscopic live donor nephrectomy, however, the technical difficulty of the operation is orders of magnitude greater than that of most other commonly performed "advanced" laparoscopic procedures. Laparoscopic donor nephrectomy differs from nearly all other laparoscopic procedures in three important respects. First, the kidney must be harvested in perfect condition. Unlike the removal of a diseased organ, no parenchymal damage is permissible during the dissection or extraction. Second, the procedure requires a delicate major vascular dissection, with the additional risk factor of complete systemic anticoagulation during the most critical step: division of the renal vessels.

Though vascular division is performed without anticoagulation by some during open donor nephrectomy, we have been reluctant to adopt this approach during laparoscopic harvests due to the somewhat longer extraction times. Finally, extraction must be rapid and atraumatic to minimize warm ischemia to the donor kidney. The successful laparoscopic donor surgeon must have thorough knowledge of basic principles of open donor surgery, commonly encountered vascular anomalies (34% of patients in this series had vascular anatomy other than a single artery and vein), and a high level of operative skills and comfort with advanced laparoscopy.

The technical difficulty and long learning curve of laparoscopic live donor nephrectomy are illustrated by the complications in this series. Both major vascular injuries (one renal artery and one external iliac artery) were basic and avoidable errors in operative technique due to relative inexperience with advanced laparoscopy on the part of the operating surgeon. Splenic injury as a result of excessive traction or inadequate mobilization during laparoscopic dissection was the reason for transfusion in three of four patients requiring blood products. There was no significant difference in morbidity, however, between the open and laparoscopic groups in this series. The total laparoscopic morbidity of 14% compares favorably with other large series of open donor nephrectomy, in which total morbidity ranges from 10 to 20%.[4,5,9,12–16] No unique types of morbidity appear to arise from the laparoscopic technique. Wound complications have been notably absent from the laparoscopic group in this series, and no cases of deep venous thrombosis or pulmonary embolism have occurred.

Several technical limitations and unanswered physiologic questions regarding laparoscopic live donor nephrectomy presently exist. The procedure is quite difficult in very obese patients, which is a group that could benefit most from the laparoscopic approach by avoidance of a large incision. Laparoscopic vascular dissection and hemostasis remain relatively crude, although laparoscopic vascular instrumentation is in development. Warm ischemia time is longer than it is for open donor nephrectomy, but it is not entirely clear what constitutes an acceptable limit. Most series of open donor nephrectomy do not quote times for warm ischemia. Mean warm ischemia for the laparoscopic patients in this series was 3.0 minutes. Although the mean time was reduced to 2.25 minutes for the last 20 cases in the series, it is unlikely that warm ischemia will drop much below 2 minutes using current techniques. Finally, the effects of kidney harvest in a positive-pressure environment are unknown at the present time. Data suggest that arterial and venous flow is decreased, and we observed that intraoperative urine output was lower and initial postoperative serum creatinine higher with early laparoscopic donors than for open donors. These observations have been corrected with improved dissection techniques, careful attention to volume status by the anesthesiologist, aggressive preload administration, and use of dopamine and topical papaverine during the arterial dissection. More study is necessary, however, to characterize and quantify the physiologic changes that occur during laparoscopic live donor nephrectomy accurately.

References

1. Cosimi AB. The donor and donor nephrectomy. *In*: Morris, PJ (ed.). Kidney transplantation: principles and practice. WB Saunders Co., Philadelphia, 1994, pp 56–70.
2. Cecka JM. Living donor transplants. *In*: Cecka JM, Terasaki PI (eds.). Clinical transplants 1995. UCLA Tissue Typing Laboratory, Los Angeles, pp 363–377.
3. Blohme I, Fehrman I, Norden G. Living donor nephrectomy. Complication rates in 490 cases. Scand J Urol Nephrol. 1992;26:149–153.
4. Dunn JF, Richie RE, MacDonnell RC, et al. Living related kidney donors. A 14 year experience. Ann Surg 1986; 203:637–642.
5. Kerbl K, Clayman RV, McDougall EM, et al. Transperitoneal nephrectomy for benign disease of the kidney: a comparison of laparoscopic and open surgical techniques. Urology 1994;43:607–613.
6. Flowers JL, Lefor AT, Steers J, et al. Laparoscopic slpenectomy in patients with hematologic diseases. Ann Surg 1996;224:19–28.
7. Gagner M, Lacroix A, Prinz RA, et al. Early experience with laparoscopic approach for adrenalectomy. Surgery 1993;114:1120–1125.
8. Terasaki PI, Cecka JM, Gjertson SW. *In*: Terasaki PI and Cecka JM (eds.). Clinical transplants 1994. UCLA Tissue Typing Laboratory, Los Angeles, pp 341–380.
9. Rosenberger WF. Dealing with multiplicities in pharmacoepidemiologic studies. Pharmacoepidemiol Drug Safety 1996;5:95–100.
10. Streem SB, Novick AC, Steinmuller DR, et al. Flank donor nephrectomy: efficacy in the donor and recipient. J Urol 1989;141:1099–1101.
11. Parra RO, Perez MG, Boullier JA, et al. Comparison between standard flank versus laparoscopic nephrectomy for benign renal disease. J Urol 1995;153:1171–1174.
12. Yasumura T, Nakai I, Oka T, et al. Experience with 247 living related donor nephrectomy cases at a single institution in Japan. Jap J Surg 1988;18:252–258.
13. Liounis B, Roy LP, Thompson JF, et al. The living, related kidney donor: a follow-up study. Med J Aust 1988;148:436–444.
14. Streem SB, Novick AC, Steinmuller DR, et al. Results of living-donor nephrectomy: considerations for the donor and recipient. Transplant Proc 1989;21:1951–1952.
15. Waples JM, Belzer FO, Uehling DT. Living donor nephrectomy: a 20-year experience. Urology 1995;45:207–210.
16. Schulam PG, Kavoussi LR, Cheriff AD, et al. Laparoscopic live donor nephrectomy: the initial 3 cases. J Urol 1996;155:1857–1859.

Part IV
Education and Training

20
The Yale Curriculum for Laparoscopic Surgery

James C. Rosser Jr.

We live in an age of technological revolution. With the help of technology, medical care previously thought to be miracles not within the grasp of mortals are routinely performed on a daily basis. The challenge does not seem to be what we can do, but rather how quickly can we assimilate these new modern day miracles into the mainstream of society. The assimilation of technology is not the only challenge. The other challenge is to handle the information explosion that is necessary to stay current and confident in all of the new treatment options that are being procured on a daily basis. These are the challenges that the Yale Curriculum for Laparoscopic Surgery is meant to overcome. The foundation of our focused efforts supports the interface of cost-effective, technological advances with patient care objectives.

There are three components to our program that together form a triangular effort to achieve these goals. The first component involves objective-based skill acquisition with standardized training protocols. This is the necessary first step that serves as a foundation to proliferate any new procedural advances in surgery. Standardized skill acquisition programs are mandatory in order to train large numbers of individuals cost effectively. You also must be able to offer a "yard stick" for new recruits to have an idea of their level of initial proficiency, as it relates to their peers. As the student proceeds with the program, progress can be monitored and tailored adjustments can be recommended to the student to assure mature proficiency. This is a tool that has been absent in the art of surgery and is long overdue.

The second component of this triangular-shaped effort involves computer based training (CBT) strategies. With the advent of CD-ROM and now emerging DVD technology, we must harness these new knowledge transfer vehicles in order to expand the educational deployment and to increase the effectiveness of knowledge transfer by utilizing these innovative tools. Computer based training with a high level of entertainment allows participants to learn with an accelerated knowledge transfer rate with greater enjoyment. These types of education tutorials are much more

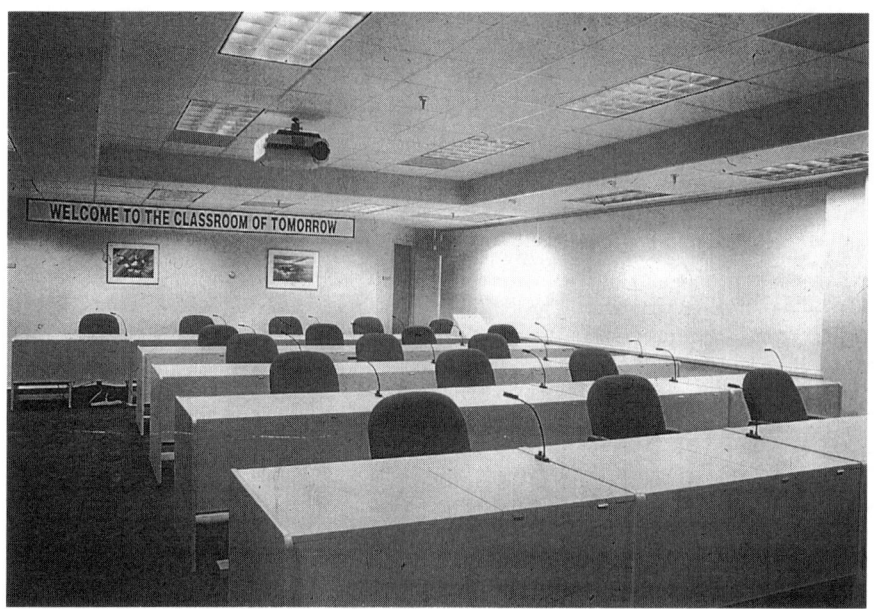

A

Figure 20.1. (A, B) Photograph of classroom of tomorrow. This is where twenty-first century technology is blended together with "content" to transform this classroom into a knowledge transfer organism. All components, both mechanical and human, work together to give the education experience a new level of effectiveness. This state-of-the-art classroom contains 20 multimedia learning stations that feature our computer-based training modules (B). Training sessions are conducted under the watchful eye of the knowledge transfer officer. All of these computers are networked and feature two-way communications. All functions are controlled from a unique command module. This allows self-paced training to be accomplished with the unique feature of individualized tutorials when needed. In addition, all of the computers in the classroom are connected to the Internet, and the entire classroom can be connected to points around the world on demand by way of digital video conferencing systems.

attractive than sitting in a room and listening to a stand-up tutorial. This educational packaging array provides us with a vehicle to achieve more effective distant education.

The third component involves the use of state-of-the-art telecommunications in the emerging arena of telemedicine. This allows the participants adopting new procedures to have pre-, intra-, and postoperative consultative support. In addition, a cost-effective continuing tele-education program can be matured so that advanced information does not have to go through a "trickle-down" filter. It can be directly distributed to all institutions regardless of the size or geological location.

The Yale Endo-Laparoscopic Center is a 7,000-square-foot facility that is dedicated to the development of education and clinical execution of

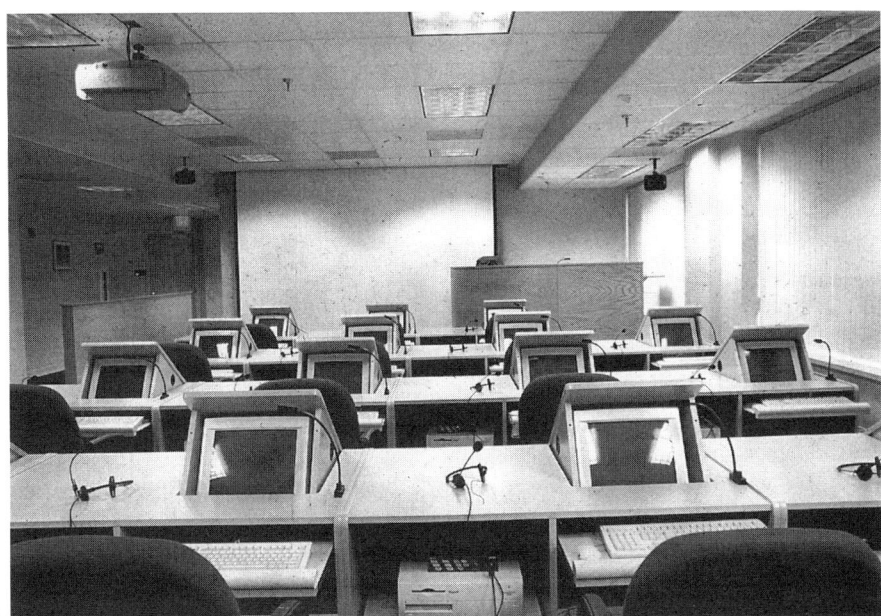

B

FIGURE 20.1. *Continued*

procedures performed in the minimally invasive environment (Figs. 20.1 and 20.2). It also serves as a reservoir of templates to be applied for other disciplines as medicine tries to interface with technology effectively. This facility houses the laboratory environment that brings together all three components of our triangular program. This center, along with its operating suites, multidisciplinary support, hotel, and recreational facilities, is dedicated to provide minimally invasive procedure-specific services to patients with maximum convenience. This joint hospital–university venture enables the delivery of cutting-edge surgical health care both to the region and to the rest of the world.

Objective-Based Skill Acquisition

Laparoscopic surgery affords opportunities for access and surgical manipulation that may replace traditional surgical approaches and permit new approaches that were previously impossible because of mechanical, anatomical, or physiologic considerations. Skills that permit competence and mastery in laparoscopic procedures are not directly acquired from skills used in open surgery. The effective acquisition of those skills by trainees is a matter of some importance to abbreviate the training period, minimize reliance on animal models, decrease operating room time, prepare surgeons

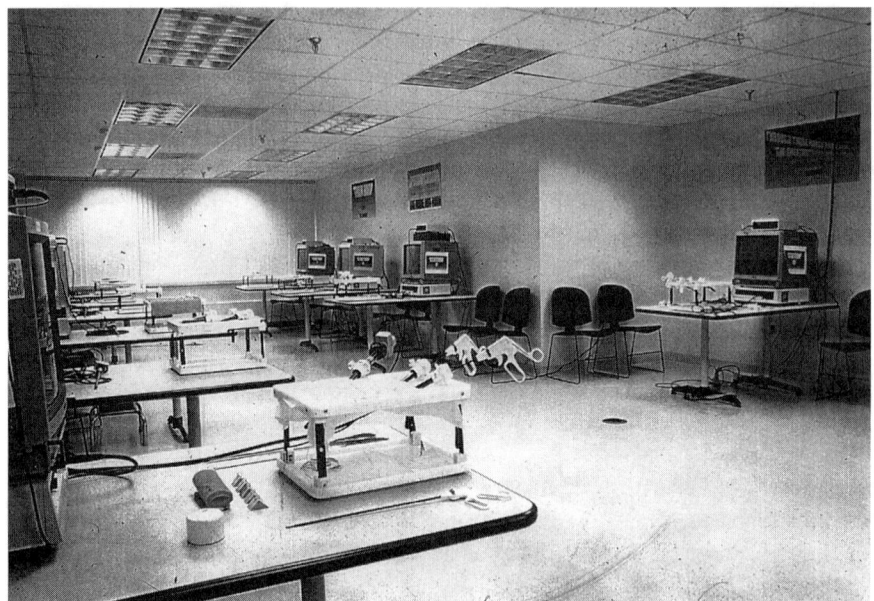

FIGURE 20.2. Yale Laparoscopy Center. Part of 7,000 square feet that has been utilized to train more than 700 medical students and physicians in new laparoscopic techniques.

for independent operations, and reduce complications. Intracorporeal suturing is perhaps the most difficult of advanced laparoscopic skills. It allows surgeons to perform almost any maneuver through the laparoscope that can be achieved through an open incision. Suturing requires depth perception in the two-dimensional image of the laparoscopy screen, accuracy with instruments beyond that necessary for dissection, and dexterity. At Yale, dexterity drills that correlate with incremental skill acquisition and the ability to perform intracorporeal suturing have been standardized. This is embodied in the Yale Laparoscopic Skills Boot Camp.[1]

It features training methods with objective evaluation to enhance laparoscopic surgical skills, provide training in laparoscopic suturing techniques, and assess whether specific training exercises were helpful in the attainment of intracorporeal suturing skills.

All exercises, including intracorporeal anastomosis, were performed in a laparoscopic trainer (Surgical Trainer, US Surgical Corporation, Norwalk, CT) (Fig. 20.3) using a monitor (Trinitrom model No. PVM-1943MD, Sony, Tokyo, Japan), a telescope (three chips, 0 degrees, 10mm) (Stryker Endoscopy, Santa Clara, CA), and a medical video camera (model No. 777, Stryker Endoscopy). The use of the nondominant hand was emphasized. The participants performed three types of drills to improve their dexterity, depth perception, instrument-targeting accuracy, visual and spatial abilities,

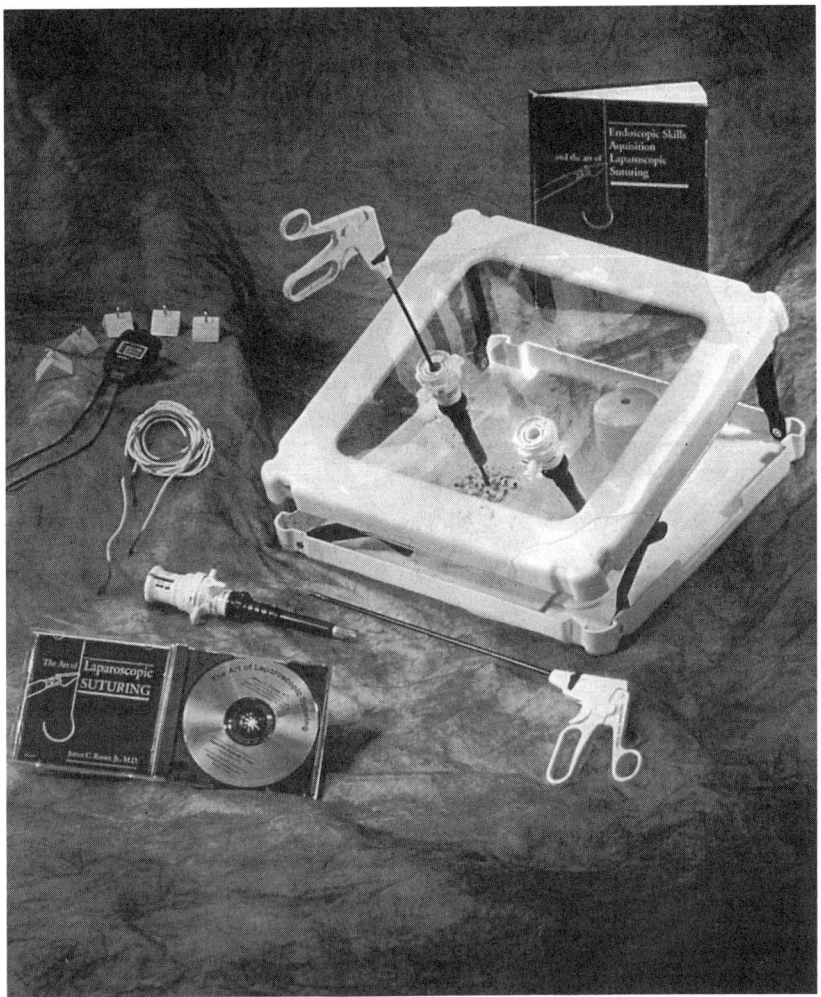

FIGURE 20.3. Photograph of all equipment necessary to training of laparoscopic exercises to increase proficiency in the laparoscopic arena.

and hand–eye coordination. These are generalized skill abilities and hand–eye coordination.

Rope Pass Drill

This drill required ambidexterity, depth perception, fine control of the instruments, and rhythmic, coordinated movement. The 60-in. 1/8-in. rope with colored bands that were 1-in. long and 4-in. apart is used for this drill (Figs. 20.4 and 20.5). The rope is passed from one hand to the next in a

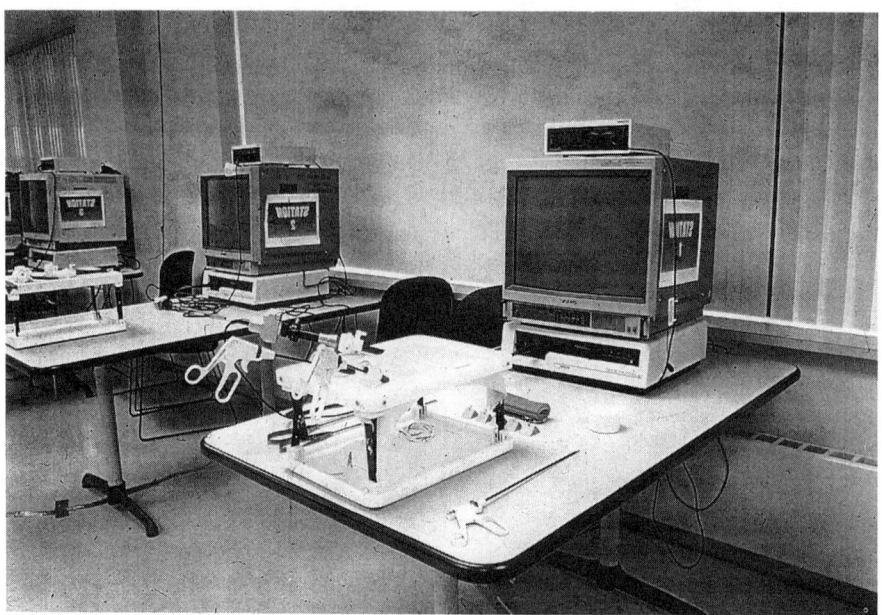

FIGURE 20.4. Photograph of laparoscopic trainer. Stryker camera projects onto screen/monitor. All exercises (e.g., cobra rope, terrible triangle, and dropping of beans in cup) are done by utilizing the nondominant hand.

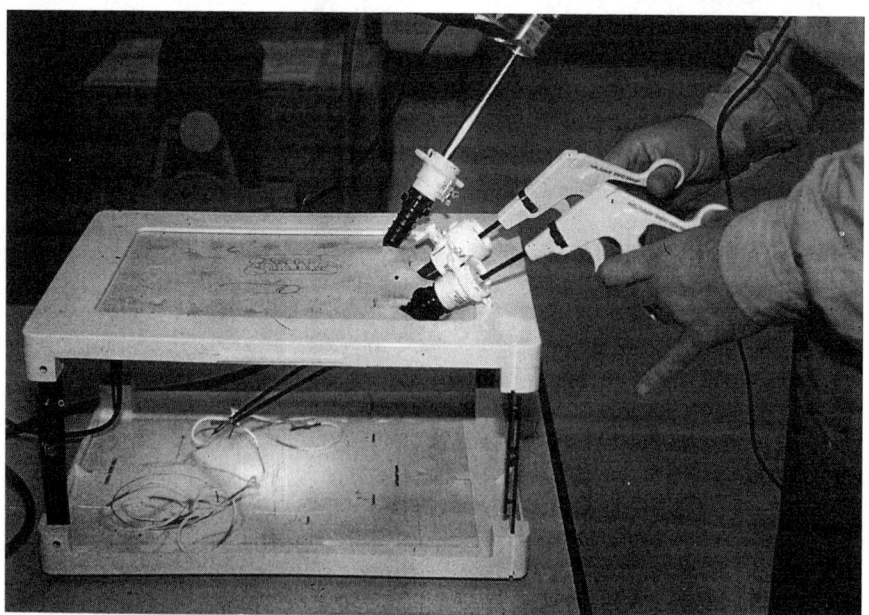

FIGURE 20.5. Photograph of cobra rope. Practice with this procedure in the laboratory lends expertise to the surgeon in the ability to manipulate bowel during laparoscopic procedures.

manner that maintains control of the instruments and manages the rope material without tangling. The rope is initially coiled on a template and lifted away serially, using the instruments with the nondominant and then the dominant hand. Each event is timed from the first grasp with the nondominant hand until the last grasp with the dominant hand.

Cup Drop Drill

This drill requires the nondominant hand to transfer a smooth object to an aperture in a cylinder and to drop the object from a height of 1 cm into the aperture. The event is timed from the voice command of *go* by the instructor. The drill requires nondominant hand dexterity, depth perception in a two-dimensional field, hand–eye coordination, and fine control of the instrument using a rhythmic motion.[2]

Triangle Transfer Drill

This exercise calls for engaging a curved needle mounted on a needle holder into a plastic loop at the apex of a triangle. The loop is seen only straight on, and its opening must be anticipated by depth perception. With the needle in place, the triangle is transferred across the field where the needle must be removed by abduction of the elbow and flexion of the wrist. This series of movements closely correlates with those necessary to establish initial penetration and recovery of the needle during the tissue penetration phase of the intracorporeal suturing process. The drill also establishes ambidexterity, depth perception, fine control of instruments, and coordinated, rhythmic motion. Five triangles are transferred in this timed event. The time begins when the instructor gives the *go* signal.[2]

Intracorporeal Suturing

A silk suture on a curved needle is used to approximate a small intestine from pigs harvested at the abattoir and stored frozen until thawing for use.[2] An interrupted Lembert suture is placed, and an instrument tie is performed.[2] This skill calls for depth perception in two dimensions, accurate instrument handling, management of the materials, and ambidexterity. The steps for the suture technique are[2]:

1. Use the nondominant hand to grasp a 0–0-silk suture 2 or 3 cm from the tip of an SH needle.
2. The suture and needle are advanced through the port into the trainer.
3. Grasp the needle at the juncture of the proximal and middle third by a needle carrier in the dominant hand.
4. Pull on the suture to adjust the needle.

5. In order to penetrate the tissue the arm is abducted at the shoulder in order to place the needle perpendicular to the tissue. The nondominant hand utilizes an empty needle-carrier to stabilize the tissue. Extension of the arm at the elbow causes lateral displacement of the wrist, and the needle pierces the tissue. Rotate the wrist of the dominant hand in order to have the needle tip emerge from the tissue.

6. Grab the needle tip with the carrier in the nondominant hand. Next, pull the needle tip in rotation through the tissue, exaggerating the rotation with a dip of the wrist to avoid traction on the tissue. The needle carrier in the dominant hand is used to stabilize the tissue, and the thread is pulled through.

7. A short tail (i.e., 2–3 cm) is left at the needle entry site.

8. Use the nondominant hand to adjust the needle by gripping its tip such that the needle tip is perpendicular to the needle-carrier. Traction on the suture is helpful. Place the swaged suture to the left of the needle-carrier in the dominant hand.

9. Rotate the nondominant hand with the needle for two more throws around the needle-carrier in the dominant hand. The tail of the suture is grasped with the instrument in the dominant hand, and the knot is pulled tight by moving the needle away and keeping the tail short. The maneuver is repeated counterclockwise for two more throws, and the sutures are cut.

10. The needle is withdrawn by grasping the suture tail and pulling the suture and needle back through the port.

Statistical Analysis

The time required to perform each dexterity drill or a single interrupted stitch was documented in seconds. The participants in the initial courses performed six dexterity drills of each type and six interrupted stitches. All of the participants were subsequently made to perform 10 drills of each type and 10 interrupted stitches. The mean time in seconds required to perform a drill was correlated (by multivariate analysis) with the mean time required to complete a suturing exercise by the participants who performed 10 of each drill and 10 of the suturing exercises. Other participants who performed less than 10 drills and/or suturing exercises were included for other analyses. Including or excluding them did not make any difference in the interpretation of the results reported in this article. An unpaired Student's test was used to compare the time required to perform the first versus the tenth drill or suturing exercise. All data are given as the mean ± SEM.

There was a significant correlation between the time required for the single interrupted stitch and the times recorded for all three drills: rope pass drill ($r = 0.62$), triangle transfer drill ($r = 0.57$), and cup drop drill ($r = 0.56$) ($n = 89$ and $P < 0.001$ for all 3 drills). These observations suggest that each drill may help to improve the skills required for laparoscopic suturing. The age of the participants (42.21 + 1.15 years) did not correlate with the mean time required to perform a single interrupted stitch.[2]

It is unclear whether drills and exercises can be used in isolation to credential surgeons. The evaluation of skill in general is subject to debate. Some studies show no relationship between an objective assessment of skills and applied clinical skill. The use of drills should be restricted to self-paced skills acquisition in analogous activities relevant to the surgical skills in question. One can ultimately only be credentialed based on actual clinical performance. The drills are designed to prepare surgeons who probably have no greater innate dexterity than other physicians. In all likelihood surgical proficiency is not a manifestation of innately superior psychomotor skills; rather, surgical proficiency is a manifestation of considerable attention to technique and good training. Conventional surgical training techniques are not necessarily applicable to laparoscopic surgery. Laparoscopic surgical training is more reasonably begun from an analogous experience, such as drills, to prepare for the real-time pace of the operating room. The experience in flight simulation as an educational tool should be taken to heart. Surgical tasks that are inefficient, impractical, slow, costly, or dangerous when taught in the operating room should be learned during an analogous experience before coming to the operating room. The initial study involved 150 participants.[2] The number has now grown to more than 1,000. A follow-up study has established a data base that allows a percentile ranking of any participant that undergoes the program.[3] A computer program has been modified to enable this process to be done quickly. An equipment package has been produced so that that the program can be exported globally in its standardized format. (Available through Cine-Med, Fig. 20.3). This training project has also spawned a competitive program called the "Top Gun Laparoscopic Skills Shootout" that has been featured at the American College of Surgeons fall meetings starting in 1996. Representatives from more than 10 training programs both domestic and abroad compete to see who has the best laparoscopic skills. The winners receive prizes and trophies and the right to wear the "Top Gun" jacket.

This serves as a fun way to encourage the importance of the need to acquire superior skills in the minimally invasive arena.

Our inanimate laboratory contains 10 stations designed to provide hands-on experience in the laparoscopic setting before going to the operating theater. This is the site of our laparoscopic skill "boot camp" that was previously described. This has been featured on the CBS morning show, the Discovery Channel, and in *Scientific American*.[4] Other training sessions can be done for advanced techniques in the same setting. This is also the site of our telementoring simulator that allows surgeons to adapt to being controlled by a specialist from a remote site while they embark on their initial exploits with a new procedure (Fig. 20.5).

Computer-Based Training

Applications developed using key multimedia elements are finding their way into a number of training and information exchange environments, including the laparoscopy training market. Emerging multimedia-based applications range from procedural information for patients to interactive CD-ROM–based applications used to train highly skilled surgeons. These products are designed with a high level of interactivity that allows the surgeon to plan a surgical procedure, review detailed patient information, and then merge that information into the surgical planning process. Using this new technology, a surgeon now has the ability to review CD-ROM–based course materials and efficiently meet continuing education requirements. The factor found most limiting in the development of multimedia-based applications for laparoscopic training is generally not the technology; rather, the limits are placed on the technology because of one's reluctance to think beyond what is accepted as the norm. When implemented properly, multimedia applications developed for laparoscopic training can reduce the cost and time associated with learning new materials, assist in retaining more of the information, and in many cases make the learning experience much more enjoyable.

We are presently living in an era of heightened technological awareness. Desert Storm with its effective display of our military's (SMART) weapons has encouraged a belief that technology can assist in efficiently accomplishing superhuman feats. This mindset, when combined with the technological presence in laparoscopic surgery, has nurtured a desire for the application of more and more "Star Wars" technology to assist in the advancement of the "new frontier" of surgery (i.e., minimally invasive surgery). Virtual reality is a component of this "Star Wars" technology, and it has become a household word with respect to the future of surgical training. It potentially offers many advances that must be explored, if we are to train surgeons and residents in new procedures while maintaining competent skills in slowly disappearing open procedures. In addition, the use of robotic and telepresence surgery suggests an even more prospective impact on the field of surgery.

In the midst of this enthusiasm, we have overlooked a cost-effective technology that is now available: computer-based training (CBT) or computer-assisted instruction (CAI) utilizing CD-ROM multimedia interactive technology.[4] Computer-based training, which uses currently available technology, offers documented advances over customary standup tutorials. With the advent of modern CD-ROM multimedia interactive programs, modern computer-based training is poised to significantly meet the challenges we face in today's surgical training dilemma.[5]

Evidence of the potential impact of CBT has been documented academically with earlier systems utilizing videodisk technology. One of the first applications of computer-based training included clinical simulations. Friedman[6] noted several potential advantages:

All students are given experience with a core group of disorders regardless of patient population or service in the hospital.

All students are given an opportunity to see the importance of cost and test availability in determining what tests are truly valuable.

Since all students can work up the same case, simulation is the ideal vehicle for teaching diagnosis skills.

Students are given detailed self-evaluation feedback so that mistakes can be rapidly corrected.

Mistakes are made on the computer, not on the patient.[6]

Those surgeons who are in the forefront of medical training, especially training as it relates to the laparoscopic surgical arena, have a tremendous opportunity to define the environment in which surgeons will be trained. In good conscience, it is bad to ignore the explosion of new information available to surgeons today; rather, surgeons must define the methods by which to gain access to this information and harness its potential for later use. Surgeons must become more proactive in all areas of medicine, especially in medical education.

As we move forward in our efforts to train surgeons for the next century, we must realize our responsibility to include as many of our colleagues as possible in this information revolution. Economics is one key consideration in reaching this lofty goal. Can we deliver this information cost effectively? Can it assist in correcting the shortcoming of our present system? The need for adjustment in our present educational strategy was illustrated with the tabulation of impressions from exit interviews after courses in 1993 on advanced laparoscopic surgical techniques. The majority of surgeons stated that they would prefer to have more laboratory time. You must do one of two things in order to implement this: shorten the didactic portions of the course and subsequently fail to go over important information, or extend the course to multiple days. The first option leads to a huge gap in the transference of information, subsequently leaving a surgeon academically unprepared and patients in potential danger. The second option drastically increases cost. With CD-ROM multimedia interactive computer modules, the surgeons could review all of the academic information before the course. This also would include pre-and posttests to evaluate the success of retention of material. We then would have a round-table discussion of the course information with clarifying questions and answers between the class and the experts. This would allow a more effective and complete review of vital information while establishing more laboratory experience without the cost-escalating increase in the length of the course.

It is believed CD-ROM–based interactive programs that are designed with the specific training requirements for laparoscopic surgery can provide a major benefit to all educators striving to disseminate accurate and timely information. This technology is here today and allows us to take the first step in this new medical information age. The reality of the matter is that we must learn to use the tools available today effectively. It is possible to better understand and apply new technology with the skills acquired using these tools. Virtual reality in medical training offers tremendous opportunity, but the reality is that we need to deploy cost-effective and widely available systems that will assist us in meeting present and current challenges.

With one of our primary mission statements being to mature full-featured multimedia tutorials for both health care providers and patients, we debuted six laparoscopic surgical educational titles (Springer-Verlag) at the 1997 American College of Surgeons. These titles are suited for attending surgeons and residents alike. They are full featured with more than 1 hour of digitized video, primary-level simulation, and full interactivity. We also debuted the first-ever patient-oriented multimedia tutorials that usher in a new era of informed consent and medical–legal risk management. These titles were procured from our tactical–digital conversion center that exists within the Yale Endo-Laparoscopic Center. With content production having been secured, we were then free to design a unique classroom setting. This is called the "Classroom of Tomorrow." This is where twenty-first-century technology is blended together with "content" to transform this classroom into a knowledge transfer organism. All components, both mechanical and human, work together to give the education experience a new level of effectiveness. This state-of-the-art classroom contains 20 multimedia learning stations that feature our computer based training modules (Fig. 20.1B). Training sessions are conducted under the watchful eye of the knowledge transfer officer. All of these computers are networked and feature two-way communications. All functions are controlled from a unique command module. This allows self-paced training to be accomplished with the unique feature of individualized tutorials when needed. In addition, all of the computers in the classroom are connected to the Internet, and the entire classroom can be connected to points around the world on demand by way of digital videoconferencing systems.

Finally, there is a multimedia patient information center. This facility presents a new concept in educating patients about the surgical procedures that they will undergo. Patients use personal computers and interactive multimedia programs for achieving informed consent before surgery. Prior to surgery, these patient tutorials help patients to understand as much as possible about their upcoming operation. These user-friendly programs have been designed for a variety of patients with varying education levels, including nonreaders and older people with limited education. It also may be adapted for people who speak other languages. This is a twenty-first-century "high tech" attempt at achieving an iron clad patient informed consent that will be very important in breaking down the legal cost burden that plagues medicine today.

Yale University Advanced Minimally Invasive Surgery and Technology Program

We stand at the brink of a new millennium. New and exciting ways of performing surgical procedures are rapidly emerging. The revolution that started in 1989 with the laparoscopic cholecystectomy has the potential to affect all procedures that have traditionally been performed in the open setting; unfortunately, we have a very large problem. This revolution of laparoscopic surgery has totally exposed the deficiencies in our historical technique for surgical training. The lack of a standardized skill acquisition and validation program, no targeted objective based performance goals, and the absence of a supervised enforced skills acquisition curriculum and training program are glaring shortcomings that we must overcome. In addition, it has exposed the deficiency of technological interfacing in the surgical arena. This void has left surgery far behind the power curve in the utilization of technology in providing more cost effective and global surgical healthcare.

In 1969, when man landed on the moon, not one surgeon in the United States was consistently using a computer on a daily basis for healthcare. In 1997, the surgical community is still adopting technology at a snail's pace. There is a need to access our current knowledge and skill transfer algorithms. The proliferation of the use of technology by surgical healthcare providers should be a high priority item.

Our current training programs are not outfitted to train individuals in minimally invasive surgery and establish a working knowledge of cutting-edge technology. It is more important to note that the resident that leaves these programs is not qualified to teach others. There have been efforts to develop and to design laparoscopic fellowships to train the leaders of tomorrow, but these programs last as long as 1 year and are generally in an unstructured environment that leads to inefficiencies in knowledge, judgment, and skill transfer. It is not realistic with the economic pressures that physicians face to expect them to sacrifice 1 year of their lives for further study. In countries with great need, this 1 year of education exile can leave the needs of the country unaddressed.

In order to improve upon this dilemma, we must blend new modern knowledge and skill transfer techniques with our traditional educational heritage. This can be done within the context of a 6-week structured, concentrated effort that is meant to expose a surgeon to a full range of advanced laparoscopic clinical procedures and establish a comfort level with the cutting edge of technology. The trainee will be taught how to instruct others in the nuances of this developing surgical art form. This is the old "train and trainer" educational motto that has proved to be quite effective in establishing advanced procedural capabilities in the past.

This program will feature an objective evaluation of skill and cognitive knowledge. Data bases have been prepared from more than 1,000 surgeons around the world, with thousands of data points to document technical ability effectively. Objective-based clinical competency evaluation scenarios (OCCES) are designed to enable the use of computer technology to evaluate a surgeons' ability to make an accurate judgment in a clinical setting. Trainees will undergo computer training to improve their computer literacy and to develop production capability in multimedia curriculums. Instruction will also be given on the proper use of telemedicine and how to implement this capability at their home hospitals. More than 17 different advanced laparoscopic surgical procedures with animal lab experience will be given. Exposure to clinical cases will be assured by utilizing local sources and by the use of modern telecommunications. Procedures from distant sites, under the supervision of "teleprofessors," will be broadcast to the Endo-Laparoscopy Center.

In order to make this program extremely cost effective, a total package will be offered that covers accommodations in a four-star hotel, three meals per day (7 days per week), course materials, parking, and exercise club membership. A trainee, therefore will only have to arrange transportation (to and from Yale). For the next 6 weeks, all other arrangements will be taken care of within the global fee.

In conclusion, we have recognized the dilemma of slow proliferation for the modern day miracle of minimally invasive surgery around the world. For this approach to surgical procedures to reach its full potential with patient quality assurance being maintained, we must utilize technology and modern day knowledge transfer techniques to stimulate a more efficient proliferation rate globally. This 6-week minifellowship offered by the Department of Surgery at Yale University School of Medicine, allows a cost effective vehicle for training the surgical leaders of the next millennium.

Telemedicine

Telemedicine is the third component of our triangular program. It is the glue that brings all the other components together as one unit by allowing preemptive distant education and continuous surveillance and support. Telemedicine has previously been defined as "live two-way interactive video communication between a physician and a patient and/or another physician, where all participants are able to see and hear one another much like a face to face encounter." This constitutes the remote practice of medicine. This concept has gained notoriety because of the great advances in telecommunication and the increasing cost-effectiveness associated with its utilization. If the subject is more closely reviewed, then it will be revealed that telemedicine is not a recent concept. Telemedicine began in the 1950s during the early days of television. Forty years later, we now have a resurgence of the telemedicine initiative. Most of the current applications are based on teleconferencing, utilizing interactive vocal communication, high-quality clinical still photographs, and video images that are not of full-motion quality.

Telementoring is a telemedicine technique that involves the remote guidance of a treatment or investigational procedure (Fig. 20.1A) where the student has no or limited experience with the featured technique. These multiple educational and technological requirements place telementoring in a much more sophisticated and higher-risk category than standard telemedicine applications. These factors dictate that a standard training protocol be formulated so that quality assurance can be maintained.

The technology that makes telementoring possible may seem to be futuristic and to require Star Wars technology, but in fact the technology is obtainable today as a cost-effective system of transferring skill by guiding actions. The heart of this technology is the coder/decoder (CODEC), an image-processing computer with the ability to digitize analog signals and compress video, audio, and other data for transmission through a digital network. The CODEC (CLI Rembrandt, Computer Labs, Inc., San Jose, CA) manages enormous amounts of information in real time, which requires a high level of compression technology. Two of these units are needed. One is placed at the control site and the other in the operating theater. The ultimate test of the development of any telementoring technique is the ability to complete a mission with the use of this technology at great distances, in spite of inherent data transmission shortcomings.

Tactical information deployment (TID) of clinical reference material is achieved by using a Power Macintosh 7200/90 Macintosh (Apple Computer, Inc., Cupertin, CA) Power PC with quadruple-speed CD-ROM drive, 16 MB of RAM, and a 500-MB hard drive. A CD-ROM on laparoscopic colon resection and Nissen Funcoplication (Yale Laparoscopic Series Procedure Specific Interactive Multimedia CD-ROM—Nissen Funcoplication and Colon Resection, New Haven, CT) can provide the less-experienced surgeon with fast and easy access to reference information about a specific laparoscopic procedure.

The utilization of a VCR (Sharp VHS VC-A543U, Sharp, Inc., Mahwah, NJ) to record the operative procedure is advantageous to clarify any inaccuracies by using "instant replay," thus avoiding them in the future. Along with this apparatus, the mentor must be able to guide the novice surgeon by utilizing a surgistrator [i.e., a telestrator (ACECATII, Boecker Instruments, Tucson, AZ)], which is a necessary component that allows the mentor to direct the learning surgeon by placing marks on the screen and pinpointing an exact location for dissection or avoidance

Finally, wireless headphones and microphones (Clear-Com CS 222, Intercom Systems, Berkeley, CA), must be worn by the operative team and the mentor to complete the two-way communication. No cameras were placed at the control site, but there was a tripod-mounted unit (Sony CCD-V5000, Sony, Corp., Tokyo, Japan) in the operating room to survey the outside of the abdomen and the team's movements. The external camera was mounted to view the abdomen for assistance on trocar placement and the hand movements of the student surgeon.

Telemedicine is not a recent innovation. It began in the United States at the University of Nebraska in the late 1950s. In 1959, the University of Nebraska implemented a telemedicine network to support clinical continuing medical education and training, as well as research collaboration applications in geographically remote areas of Nebraska. The majority of the early experiments in telemedicine were eventually closed down. At the same time during the investigation of the remote delivery of health care, there was an increase in the efforts to expand the health care delivery system in the United States, and telemedicine entered a period of stagnation.

The potential advantages of telemedicine were revisited as a result of the health care delivery crisis, ever tightening budgetary concerns, and the impact of managed care. Telecommunication and other technological breakthroughs also fueled renewed enthusiasm. Credible, financially sound programs have now been established. In 1986, the Mayo Clinic implemented a two-way satellite program between their Rochester, Minnesota, campus and remote clinics in Scottsdale, Arizona, and Jacksonville, Florida. In 1991, the Medical College of Georgia established a telemedicine link between its Augusta, Georgia, campus and Dodge County Hospital in Eastman, Georgia, to provide consultation and continuing education to the 87-bed hospital.[7]

Telementoring is an advanced application of telemedicine. It adds new dimension to current educational and clinical practices. It involves the remote guidance of a procedure when the student has no or limited experience.

Others have also begun investigating this new application. Go et al. used videoconferencing applications to evaluate early technology.[8] Ranshaw et al.[9] teleproctored a Georgia rural surgeon in more than 24 cases. All cases were successfully completed laparoscopically without any complications. They utilized one-half and full T1 lines and demonstrated that they can be used for telementoring. Moore et al.[10] developed an inhouse telementoring system without the use of computer compression technology. These studies represent preliminary investigations. There is a need for further critical evaluation of this technology in clinical settings.

There are several impressions that have come from our initial experience. At this time, with current CODEC computer compression algorithms, one-half T1 bandwidth is the minimum required for maximal motion display capability with minimal delay. With new advances with compression algorithms this will be able to be done with one-quarter T (384 kbs) ISDN lines. The two-way audio link is best handled with individual headsets rather than by relying on one speaker and microphone for all parties in the remote OR. Well-established military and aviation communication speech patterns are crucial for prompt execution of commands. In addition to an annotator to target important landmarks, the use of "instant replay" with a VCR allows for the rapid review and critique of unsafe or unwanted operative techniques. The use of TID provides the surgeon with rapid access to reference information in the operating suite. Multimedia interactive CD-ROMs with digitized movie clips, illustration, sound bits, and the latest academic review of the literature arm the surgeon with a data base that establishes an unprecedented clinical adaptive capability.

We hope that the unique initiative that has been deployed at Yale will serve as a template for other institutions to follow. Of course, all training programs will not be able to procure the full breadth of the hardware and software configurations presented here at this time. If we can develop a few strategically placed centers, then these can support the majority of the others. The task at hand is to thin the interface between the technology, the educators, and the students. This can be accomplished only if these educational strategies are explored by increasing numbers of newcomers. With the cost of technology and software production continuing to decrease, this twenty-first-century platform will become the standard, not a unique aberration.

References

1. Stix G. Boot camp for surgeons. Scientific American 1995;273:24–26.
2. Rosser JC, Rosser LE, Savalgi RS. Skill acquisition and assessment for laparoscopic surgery. Arch Surg 1997;132:200–204.
3. Rosser JC, Rosser LE, Savalgi RS. Objective evaluation of a laparoscopic surgical skill program for residents and senior surgeons. Arch Surg 1998; in press.
4. Review of CD-ROM MO 8.1.594: aparoscopic inguinal hernia repair. Rosser J. (ed.) N Engl J Med 1995;332:352.
5. Rosser J. CD-ROM multimedia: the step before virtual reality. Surg Endosc 1995;10:1033–1035.
6. Friedman CP, France CL, Drossman DD. A randomized comparison of alternative formats for clinical simulations. Med Dec Making 1991;11:265–272.
7. Whitehead R. The evolution of telemedicine: then, now, and what will be. Teleconference 1995;14:9–11.
8. Go PM, Payne H Jr., Satava RM, et al. Teleconferencing bridges two oceans and shrinks the surgical world. Surg Endosc 1996;10:105–106.
9. Ranshaw B, Tucker J, Duncan T, et al. Laparoscopic herniorrhaphy: a review of 900 cases. Surg Endosc 1996;10:255.
10. Moore RG, Adams JB, Partin AW, et al. Telementoring of laparoscopic procedures. Surg Endosc 1996;10:107–110.

21
Current Status of Virtual Reality Surgical Simulators

RICHARD M. SATAVA

There is more than a decade of practical implementation of virtual reality for education, training, maintenance, and innovative visualization. The original research involved three-dimensional (3-D) scientific visualization in aerospace, geological survey, computer-aided design (CAD), engineering, transportation and other nonmedical fields. As both computer power and the level of visual realism increase, there are more applications relevant to the medical profession. While not comprehensive, the following is a survey of representative simulations, many of which began as military medical applications for combat casualty care, but have now migrated into civilian applications. The thread that ties these seemingly unrelated applications together is the ability to represent a person as a 3-D data set, epitomized by the accomplishments of the Visible Human project (see below). In accepting such a 3-D image as a representation of the real person (a "medical avatar"), new applications are enabled in the area of education and training (simulators), certification (simulators), and diagnosis (virtual endoscopy). Thus, those technologies that enhance the realism (visual, acoustic, and haptic) of a simulation are in the direct pathway to new products in the twenty-first century.

Out of the scientific accomplishments of flight simulators and 3-D graphics visualization, virtual reality for surgical simulation and medical training began in the late 1980s. Drs. Scott Delp and Joseph Rosen[1] created one of

---

*The opinions or assertions contained herein are the private views of the authors and are not to be construed as official, or as reflecting the views of the Department of the Army, Department of the Navy, the Advanced Research Projects Agency, or the Department of Defense.

Surgical simulation will add an entire new dimension to our ability to train and educate our surgeons. For the first time, technical skills can be evaluated with objectivity, providing a powerful tool for performance assessment. The surgical simulators of today are just the beginning of a future that promises a more personalized approach to education, with training on both generic models as well as patient specific models. The development from early simulations through current innovations is reviewed.

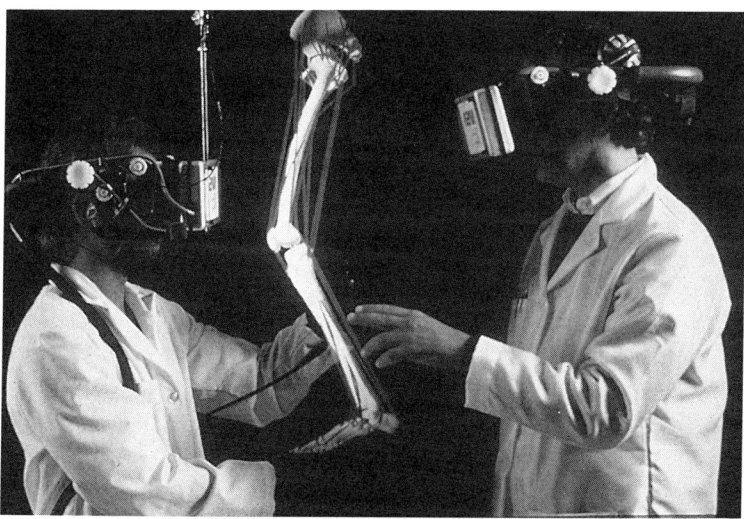

FIGURE 21.1. Lower limb simulator to evaluate tendon transplant (courtesy of Dr. Scott Delp and Joseph Rosen, Musculographics, Inc., Evanston, IL).

the first virtual reality systems to investigate alternative surgical procedures (tendon transplants) of the lower leg (Fig. 21.1). In 1991, Satava[2] created the first abdominal surgery simulator, using images of organs created in a simple graphics drawing program (Fig. 21.2). These graphics were neither realistic nor highly interactive, but the simulator provided the opportunity to fly around and through the anatomy and to "practice" a surgical procedure with virtual instruments. Within 18 months, Jonathan Merrill[3] of High Techsplanations created a highly sophisticated graphic representation of the human torso, with organs that simulated physical properties such as bending or stretching when pushed and pulled, or edges that retracted when cut (Fig. 21.3). The landmark event was the 1994 release of National Library of Medicine's "Visible Human Project" under Michael Ackerman that provided images that were reconstructed from an actual person's data. The virtual cadaver was created by Victor Spitzer and David Whitlock[4] at the University of Colorado from 1,871 slices, each 1 mm in thickness, that had been digitized and stored in the computer (Fig. 21.4). In rendering the images, there was near photorealism; however, there were no properties because the entire power of the computer was used in portraying the image.

Later that same year, Scott Delp[5] used the Visible Human leg to create a Limb Trauma Simulator (Fig. 21.5). The image did not look as realistic as the Visible Human because so much computer power was used for the tissue properties, bleeding, wounding, and instrument interaction that a less realistic visual image resulted; however, this model permitted debridement

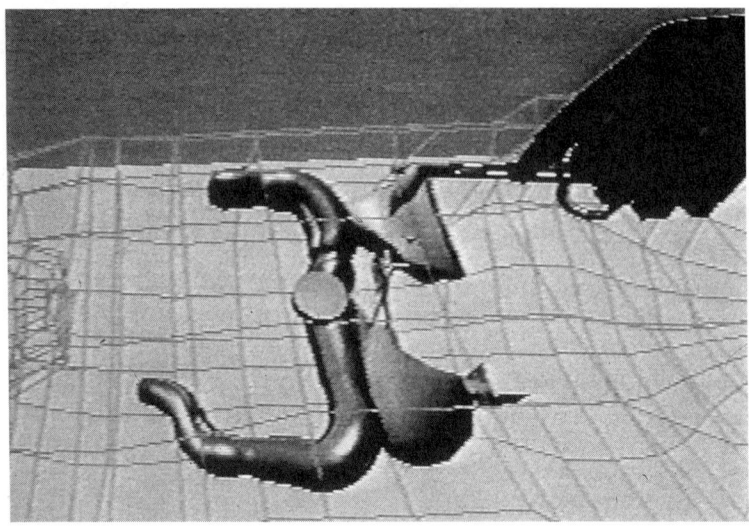

FIGURE 21.2. Early surgical simulation of the abdomen using simple graphics drawing programs (courtesy of author).

of the wound, removal of bone fragments, and stopping of hemorrhage. The purpose of this simulator is to decrease the number of animals that need to be wounded in order to train physicians and medics in the essentials of combat casualty care and trauma management.

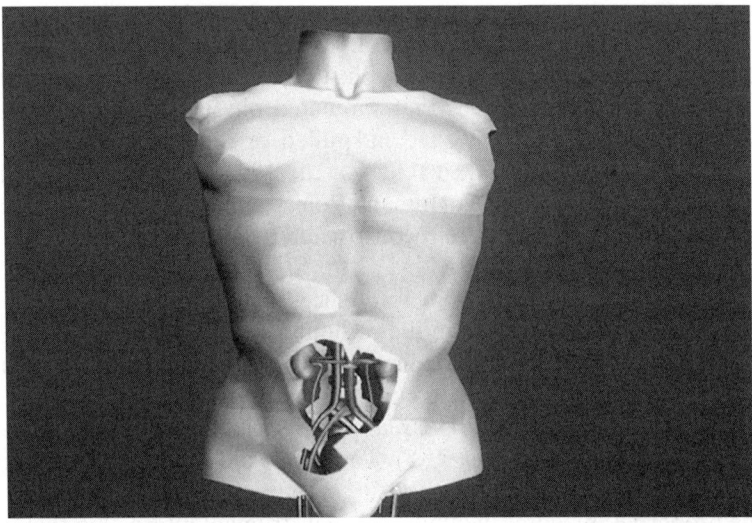

FIGURE 21.3. Improved graphic rendering of human torso that includes organ properties (courtesy Jonathan Merril, High Techsplanations, Inc, Rockville, MD).

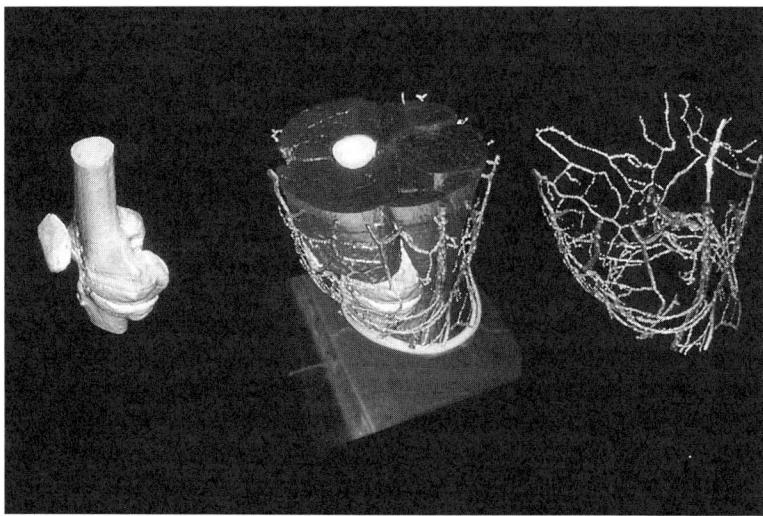

FIGURE 21.4. The Visible Human Project: full high resolution of the knee derived from actual patient data (courtesy of Dr. Victor Spitzer, University of Colorado School of Medicine, Denver, CO).

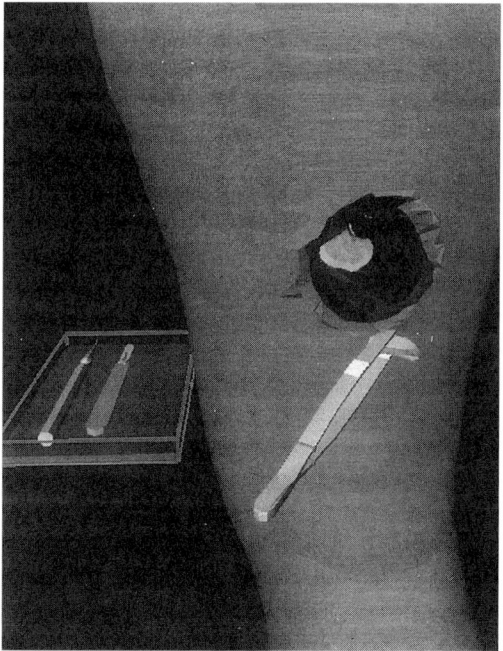

FIGURE 21.5. The Visible Human leg with less visual realism due to added properties, and accurate ballistic wounding model (courtesy Dr. Scott Delp, Musculo Graphics, Inc., Evanston, IL).

In 1995, Jeffrey Levy constructed a surgical simulator for hysteroscopy. This system incorporated a simple haptic device for the hysteroscopic instruments, and imported patient specific anatomy and pathology. Surgeons could now practice on exactly the same virtual pathology that they would encounter in their patient for the first time. When the anatomy is not extremely complex, a near photorealistic image, with full tissue properties and haptic input, can be achieved, such as the central venous catheter placement simulator (Fig. 21.6) by Higgins[6] of HT Medical Inc. In 1996 Boston Dynamics[7] introduced their task oriented surgical simulator with high fidelity haptics (sense of touch) with the Phantom Haptic Device, focusing upon individual tasks such as anastomoses, ligating and dividing, and so on, rather than on full procedures. Within the field of catheter-based endovascular therapy, simulators of catheter systems with balloon angioplasty and stent placement are being developed (Fig. 21.7).

There are four levels of simulators, and it is now time to begin implementing the simulators by matching their capabilities to the educational curriculum. The levels are: (1) Needle-type simulators, as in spinal tap, IV needle insertion, central venous catheter placement (CVP), chest tube insertion, liver biopsy, and so on, which have simple visual objects, and minimal axis of a single haptic device; (2) Catheter/scope type, in which the view on the video monitor will change in relation to movement of a control handle (in a scope) or catheter (as in angioplasty); (3) Task-oriented simulations, such as cross-clamping, ligate and divide, anastomoses, and so on, with one or two instruments; and (4) Full operative procedures. The lower

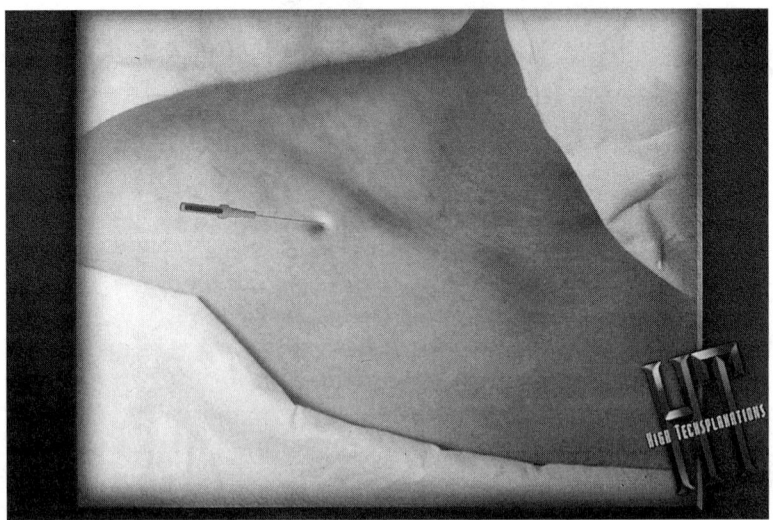

FIGURE 21.6. Central venous catheter placement (CVP) simulator for training (courtesy Dr. Gerry Higgins, HT Medical, Inc, Rockville, MD).

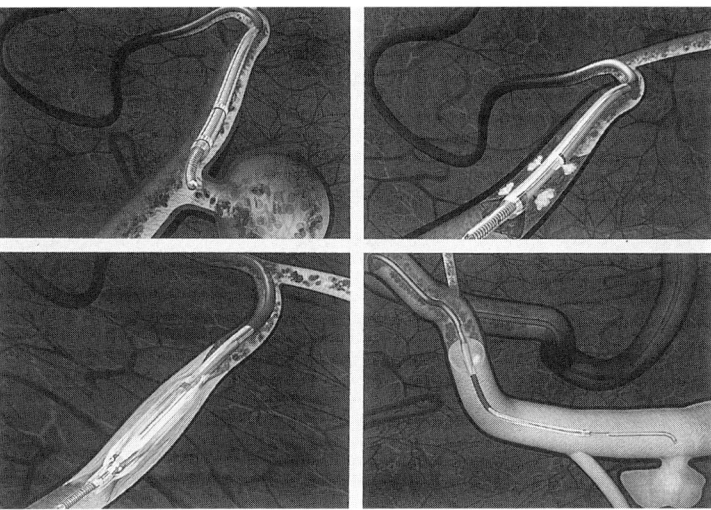

FIGURE 21.7. Angioplasty catheter in blood vessel (courtesy of Greg Merrill, HT Medical, Rockville, MD).

level simulators exist today with rather high levels of visual and haptic fidelity. They are capable of significant educational value, whereas the higher level simulations that exist have lesser fidelity, and the expectations of the educational content must be scaled back. The task level procedures have been subjected to analysis, and the training transfer (i.e., the amount of time in a simulator, which is equal to the time on actual animal or patient training) is about 25–28%. This means that every hour on a simulator is equal to 15 minutes (25% of an hour) of operating time on an animal. Based upon current standards for flight simulators, it could be expected that the training transfer for surgical simulators should achieve about 50–55% (1 hour of simulator time would equal about $\frac{1}{2}$ hour practice on an animal model).

Whereas significant improvement is needed from a technology standpoint, it is time to begin implementing the simulators at the level that will provide added value. The critical feature now is not the technology; rather, it is matching the curriculum to the level of technology. For example, in a simulation of an anastomoses (task level), a blood vessel or ureter can accurately be visualized and physically modeled to teach medical students and beginning residents the essentials of surgical skills. The content focuses upon how to perform an anastomoses and basic instrument techniques. The expectation of the student is that the model will behave as realistically as a real structure, not that they will suture organs that are indistinguishable from a real structure—the educational content is tailored to the technology. The level of realism will increase as computer power increases.

Hand in hand with the development of surgical simulation is the use of real patient data from CT or MRI scans to perform diagnostic procedures on the data set instead of inserting invasive or minimally invasive instruments into the patients. The currently accepted term is *virtual endoscopy*. This can be applied to those areas where endoscopic procedures are performed, but it also has the opportunity to explore areas not amenable to endoscopic procedures, such as parts of the body that are too dangerous (e.g., inside the eye) or too small (e.g., inner ear) to be accessible to real instruments. The process of virtual endoscopy consists of performing a standard helical CT scan of the area of the body of concern and "segmenting" the various organs and tissues. By applying sophisticated "flight path" algorithms (derived from terrain following algorithms for military aircraft), the organ can be "flown through," with the resulting image being comparable to performing the examination with a videoendoscope.[8] Areas providing initial success are the lungs, colon (Fig. 21.8), stomach, kidney-ureters-bladder, uterus, sinuses and ventricles of the brain. Other areas, such as the inner ear (Fig. 21.9) and ganglion, are being explored.[9]

The level of resolution of structure is now at 0.3 mm, which is adequate for diagnosing structural abnormalities that cause distortion of a surface, such as polyps, cancers, or ulcers. The surface renderings are generic texture maps; therefore, the many disease states that do not distort the anatomy (i.e., many infections, very flat and superficial cancers, ischemia, etc.) are not able to be diagnosed at this time. An attempt to provide a

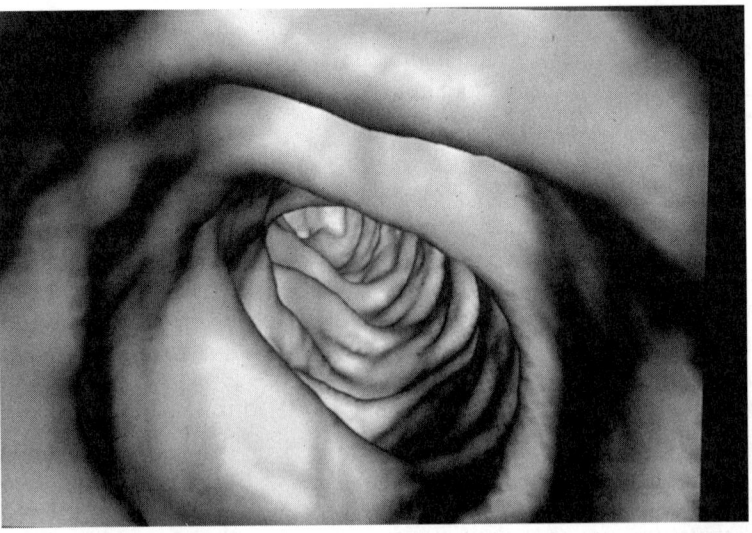

FIGURE 21.8. Virtual colonoscopy with internal view of the transverse colon (courtesy of Dr. Richard Robb, Mayo Clinic, Rochester, MN).

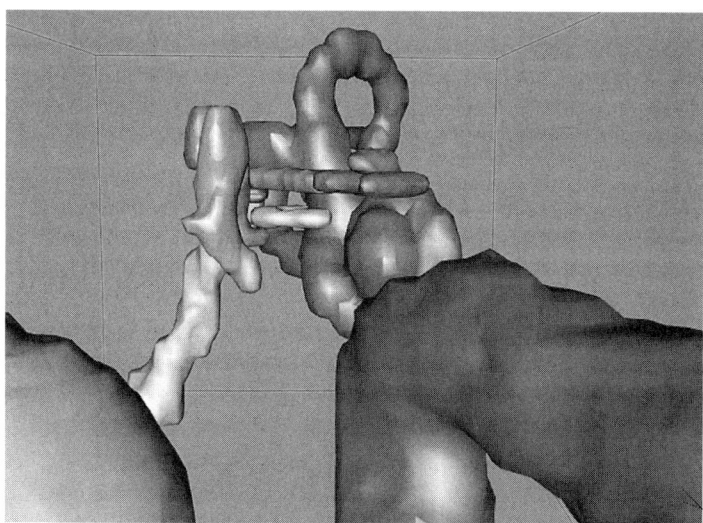

FIGURE 21.9. Virtual endoscopy of the inner ear with view of semicircular canals, chochlea, and associated structures (courtesy of Dr. Richard Robb, Mayo Clinic, Rochester, MN).

"look-up table," however, that correlates Hounsfield units of a CT scan to organ-specific color and texture has been successfully demonstrated. Thus, once the problem of accurate, real-time registration is solved, it will be possible for the virtual organs to not only be anatomically correct, but have precisely accurate coloration. With these capabilities, virtual endoscopy can be used for diagnosis, not therapy. There are, however, a number of energy-directed methods, such as high-intensity focused ultrasound or laser or cryotherapy, that will permit precise localization of diseases that can then be destroyed (through coagulation, protein denaturing or freezing) totally noninvasively. By using the patient's image during the procedure (i.e., by data-fusion) the physician can intraoperatively augment in real-time preci-sion localization through data fusion and stereotaxis. The result is providing a higher level of patient care by enhancing the physician's capabilities above trail human limitations.

The potential of these examples (and similar information and 3-D visualization-based innovative and nontraditional approaches to medicine) can be best illustrated by the results of a "blue sky" brainstorming session in late 1995. This rudimentary idea is referred to as the "Doorway to the Future," and it touches upon how information representation of actual anatomy (referred to as "information equivalents" of the actual organs and tissues) tie the fabric of medicine together. It was inspired by the many technologies under investigation, and it integrates them into a meaningful system of complementary technologies. The following scenario is used to illustrate one possible portion of the future of 20, 50, or, perhaps, 100 years from now.

A patient enters a physician's office and passes through a doorway, the frame of which contains many scanning devices, from CT scan to MRI to ultrasound to near infrared, and others. These scanners acquire anatomic data as well as physiologic and biochemical (like the pulse oximeters) data. When the patient sits down next to the physician, a full 3-D holographic image (Fig. 21.10) of the patient appears suspended upon the desktop—a visual integration of the information acquired just a minute before by the scanners. When the patient expresses the complaint of pain over the right flank, the physician can rotate the image, make various layers transparent, and query the representation of the patient's liver or kidney regarding the LDH, SGOT, alkaline phosphatase, serum creatinine, or other relevant information. This information and more is stored in each pixel of the patient's representative image (a medical "avatar") such that the image of each structure and organ (e.g., the liver) stacks up all the relevant information about the structure into a "deep pixel". Each pixel contains anatomic data as well as biochemical, physiologic, past historical, and so on, so that information can be revealed directly from the image rather than through a search of volumes of written medical records or a prolonged computer database. If a problem or disease is discovered, then the image can be immediately used for patient education, instantly explaining to the patient on their own avatar what the problem might be. If a surgical problem

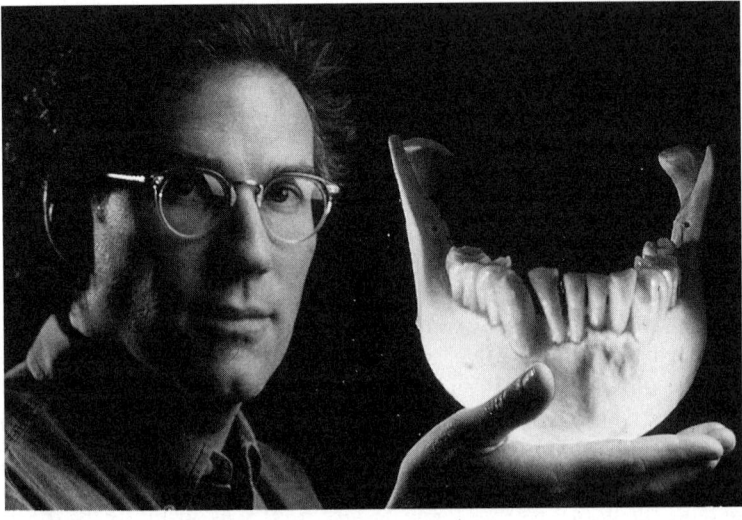

FIGURE 21.10. Full 3-D suspended holographic image of a mandible (courtesy Jonathan Prince, Dimensional Media Associates, New York, NY).

is discovered, then this same image can be used by the surgeon for preoperative planning, or imported into a surgical simulator to practice a variety of different approaches to a difficult surgical procedures that will be performed upon the patient the next morning. At the time of operation, the image can be fused with a video image and used for intraoperative navigation or to enhance precision, as in stereotactic surgery. During the postoperative visits, a follow-up scan can be compared with the preoperative scan, and, using digital subtraction techniques, the differences can automatically be processed for outcomes analysis. Because the avatar is an information object, it can be available and distributed (through telemedicine) anytime and to any place. Thus, this single concept of replacing the written medical record (including X-rays and other images) with the 3-D visual record of a medical avatar permits the entire spectrum of health care to be provided with unprecedented continuity.

It is certain that not all of these technologies will be developed in precisely the manner indicated, and many other technologies not mentioned will impact even greater than those currently envisioned. We now have information tools that can fundamentally and totally revolutionize our approach to patient care—tools that are existent today and are based upon known and provable science. While it is true that we must stringently evaluate the technologies and concepts with all known scientific rigor, we must not discard these powerful ideas because of our Industrial Age preconceptions.

References

1. Delp SL, Zajac FR. Force and moment generating capacity of lower limb muscles before and after tendon lengthening. Clin Ortho Rel Res 1992;284:247–259.
2. Satava RM. Virtual reality surgical simulator: the first steps Surg Endosc 1993;7:203–205.
3. Merril JR, Merril GL, Raju R, et al. Photorealistic interactive 3-D graphics in surgical simulation. In: Satava RM, Morgan K, et al. Interactive technology and the new medical paradigm for health care. IOS Press, Washington, D.C., 1995, pp. 244–252.
4. Spitzer VM, Whitlock DG. Electronic imaging of the human body. Data storage and interchange format standards. In: Vannier MW, Yates RE, Whitestone JJ. Proc electronic imaging of the human body working group, March 9–11, 1992; pp. 66–68.
5. Piper S, Delp S, Rosen J, Fisher S. A virtual environment system for simulation of leg surgery. Proc of stereoscopic display and applications II, SPIE Vol. 1457, pp. 188–196.
6. Meglan DA, Raju R, Merril GL, et al. Teleos virtual environment for simulation-based surgical education. In: Satava RM, Morgan K, et al. Interactive technology and the new medical paradigm for health care. IOS Press, Washington, D.C., 1995, pp. 346–351.
7. Raibert, MA Personal Communication.

8. Lorensen WE, Jolesz FA, Kikinis R. The exploration of cross-sectional data with a virtual endoscope. In: Satava RM, Morgan K, et al. Interactive technology and the new medical paradigm for health care. IOS Press, Washington, D.C., 1995, pp. 221–230.*
9. Geiger B, Kikinis R. Simulation of endoscopy, AAAI spring symposium series: applications of computer vision in medical images processing, Stanford University 1994, pp. 138–140.

22
Problem-Based Learning: The Live Animal Model

Spyros G. Condos

The resolution of problems derived from the world of reality surpasses any mode of simulation in the learning process.

JS Felton. Problem-based learning as a training modality in the occupational medicine curriculum. Occup Med 1996;46(1):5–11.

More than 82% of U.S. medical schools teach basic science using problem-based learning (PBL) in various degrees.[1,2]

PBL was initiated at McMaster University in Hamilton, Ontario, Canada. It forbids lectures and other forms of formal instructions. The objective is to force the students "to find out for themselves."[3] PBL is well suited to medical education because it avoids overteaching subject matter, the pitfall of incongruence between basic and clinical subjects, and the problems created by natural decay of knowledge.[4] PBL is commonly thought of as a means to cope with the rapidly increasing and changing information base of any discipline.[5]

The essential characteristics of PBL include curricular organization around the problems rather than the disciplines, an integrated curriculum rather than one separated into basic science and clinical science componets, and an inherent emphasis on cognitive skills as well as on knowledge. Second, there are situations that facilitate PBL, such as small group tutorial instruction, student-centered instruction, active learning independent study, and simulation of relevant, high-priority community-oriented issues. Third, there are outcomes that are facilitated by PBL, such as enhanced functional knowledge, development of skills and motivation required for a capacity for continued learning, and the development of self-assessment.[6] Twelve basic steps are generally followed in PBL:

- clarification and definition of the problem
- analysis of the problem
- development of hypothesis(ses)/plausible explanation
- identification and characterization of the knowledge needed
- identification of what is already known

- identification of appropriate learning resources
- collection of new information/knowledge
- synthesis of old and new information, and understanding of it by application to the problem (i.e., how much of the problem can now be explained)
- repetition of all or some of the previous steps, as necessary
- identification of what was not learned
- summary of what was learned
- test the knowledge comprehension by its application to another problem[7]

Rosser et al.[8] have shown that in an effort to train surgeons on new skills that will permit them to perform laparoscopic procedures they had to devise simple drills that the surgeons could master before advancing to the new technology. Such drills include the rope pass, triangle transfer, and the successive cup drop. Each drill required a learning period of approximately 10 controlled attempts.

The same group has shown that in the case of intracorporeal suturing, which is the most difficult of advanced laparoscopic skills, the necessary learning period requires about the same number of attempts, after the technique had been precisely taught.[8] The hypothesis of this work was that what was proven to be true in the case of the simple laparoscopic drills as well as in the case of the intracorporeal suturing should also be true for a complex laparoscopic procedure.

The procedure chosen was the laparoscopic Nissen fundoplication. The surgeon was experienced in open surgery of the same procedure and had taken the training course of performing it laparoscopically,[9] and also attempted to perfect skills in the animal (pig) model without measurable improvement (see phase I, Table 22.3) in the time needed to complete the operation, as well as quality of the operation performed. The surgeon agreed to participate in a PBL approach to training in an effort to perfect skills in this procedure.[7]

The problem was defined as: to complete a quality, functional laparoscopic Nissen fundoplication on a live pig. The conditions, prerequisites, and the evaluation of the performance were defined precisely as is shown in Table 22.1. The operation was always performed the same way following the steps of the procedure[9] (see Table 22.2). In such a controlled environment, the surgeon performed nine operations (see Table 22.3, phase II) with a gradual improvement in both quality of the operation and time needed to complete the operation. It was the surgeon's opinion that he was able to perform the operation well, comfortably, and safely for the patient.

A phase III (Table 22.3) was designed to evaluate the hypothesis that additional training might result in shorter operative times and improvements in skill levels. The results of phase III support the findings of both the simple drills and the intracorporeal suturing scenario that we are reaching a plateau of competence after 10 attempts in a control environment that can be sustained with additional maintenance practice.

TABLE 22.1. Problem: To complete a quality, functional laparoscopic Nissen fundoplication on a live pig.

Conditions
   The animal should be a 50–60-pound pig.
   The animal should be anesthetized, on the respirator with a dilator in the esophagus, and
      advanced into to the stomach.
   Nothing by mouth for 18 hours.
   Establish pneumoperitoneum.
   Trochars in place.
   Use of a 30-degree laparoscope.
   Two assistants, one anesthesiologist, and one circulating nurse (the team should always
      be the same).

Prerequisites
   Experience in open Nissen.
   Laparoscopic skills enhancement and suturing course.
   Laparoscopic Nissen fundoplication course.

Evaluation of Performance
   The operation should take place on a live animal.
   Examine damage on surrounding organs.
   Evaluate bleeding.
   Quality of the placement of the sutures.
   Constriction of the esophagus.
   Time for completion of the operation.

Other
   The operations should be videotaped.
   The evaluator should be the same.
   The evaluation should be based on observations during surgery, review of the video, and
      posteuthanasia examination.

TABLE 22.2. Laparoscopic Nissen fundoplication—steps of the procedure.

1. Establishment of the pneumoperitoneum.
2. Elevation and retraction of the liver if necessary.
3. Division of gastrohepatic and phenoesophageal ligament to gain exposure of the
   esophageal hiatus, abdomen esophagus, and proximal stomach.
4. Mobilization of the lower esophagus and hiatal hernia (if present).
5. Identification of the anterior and posterior vagus nerves.
6. Establishment of a window behind the esophagus for the fundic wrap. A penrose drain
   may be used to facilitate esophageal retraction.
7. Closure of the esophageal hiatus by approximation of the crura with nonabsorbable
   suture (if necessary).
8. Mobilization of the greater curvature of the stomach with division of short gastric veins
   (if necessary).
9. Placement and fixation of the fundic wrap around the lower esophagus with
   nonabsorbable suture.

Yale University School of Medicine: Laparoscopic Nissen fundoplication course, James C. Rosser, Jr., course director.

TABLE 22.3. Quality of operations.

Date of operation	Animal number	Duration of operation	Quality of operation*
Phase I			
2-13-1995	P-297	7.5 Hours	F
2-27-1995	P-971	4.0 Hours	D
3-27-1995	P-974	4.0 Hours	D
4-3-1995	P-982	5.0 Hours	F
6-5-1995	P-17	3.5 Hours	D
6-19-1995	P-40	3.5 Hours	C
6-26-1995	P-51	3.0 Hours	C
Phase II			
7-10-1995	P-52	3.0 Hours	B
7-31-1995	P-53	5.0 Hours	B
9-27-1995	P-88	3.5 Hours	B
10-02-1995	P-87	5.0 Hours	B
10-09-1995	P-91	3.75 Hours	C
10-12-1995	P-90	4.5 Hours	A
10-16-1995	P-98	3.0 Hours	B
10-16-1995	P-99	3.0 Hours	A
11-02-1995	P-108	5.0 Hours	B
Phase III			
2-05-1996	P-147	2.5 Hours	A
4-22-1996	P-198	2.5 Hours	A
5-20-1996	P-213	2.7 Hours	A
7-08-1996	P-254	3.0 Hours	A
7-29-1996	P-263	2.0 Hours	A

* C. Elton Cahow series.

In conclusion, we have proven that the PBL approach to learning a complex, new surgical procedure on the live animal model is successful, measurable, and necessary. We can therefore safely suggest that PBL should become an integral part in the surgical training of the new laparoscopic complex procedures. This training should occur following the formal training process, but before the surgeon performs the operation on a patient.

References

1. Jonas HS, Etzel SI, Barzasky B. Undegraduate medical education. J Am Med Assoc 1989;262:1011–1019.
2. Branda LA. Implementing problem-based learning. J Dental Ed 1990;54:9.
3. Gardner AW. A discussion paper for the Workshop on Guidelines for Teaching Occupational Health. Kitakyutsu, Japan, University of Occupational and Environmental Health, October 27–29, 1988:1.2–24–26.
4. Mitchel G. Problem-based learning in medical schools: a new approach. Med Teacher 1988;10:1.

5. Ferrier BM. Problem-based learning: does it make a difference? J Dental Ed 1990;54:9.
6. Walton JH, Matthews MB. Essentials of problem-based learning. Med Ed 1989;23:542–558.
7. Tedesco LA. A discussion paper presented at a symposium entitled, "Problem-based learning and information technology: maching methods and tools for teaching in the 21st century," at the 67th Annual Session of the American Association of Dental Schools, Cincinatti, OH, March 4, 1990.
8. Rosser JC, Rosser LE, Savalgi RS. Skill acuisition and assessment for laparo-scopic surgery. Arch Surg 1997;132:200–204.
9. Rosser JC, course director. Laparoscopic Nissen fundoplecation. Yale University School of Medicine, 1995.

Part V
Laparoscopic Surgery in the Future

23
Generalist versus Specialist in Laparoscopic Surgery

Ronald C. Merrell and Robert M. Olson III

The rapid emergence of laparoscopic surgery in recent years has radically changed the surgical approach to abdominal disease. General surgery in the abdomen, now performed via the laparoscope, is so different that special training and credentials are required for even the most mature and accomplished general surgeon. Does laparoscopic surgery constitute a new specialty, leaving the head of general surgery Zeus as its offspring Athena aided by the blow of Hephraistos not with an axe but a fiber optic scope?

To answer this question we must first ask: Is laparoscopy especially different as a surgical event? Laparoscopy certainly challenges the traditional general surgeon. Hand–eye coordination is replaced by manipulation of a television image by hand motions via long instruments in an environment we can know intuitively only rather than by direct engagement. The laparoscopic surgeon works without depth vision, cannot palpate the operative anatomy, and only imperfectly perceives through long instruments the tissue properties during dissection. Is this new to surgery?

Hippocrates described an early scope was for anoscopy.[1-3] Open tubes with reflected light were ingenious for monocular access to distant body cavities. Desmoureaux presented a reasonable cystoscope in 1865.[2] Nitze put Bruck's heated platinum wire on the end of his cystoscope in 1879.[4] Edison's incandescent bulb was applied successfully to a gastroscope by Mickulicz in 1881 and to a cystoscope by Newman in 1883.[3] All three scopes were monocular and permitted no palpitation or hand–eye coordination for their use, which was almost entirely diagnostic.

The laparoscope was named by Jacobaeus from Sweden in 1901[5] drawing from Greek to describe a viewing instrument for the soft abdomen bordered by ribs, hips, and flanks. When Veress described his retractable needle in 1938, safe and effective pneumoperitoneum invited operative work through the scope. The dominant use was in gynecology. Thus by 1960, urologists, proctologists, gynecologists, and pulmonologists were all working briskly through long tubes in otherwise inaccessible places. No one supported specialization with the disease categories and anatomical confines within these surgical specialties. It is possible that skill with endoscopes accelerated the departure of certain specialties from the general surgery parent, which persisted in open anatomic approaches.

Hirschowitz adapted fiberoptic principles to permit flexible endoscopy. His 1961 article inaugurates an era of rapid realization of surgical possibilities.[6] Flexible endoscopy brought medical gastroenterologists into the role of intervention of surgical therapy. Between 1960 and 1980 highly creative work in electrocautery, instrumentation, computing, lasers, photography, and fiberoptics saw a great expansion in the field of gynecology, otolaryngology, pulmonary, critical care, urology, and gastroenterology. General surgery seemed to wait.

In various laboratories including, principally, Cushieri at Dundee,[7] and Frimberger,[8] laparoscopic biliary surgery was studied. Lukichev described cholecystectomy in 1983.[9] Events, however, overwhelmed incremental science in 1987,[10] when Mouret removed the gallbladder from a patient after forcefully retracting the gallbladder toward the diaphragm to facilitate dissection. The procedure was rapidly reproduced and improved,[7,10] and patients afflicted with symptomatic cholelithiasis had made their choice within only months. Almost every patient considering cholecystectomy has some clear familial memory or general impression of open cholecystectomy that made laparoscopic cholecystectomy obviously superior. Cries for randomized trials were drowned by the cries for improved care, and traditional general surgeons were faced with extermination or adaptation. Courses proliferated, and thousands of general surgeons in the United States were retrained in a matter of months to meet patient demand.[11] New operations via laparoscope followed by patient demand and professional response slowed sharply. Fundoplication,[7] splenectomy,[12,13] adrenalectomy,[14,15] choledochoscopy,[16,17] common duct surgery,[18] colectomy,[19–21] and hemorrhoidectomy[22] have only been available to a limited number of patients at rather specialized centers.

We will now return to the definition of specialized versus generalist surgeons. There is certainly no movement to make cystoscopic surgery a subspecialty of urology, or laparoscopic gynecology a subspecialty of gynecology, or to split orthoscopy from orthopedics, or endoscopy from gastroenterology. The use of scopes for diagnosis and treatment in these specialties evolved perhaps more slowly than did laparoscopy in general surgery, but there have never been any serious attempts to divorce a specific methodology from the discipline treating a group of diseases. There has been substantial differentiation within general surgery, which has ignored any barrier that might be defined by the laparoscope. Some general surgeons restrict their efforts to GI surgery or, further, to hepatobiliary surgery. Others stay limited to surgical oncology, and still others to trauma. The laparoscope is finding utility in all these arenas. A clinical discipline should be defined by the diseases treated, not by methodology. A scientific discipline in general is defined by what it does, by what it knows, and by what questions it asks. These three requirements for old or new disciplines are helpful in the identification of a new discipline or in pronouncing the end of an old science. For example, when a discipline no longer has unique questions, its subject is sterile and cannot be considered a vital part of science. A clinical discipline should be further defined by the patients treated rather than by the technology used. It is reasonable to define radiology by the technical use of various energies to produce an image because it is not a clinical discipline, having no defined patient population to treat.

When specialists are trained in their clinical or nonclinical disciplines after medical school, a curriculum is applied over several years of incremental acquisition of skills and experience. That curriculum contains all the didactic technical material to prepare a resident to practice the discipline of note. Fellowships split further to a smaller but more intense set of skills. Practitioners in many disciplines must demonstrate their currentness in the discipline by maintaining educational credits or being recertified, taking the qualifying examination again. This process works well in the United States. New technology should not automatically imply neither a new discipline nor a new specialty. A new technology with a discipline or specialty calls for new credentials appropriate for the care of an existing group of patients.

Is laparoscopy, then, a new specialty? The laparoscope is a tool, not a discipline. The tool has been around for a while, yet was discovered quite late by general surgeons for the care of their patients. Laparoscopy is a technical jolt for general surgeons, and the proliferation of technology associated with the laparoscope is changing almost every aspect of surgery toward nominally invasive surgery. Surgery is evolving so quickly that it will not be recognizable in its technical aspect by our predecessors. They would immediately recognize the patients associated with their discipline, but the technology would be a barrier to their active involvement in the care of those patients. The new surgery will be practiced by a new surgeon. That surgeon will be masterful in the use of technology to treat those patients associated with his or her clinical discipline. The laparoscope is one of the defining tools of the new surgeon.

To enrich the care of our patients with new technology, therefore, we must prepare the practitioner. Laparoscopy should be taught in general surgery residency just as in gynecology programs. Because laparoscopy is a relatively new skill for the faculty, serious attention must be paid to the preparation of the faculty. Because laparoscopy is replacing many traditional surgical approaches such as an open cholecystectomy, there is no practical way to teach the tradition and then the replacement (Fig. 23.1).[23] Because the laparoscopic operative field is more difficult to share with trainees than the open abdomen, a place outside the OR is needed to initiate laparoscopic training.[23] That teaching laboratory should employ an effective and validated curriculum, that will bring surgical trainees to the OR ready for meaningful participation in the operative care for patients via the laparoscope. Such a curriculum is used at Yale and has now restored

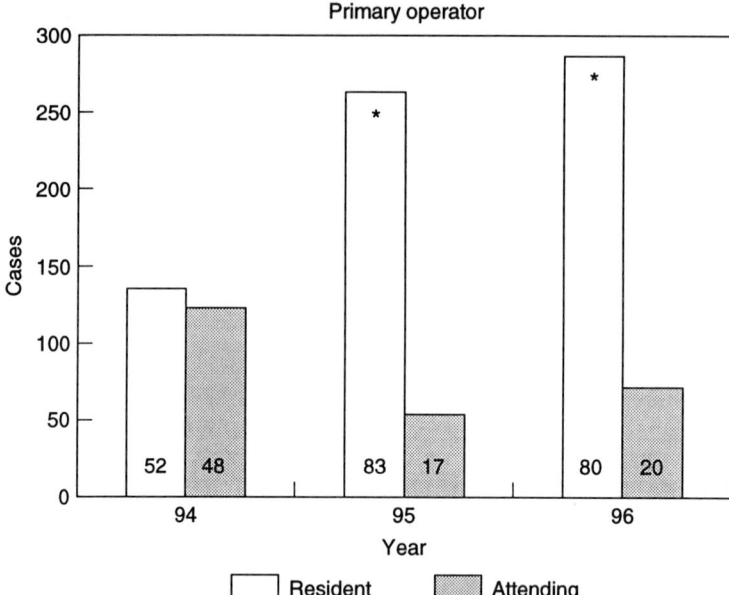

FIGURE 23.1. Role of surgeon in laparoscopic cholecystectomies by year. Columns are labeled with the percentage of cases they represent. *$p < 0.001$ compared with 1994.[24]

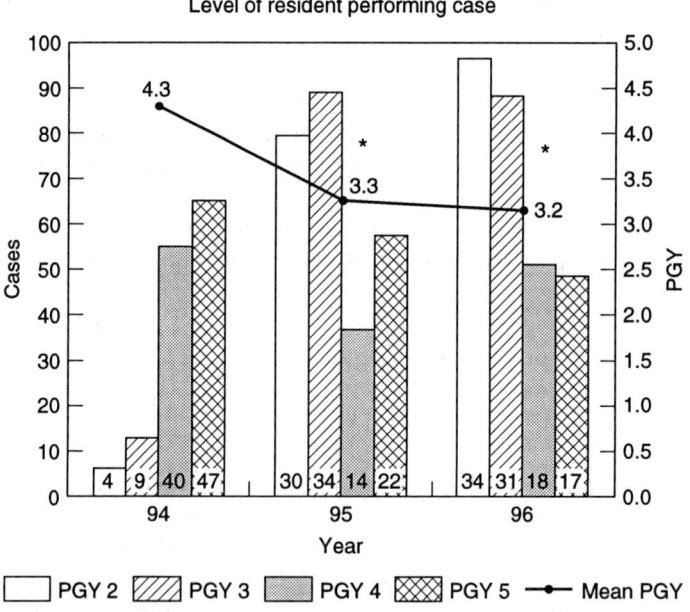

FIGURE 23.2. Postgraduate year (PGY) of resident performing laparoscopic cholecystectomies each year. The gross number of cases is represented by the height of the columns, the percentage of cases done by each level of resident labels each column, and the mean PGY level for each year is graphed as a line. $p < 0.0001$ by x^2 test for the change in distribution over the 3 years. *$p < 0.0001$ by Student's t test compared with 1994.[24]

cholecystectomy to the second postgraduate year in terms of incremental operative skills (Fig. 23.2).[24] General surgery in the future without laparoscopy will be a discipline without patients. We must teach laparoscopy as a primary surgical skill, not as a specialty.

References

1. Rosin D. History. In Minimal access medicine and surgery. Oxford, Radcliffe Medical Press, 1993, pp. 1–9.
2. Gorden A. The history and development of endoscopic surgery. In Endoscopic surgery for gynecologists. Sutton C, Diamond MP, eds. London, Saunders, 1993, pp. 3–7.
3. Lau WY, Leow CK, Li KC. History of endoscopic and laparoscopic surgery. World J Surg 1997;21:444–453.
4. Nitze M. Beobachtung-und Untersuchungsmethode fur und untersuchungs-methode Harnohre, Harnblase, und Rectum. Wien Med Wochenschr 1879; 29:649.
5. Jacobaeus HC. Kurze Ubersichtuber meine Efahrungen mit der Laparothora-koskopie. Munchen Med Wochenschr, 1911;58:2017.
6. Hirschowitz BI. Endoscopic examination of the stomach and the duodenal cap with the fiber scope. Lancet 1961;7:1074.
7. Cuschieri A, Buess G. Introduction and historical aspects. In Operative manual of endoscopic surgery. Cushieri A, Buess G, Perissat J, eds. Springer-Verlaug, Berlin, 1992, pp. 1–5.
8. Frimberger E, vonSanden H, Wersdorfer C, et al. Laparoskopischo cholecystotomie. Fortschr, Gastroenterol Endosk 1987;17:100.
9. Lukichou OD, Filimonov MI, Zybin IM. A method of laparoscopic cholecystectomy. Khirargiia 1983;8:125.
10. Filipi CJ, Fitzgibbons RJ, Salerno GM. Historical review: diagnostic laparoscopic cholecystectomy and beyond. In Surgical laparoscopy. Zucker KA, ed. Quality Medical Publishing, St. Louis, 1991, pp. 3–21.
11. Gotz F, Pier A, Schippers E, et al. The history of laparoscopy. In Color atlas of laparoscopic surgery. Gotz F, Pier A, Schippers E, et al. eds. Thieme, New York, 1992, pp. 3–5.
12. Delaitre B, Maignien B. Splenectomie par voie coelioscopique: 7 observation. Presse Med 1991;20:2263.
13. Delaitre B, Maignien B, Icard, P. Laparoscopic splenectomy. Br J Surg 1992;79:1134.
14. Higasihara E, Tanaka Y, Horie S, et al. A case report of laparoscopic adrenalectomy. Nipon Hinyokika Gakkai Zasshi 1992;83:1130.
15. Gagner M, Lacroix A, Bolte E. Laparoscopic adrenalectomy in Suching's syndrome and pheochromocytoma. N Engl J Med 1992;327:1033.
16. Sockier JM, Berci G, Paz-Partlow M. Laparoscopic transcystic choledocholithotomy as an adjunct to laparoscopic cholecystectomy. Ann Surgy 1991;57:323.
17. Carroll BJ, Phillips EH, Daykhovsky L, et al. Laparoscopic choledochoscopy: an effective approact to the common duct. J Laparoendosc Surg 1992;2:15.
18. Jacobs M, Verdeja JL, Goldstein HS. Laparoscopic choledocholithotomy. J Laparoendosc Surg 1991;7:79.

19. Schlinkert RT. Laparoscopic-assisted right hemicholectomy. Dis Colon Rectum 1991;34:1030.
20. Monson JRT, Darzi A, Carey PD, et al. Prospective evaluation of laparoscopic-assisted colectomy in an unselected group of patients. Lancet 1992;340:831.
21. Coperman AM, Katz V, Zimmom D, et al. Laparoscopic colon resection: a case report. J Laparoendosc Surg 1991;1:221.
22. Ger P. Lapaaroskopische hernienoperation. Chirurg 1991;62:266.
23. Rosser JC, Rosser LE, Savalgi RS. Skill acquisition and assessment for laparoscopic surgery. Arch Surg 1997;132:200–204.
24. Coppola LP, Merrell RC. Effect of a training program on performance of laparoscopic cholecystectomy. Best Pract Benchmarking Healthcare 1997; 2:24–27.

24
Beyond Laparoscopic Surgery: Robotics and Telepresence Surgery

Richard M. Satava

Laparoscopic surgery continues with an evolution so rapid that before one change has been accepted and perfected, another even more dramatic change promises to replace it. Flexible endoscopy and laparoscopic surgery have just become accepted standards of surgical practice, and even more advanced technologies promise to further improve the practice of surgery. It is essential that surgeons understand these changes and are prepared to adapt and improve all their surgical and cognitive skills. These technologies enable entirely new capabilities in the generation of surgery beyond laparoscopic surgery, which includes computer assisted surgery and telepresence surgery. These applications are mediated through the computer and information networks. As such, they are the essence of the paradigm shift in the field of medicine.

These new technologies are a subset of *telemedicine*, which covers a wide range of remote medical capabilities, whereas *telesurgery* refers primarily to a surgical operation over a telemedicine network. One of the first systems emphasizes remote surgery and consists of two components: the surgical workstation [with a three-dimensional (3-D) monitor and dexterous handles with force feedback] and remote work site (with a 3-D camera system and responsive manipulators with sensory input). Other systems focus upon dexterity enhancement to improve human performance beyond physical limitations.

Introduction

Laparoscopic surgery has changed both the technical and the cognitive approach to surgery. Surgeons think in terms of minimal access, constrained surgical abilities, and novel surgical instruments. The fields of robotics and

---

*The opinions or assertions contained herein are the private views of the authors and are not to be construed as official, or as reflecting the views of the Department of the Army, Department of the Navy, the Advanced Research Projects Agency, or the Department of Defense.

telepresence surgery introduce yet another level of thinking about the practice of surgery, one in which there is enhancement of human performance as well as the ability to project surgical expertise to remote and distant places. These new capabilities share the fact that they use information age technologies and represent the real world with "information equivalents" in order to accomplish a task not otherwise possible.

The information equivalent of vision is a video image, of motion is telemanipulation and of X-ray film is digital images (like CT or MRI). Robotics takes the surgeon's motions and converts them into electronic signals that can be enhanced through a controlling computer, integrated, scaled, and sent over networks to places hundreds of miles away. Coupling the electronic motion with video allows the procedures to be performed anywhere by transmitting them over communication lines, whether for actual procedures with telepresence surgery or for education with tele-mentoring. The fundamental precept for surgeons of the next century is to learn to use information to enhance their natural capabilities in order to provide better patient care.

While robotics and automation have been used in science and industry for more than three decades, there are precious few applications within the medical field. The introduction of laparoscopic surgery, however, which requires operating inside a patient while observing a video monitor, will rapidly and dramatically increase the demand for robotic and telepresence manipulation. Laparoscopic surgery has more in common with remote manipulation than with open surgery. It is more important, however, that these technologies are electronically controlled; as such, they are the final piece for the total revolution of medicine. The circle is complete: much of medicine can be described as digital input or output. This is medicine's wake-up call to the digital information age.

The time could not be more perfect, for we now have the right type of doctor to take advantage of this new technology. First it was the "Nintendo surgeon" for laparoscopic surgery; now it is the "Digital Physician" for telepresence surgery and robotics. These are our younger physicians who have grown up in the video/electronic generation—they are both comfortable with the new technology, and they are now demanding it. They play video games, "surf" over the Internet and the "information super highway," or become educated with computer-aided instruction, multimedia, and virtual reality. To them, the future is now, and it is all digital.

The Paradigm Shift

Now is the time that all of these separate elements (i.e., laparoscopic surgery, telepresence, virtual reality, digital imaging, and networking) are coming together, and the common focal point is the video monitor at a physician's workstation.[1] The video monitor is the portal into the entire world of information; this "electronic interface" will bestow power beyond imagination. Although the current portal into this information-rich arena is the video monitor, in the future other display technologies, such as head mounted displays (HMD), video glasses, holograms, and palmtop computers, may be the interface. This interface is also the point of intellectual enhancement, for it is here that all the information can coalesce and be presented to the individual as knowledge, not data. This interface can bring in information, and it can also send out information or commands for action in the real world (teleoperation or remote manipulation enables a person to work at a distance). For example, a surgeon could be at the monitor during a real operation, doing a surgical procedure in the next city, and collaborating with another surgeon on the same patient. It might eventually be possible to operate at a place that is too distant or dangerous, such as the space station or third world country. In taking this approach, we are able to "dissolve time and space," the physician can "be" at a distant place at the same time as another person without needing to travel there. Of utmost importance, however, is the fact that the physician can simultaneously bring in many different digital images, such as the patient's CT or MRI scan, and fuse them with real-time video images, giving the surgeon "X-ray vision." Before performing a surgical procedure, the surgeon could sit at the workstation and practice on a virtual patient (see Chap. 21 on virtual reality surgical simulation) to simulate the operation, then flip the switch and begin operating on the real patient with precisely the same workstation—this is the power of the electronic interface and the core technology for the medical revolution. The following represents the current status of a number of the new information-based surgical innovations such as telesurgery and enhanced dexterity surgery.

Surgical Applications

In the area of remote surgery, Dr. Philip Green[2,3] of SRI International has invented the Green Telepresence Surgery System. This system restores to the surgeon those native and intuitive abilities that have been lost with laparoscopic surgery: 3-D vision, dexterous precise surgical instrument manipulation, and the sense of touch from input of force feedback sensory information. The system consists of a surgical workstation (Fig. 24.1) that has a 3-D monitor, responsive instrument handles, and force feedback for touch (Fig. 24.2), whereas the remote work site has a 3-D camera system, dexterous manipulators, and sensory input (Figs. 24.3 and 24.4). The surgeon's abilities are enhanced and surgery can be performed with greater skill and precision. The current generation system is a two-handed very dexterous system with paired cameras for stereovision; the next generation will have a stereoscopic laparoscope to replace the fixed cameras. The system is engineered in such a way that the surgeon actually feels as if the

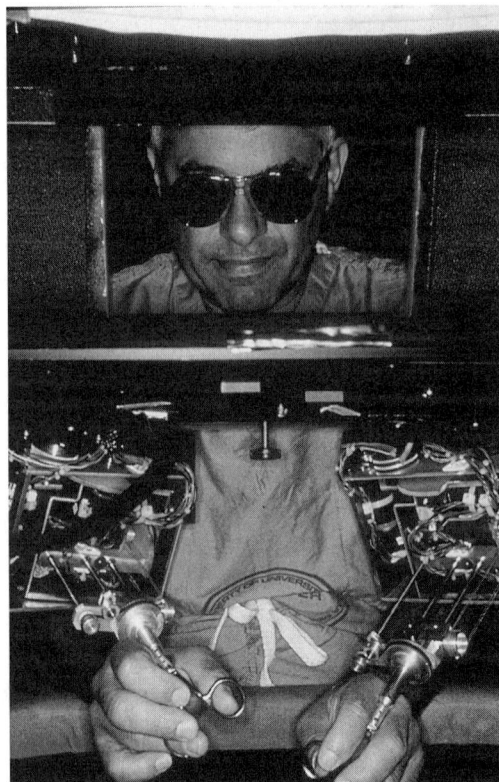

FIGURE 24.1. Surgeon seated at the surgical workstation of a Green Telepresence Surgery System (courtesy of SRI, International Menlo Park, CA).

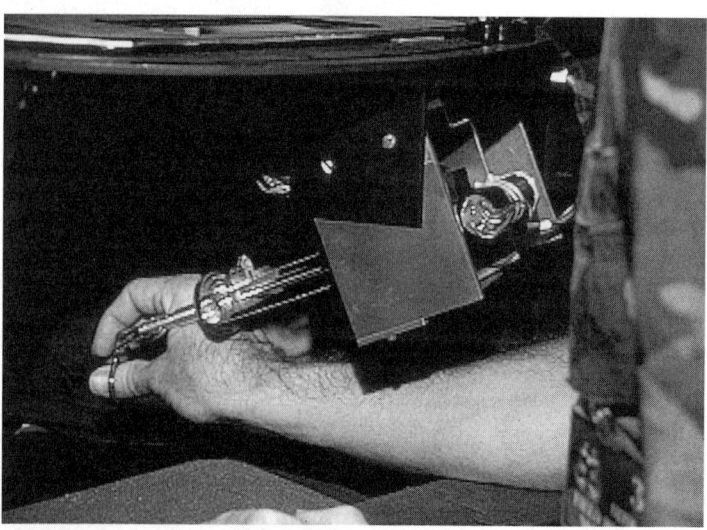

FIGURE 24.2. Instrument handle device for the surgical workstation of a Green Telepresence Surgery System (courtesy of SRI, International, Menlo Park, CA).

FIGURE 24.3. Close up of the handle of the surgical interface (courtesy of SRI, International).

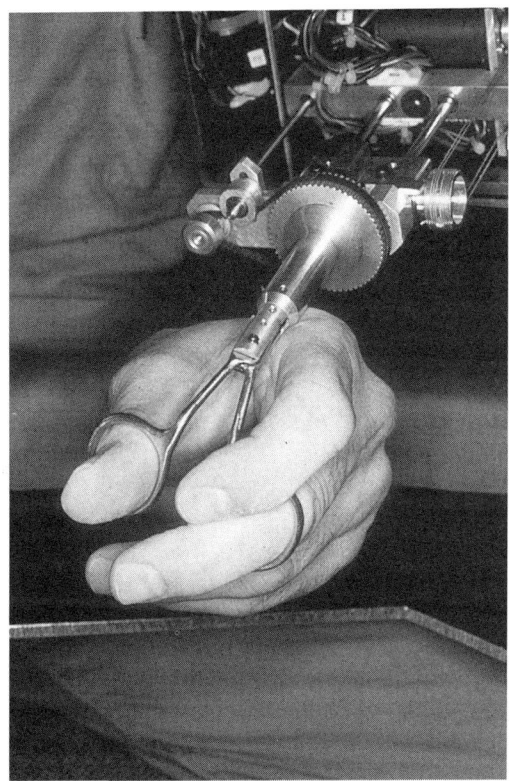

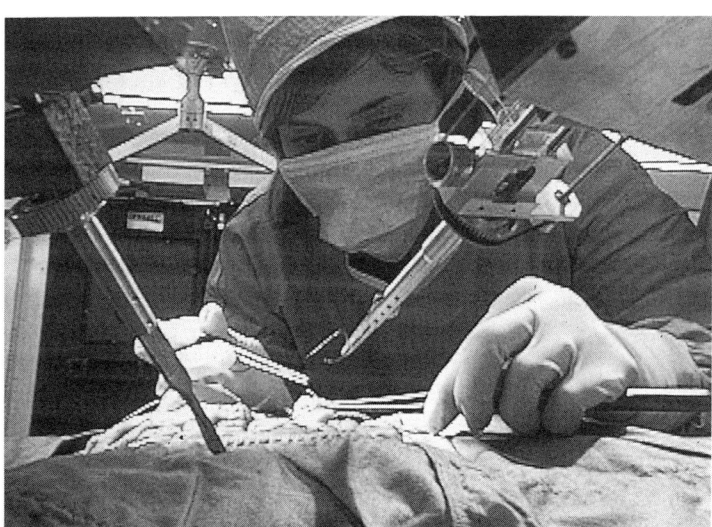

FIGURE 24.4. Remote manipulators of a Green Telepresence Surgery System across from the assisting medic (courtesy of SRI, International Menlo Park, CA).

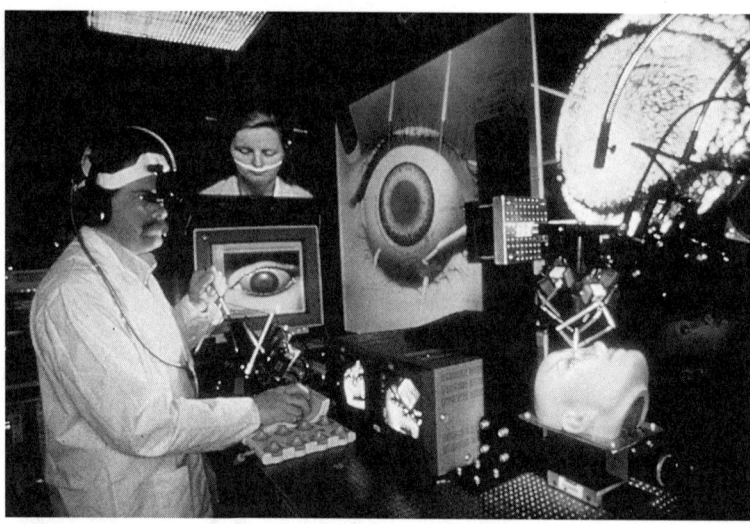

FIGURE 24.5. Enhanced dexterity system for retinal laser microsurgery (courtersy of Ian Hunter, PhD, Massachussets Institute of Technology, Cambridge, MA).

surgery were being performed directly in front of him/her, when in reality the remote site (and patient) could be feet, miles, or even hundreds of miles away. Because the system was designed to mimic open surgery, there will be essentially no training required, thus permitting surgery with all the feeling, dexterity, and 3-D vision of open surgery.

Another advanced surgical system that has been created by Hunter et al.[3] focuses upon enhanced dexterity through the use of a computer-aided or robotic system (Fig. 24.5). In laser retinal surgery, the blood vessels of the retina are 25 μm apart. If one is injured during surgery there is bleeding and blindness. The human hand, unfortunately, is physically incapable of positioning with an accuracy of greater than 200 μm. Through Hunter's robotic and computer-aided system, however, the motion of the hand is scaled up by 100-fold, so 1 cm of the surgeon's hand motion moves the laser-scalpel 10 μm and vision magnifies the retinal vessels to the size of a finger. The involuntary motion of the eye (called *saccades*, which flicker the eye back and forth 200 times a minute) are removed by a motion compensation algorithm that tracks the eye movement at a rate of 1,000 times per minute. By applying sophisticated signal filtering techniques through the computer interface, the normal intention tremor of the human hand can be removed. The combination of applying all these sophisticated techniques through the computer provides an accuracy and precision to 10 μm, which is 20 times more accurate than the unaided hand. A similar system for other microsurgery applications is being developed by Charles et al. of MicroDexterity Inc.

3-D Visualization

The cognitive aspects of surgery are enhanced by 3-D visualization of images. By taking CT or MRI scans and generating full 3-D volume renderings of the patient's specific anatomy, the surgeon is able to conduct a number of essential surgical skills on the "information equivalent" of the patient, before actually operating on the patient. Today, diagnosis is made by looking at flat two-dimensional (2-D) films or by performing an endoscopic procedure. Preoperative planning is then done with matching templates or diagramming with pen or pencil. If the operation is extraordinary, then the only opportunity to practice the procedure would be on animal models. During a procedure there are few aids to precise navigation or positioning. With a 3-D representation of the patient, however, all these capabilities can be attained upon a single image.

The 3-D image can be used for preoperative diagnosis. This begins by taking CT or MRI 2-D slices, and reconstructing 3-D images that could be rotated, layers peeled away, and individual organs separated and isolated (referred to as "segmentation"). The result is an imaginary reconstruction of a specific portion of a patient's anatomy, in essence a virtual reality brain or colon. Based upon these successes, and taking the next generation of CT scans (spiral or helical CT scan), which can generate much more accurate images, radiologists are segmenting out even more organs, such as the aorta, ear, sinuses, esophagus, and trachea.

Before performing a procedure, a surgeon can preplan an operation with the same image (see earlier) used for diagnosis. Dr. Joseph Rosen[4] of Dartmouth University Medical Center has a virtual reality model of a face with deformable skin that allows the practicing of a plastic surgical procedure and the demonstration of the final outcome before making the incision on a patient. Dr. Scott Delp[5] has a virtual model of a lower leg upon which he can practice a tendon transplant operation and then "walk" the leg to predict the short- and long-term consequences of the surgery. Dr. Altobelli[6] of the Brigham and Woman's Hospital has developed a system that creates 3-D images from the CT scan of a child with bony deformities of the face (craniofacial dysostosis); using this 3-D model, the bones can be correctly rearranged to symmetrically match the normal side of the face, permitting repeated practice of this extremely difficult procedure. In neurosurgical applications, Dr. Ferenc Jolesz[7] of the Brigham and Women's Hospital has provided the capability for 3-D MRI scan of an individual patient's brain tumor. At the time of brain surgery, the MRI scan is fused with the video image of the patient's actual skull or brain, thus giving "X-Ray vision" of

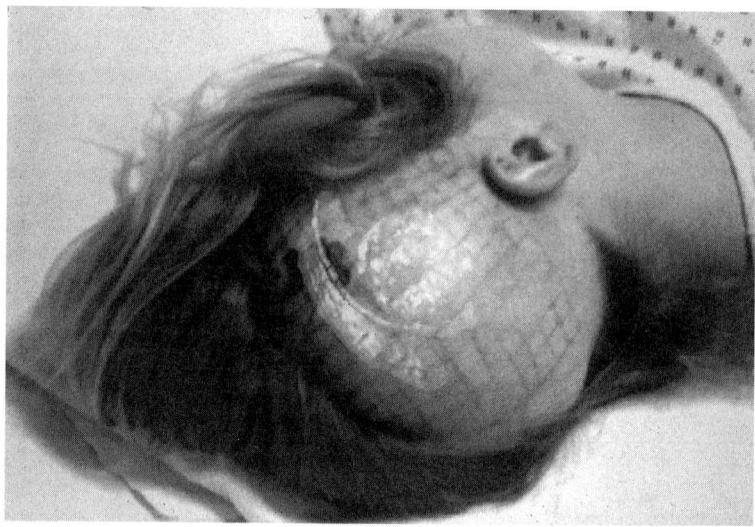

FIGURE 24.6. Fusion of the 3-D reconstruction of a brain tumor over the patient's skull preoperatively (courtesy of Drs. F. Jolesz and R. Kikinis, Brigham Women's Hospital Boston, MA).

the tumor that is not otherwise visible where it is deeply embedded in the brain tissue (Fig. 24.6). These examples are but the first of many potential applications of virtual reality for medical and surgical therapy, and they demonstrate how the computer and robotics can enhance a surgeon's ability through both the visualization and the performance of surgical procedure by using a single, seamless, integrated system.

Conclusions

Advanced technology is enabling many aspects of medicine; however, the ultimate direction and outcome will not be determined by the state of the technology, but by the intangibles of personal behaviors, social and cultural preferences, and political will. The surgeon must embrace the innovative technologies and learn how to increase his or her own surgical abilities. It must be remembered that technology is neutral—it is neither good nor evil. Technology requires human intellect and compassion to breathe the ethical and moral life into it in order to enhance the art as well as science of medicine. We must be ever mindful that, no matter how wonderful the technology might appear, it is of absolutely no value unless it provides better care for each and every patient.

References

1. Satava RM. Surgery 2001: a technologic framework for the future. Surg Endosc 1993;7:111–113.
2. Satava RM. Robotics, telepresence and virtual reality: a critical analysis of the future of surgery. Minimally Invasive Therapy 1992;1:357–363.
3. Green PS, Hill JH, Satava RM. Telepresence: dexterous procedures in a virtual operating field (Abstr). Surg Endosc 1991;57:192.
4. Rosen J. From computer-aided design to computer-aided surgery. Proceedings of Medicine Meets Virtual Reality. San Diego, CA. June 1–2, 1992.
5. Delp SL, Zajac FR. Force and moment generating capacity of lower limb muscles before and after tendon lengthening. Clin Ortho Rel Res 1992;284:247–259.
6. Altobelli DE, Kikinis R, Mulliken JB, et al. Computer assisted three dimensional planning in craniofacial surgery. Plast Reconstr Surg 1993;92(4):576–585.
7. Jolesz F, Shtern F. The operating room of the future. Proc of the National Cancer Institute Workshop, 27, April 1992, pp. 326–328.

25
Laparoscopic Surgery in the Elderly

RONNIE ANN ROSENTHAL

Over the next 60 years, the portion of the persons in the United States over the age of 65 years is expected to grow from the present 12.5% to 20.4%. The most rapidly growing segment of this aging population are those persons over age 85, whose number is expected to increase from the present 3 million to more than 20 million by the year 2050 (Fig. 25.1).[1] It is important to note that life expectancy in the elderly population is not insignificant: A male can expect to live an additional 9 years and a female approximately 11 years at age 75 years, and at 85 years a male can expect to live more than 5 years and a female for more than 6 years.[2]

This aging of the population is reflected in the age of patients requiring surgical care. In 1980 approximately 19% of operations in acute care, non–federally funded hospitals were performed on persons age 65 or more. This number had increased 31% by 1993 (Fig. 25.2).[3]

For the elderly patient, the concept of providing this major surgical treatment with minimal impact on function is most appealing. The rapidly expanding application of minimal access techniques to a wide variety of surgical procedures now makes such care possible. Laparoscopic approaches for diseases of biliary tract and colon, which are the two most common indications for abdominal surgery in patients over age 65 (Table 25.1),[4] have widely been adopted with great success. Before generally applying these techniques to older patients, however, it is important to consider the physiologic effects of laparoscopy and the limitations imposed by the disease processes in older patients.

Two issues are most important when considering any surgical care in the elderly patient (Fig. 25.3). The first is related directly to factors intrinsic to the older patient. There is an overall decline in physiological function of nearly all major organ systems with increasing age, although this decline is variable among organs and among individuals (Fig. 25.4). There is also an increase in the prevalence of cormorbid disease. The decline in physiologic function limits the reserves available when the surgical stress is increased, as in emergent operations or in cases where a postoperative complication has occurred. It is the presence of comorbid conditions other than the surgical

286

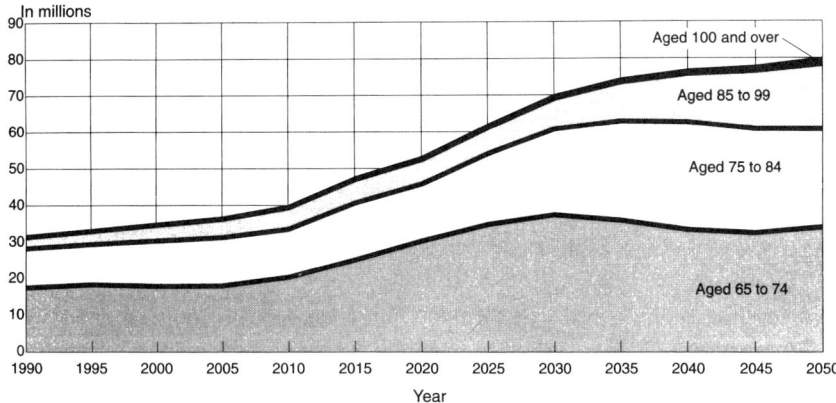

FIGURE 25.1. Projected population growth by age group in the United States. (Reprinted with permission from U.S. Department of Commerce Bureau of the Census. Population Report P25-1104. Day JC. Population projections of the United States by age, sex and Hispanic origin, 1993.)

disease, however, that impacts more directly on surgical outcome. In a series of patients over age 50 undergoing colon resection, Boyd et al. documented a clear increase in cormorbid conditions such that only 5% of patients had no disease of any organ other than the colon by age 80 (Table 25.2).[5] In a large series[6] of patients over age 65 years undergoing open cholecystectomy, Escares correlated the number of comorbid conditions

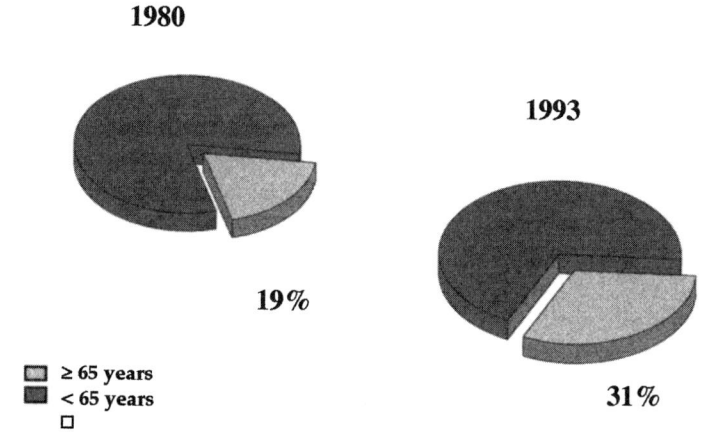

FIGURE 25.2. The proportion of operations in which the patient is over age 65 has increased from 19% in 1980 to 31% in 1993. [Reprinted with permission from Peebles RJ, Schneidman DS. (eds.). Socio-economic factbook for surgery 1993, Chicago,1993, American College of Surgeons.]

TABLE 25.1. Abdominal operations in the elderly, 1993.

	Total # ×1,000	Age > 65
Cholecystectomy	502	168 (34%)
Colon resection	207	120 (58%)
Lysis adhesions	347	90 (26%)
Inguinal hernia	109	54 (50%)
Appendectomy	250	17 (7%)

Source: CDC Advanced data No. 264, May 1995.

with operative mortality (Table 25.3). Whereas it appears that mortality increases directly with increasing age, it is cormobidity rather than chronological age that is responsible for this increase.

Second, there are issues related to the disease itself. Surgical disease in the elderly frequently presents in an acute and/or complicated manner and requires emergency operation. This may, in part, represent some changes in the natural history of these diseases in this age group, or it may be the result of delays in presentation and treatment caused by the atypical nature of signs and symptoms of surgical disease. Regardless of the cause, operations in the acute or emergent setting are associated with at least a threefold increase in mortality and morbidity.

When considering laparoscopic surgical procedures in elderly patients these two issues should be addressed (Fig. 25.5). The questions to answer before recommending this approach are, "Does the laparoscopic approach limit operative stress to lessen the impact of physiologic decline," and, "Does this approach lessen the importance of comorbid conditions by limiting the impact of these conditions in the postoperative period?" If the answer to these questions is yes, then laparoscopic approaches will clearly

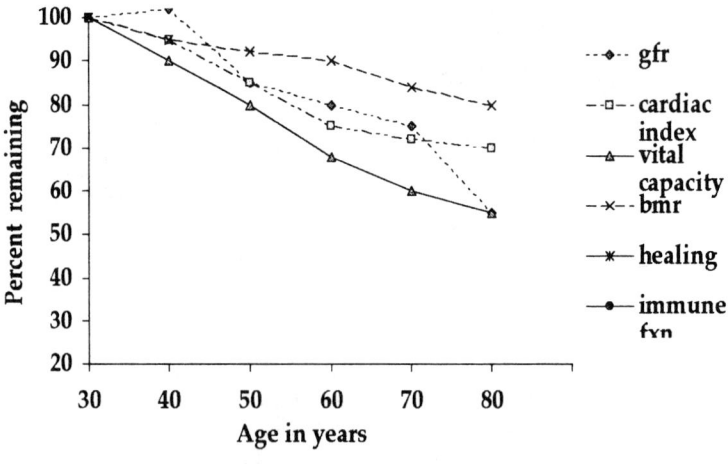

FIGURE 25.3. Age in years.

Characteristics of the Patient
Decline in physiologic reserve
Increase in comorbid illnesses
Characteristics of the Diseases
Acute and complicated presentation
Atypical signs and symptoms

FIGURE 25.4. Decline in physiologic function with increasing age. Note that wound healing and immune function decline as well, but this decline is not easily quantitated.

improve outcome. It must also noted, however, that the utility of the minimal access route in the presence of acute and complicated disease may be limited by longer operative times and the more frequent need to convert to open operation. To answer to the first question "Does laparoscopy impose less of a surgical stress" it is necessary to review the effects of the procedure on cardiovascular and pulmonary function, as well as on the hormonal, metabolic, and immune responses to surgery. In a study of the cardiovascular response to pneumoperitoneum in elderly patients undergoing laparoscopic colon resections performed at the Yale VA Hospital in Connecticut,[7] Harris et al. divided the laparoscopic procedure into three phases and measured the response to pneumoperitoneum in each phase. In response to insufflation (Fig. 25.6A) there is an increase in central venous pressure (CVP), pulmonary capillary wedge pressure (PCWP), mean arterial pressure (MAP), and systemic vascular resistance (SVR), with a concomitant decrease in cardiac index and ejection fraction. These changes suggest a systolic ventricular dysfunction in the face of the acute rise in afterload. When the patient is positioned in Trendelenburg position (Fig. 25.6B), there is a further increase in CVP, PCWP, and MAP, but a decrease in SVR along with an increase in cardiac index and ejection fraction. This suggests increased preload facilitates ventricular function and reverses some of the changes caused by insufflation. In the final phase—release of pneumoperitoneum (Fig. 25.6C)—there is a decrease in CVP, PCWP,

TABLE 25.2. Percentage of patients with comorbid conditions.

# of conditions	Age (years)				Total
	50–59	60–69	70–79	>80	
0	46	33	21	5	30
1	37	34	28	37	33
2	13	27	23	41	24
≥3	3	8	22	15	11

Source: Boyd et al., 1990.

TABLE 25.3. Effect of age and comrobidity on opertive mortality.

	Mortality (%)
Age (years)	
65–69	0.7
70–74	1.4
75–79	2.2
80–84	4.4
≥85	7.5
Comorbid index	
0	1.5
1	2.3
2	3.7
≥3	6.1

Source: Escarce et al., 1995.

MAP, and SVR with an increase in heart rate, cardiac index, and ejection fraction. This suggests a reactive type of hyperdynamic state, which is well tolerated, with no evidence of impaired coronary perfusion. These combined hemodynamic effects of pneumoperitoneum can be minimized by appropriate preoperative preloading.

The pulmonary consequences to pneumoperitoneum result from the use of CO_2 for insufflation and as a consequence of increased intraairway pressures (Fig. 25.7). Although the impact of the acidosis and increased $PaCO_2$ is usually minimal, the increased work of breathing associated with pneumoperitoneum maybe significant; however, a comparison of the postoperative pulmonary functions in patients undergoing laparoscopic versus open cholecystectomy reveals that pulmonary function declines far less significantly after laparoscopic procedure than it does after open operation (Table 25.4).[8]

Characteristics of the Patient

Decline in physiologic reserve

Less operative stress?

Increase in comorbid illnesses

Less negative impact on recovery ?

Characteristics of the Diseases

Atypical signs and symptoms

Earlier definitive diagnosis ?

Acute presentation

Greater need to convert to open ?

FIGURE 25.5. Laparoscopic geriatric surgery.

A. Insufflation

Increased $PaCO_2$ (still wnl)

Increased CVP, PCWP, MAP

Increased SVR

Decreased Cardiac Index

Decreased Ejection Fraction

Suggests systolic ventricular dysfunction in the face of acute rise in afterload

B. Trendelenburg position

Increased $PaCO_2$ (still wnl)

Increased CVP, PCWP, MAP

Decreased SVR, Core temp

Increased Cardiac Index

Increased Ejection Fraction

Suggests increased preload facilitated ventricular function

C. Release of pneumoperitoneum

Slight decrease $PaCO_2$ (still wnl)

Decreased CVP, PCWP, MAP

Decreased SVR, Core temp

Increased heart rate

Increased Cardiac Index

Increased Ejection Fraction

Resultant hyperdynamic state

FIGURE 25.6. (A) Cardiovascular responses to pneumoperitoneum in older patients (Yale-VA CT). (B) Cardiovascular responses to pneumoperitoneum in older patients (Yale-VA CT). (C) Cardiovascular responses to release of pneumoperitoneum in older patients (Yale-VA CT). [From Harris, et al. Anesth Analg 1996.]

The importance of other physiological responses to laparoscopic surgery is also best understood when compared with the response in the open operative setting. Using cholecystectomy as the model, there is a clear increase in the hormonal and metabolic responses in both the laparoscopic and the open setting (Fig. 25.8).[9] The magnitude of the increase, however,

Effects of CO_2
Hypercarbia, increased $PaCO_2$
Acidosis
Effects of increased IAP
Increased airway pressures
Decreased pulmonary compliance
Increased work of breathing

FIGURE 25.7. Pulmonary response to pneumoperitoneum.

particularly of the catecholamine response, is significantly smaller with the laparoscopic approach. The inflammatory response, as measured by IL6, IL1β, TNF, C-Reactive protein (Fig. 25.9),[9,10] and the immune response (Fig. 25.10)[11] are also increased with both approaches, but significantly less so in the laparoscopic milieu.

The answer to the second question, "Does the laparoscopic approach lessen the impact of comorbid conditions," is more difficult because data correlating these conditions directly with outcome are not yet available. The answer, however, can be inferred from the fact that postoperative pain is less, time to ambulation is shorter, time to return to normal activity is shorter, and length of hospital stay is reduced. This rapid return to the preoperative level of function is perhaps the most important means of limiting postoperative complications, thereby limiting the impact of comorbidity.

The positive impact of the laparoscopic approach on postoperative outcome is well documented for cholecystectomy. In a comparison of the postoperative complications from laparoscopic versus open cholecystectomy, Fried and colleagues[12] demonstrated a substantial reduction in

TABLE 25.4. Postoperative pulmonary function: laparoscopic versus open cholecystectomy.

	% of preop	
	Lap	Open
FVC	79	49
FEV1	76	44
FEF max	76	38
MVV	78	48
TLC	92	78

Source: Schauer et al., Surgery, 1993.

Hormonal and metabolic responses

Cortisol	Same increase
ACTH	Same increase
Epinephrine	Smaller increase (24h)
Norepinephrine	Smaller increase (24,48h)
Glucose	Smaller increase (24h)
Albumin	Same decrease

FIGURE 25.8. Physiologic response: laparoscopic versus open cholecystectomy.

postoperative complications in patients over age 65 from 18 to 35% in open cases, to 12% in laparoscopic cases (Table 25.5). Feldman et al.[13] also demonstrated a decrease in operative mortality from 1.4% in open cases to 0.3–0.6% in closed cases. It must be noted, however, that mortality for patients under age 65 years treated laparoscopically in the series by Fried et al. was 0% compared with 0.6% in those over age 65. This is in large part attributable to the higher percentage of patients treated for acute disease in the older age group (30% vs. 17%). In a larger series of 21,000 open cholecystectomies in patients over age 65 from the prelaparoscopic era,[6] two thirds of patients required urgent or emergent surgery, with the operative mortality increasing from 1% electively to nearly 3% in the emergent setting. In addition, mortality rate correlated with the type of procedure performed. Thirty-day mortality for patients requiring common duct exploration was twice that of those undergoing simple cholecystectomy. Because the incidence of common duct stones rises with increasing age, additional intervention other than simple cholecystectomy will be required more frequently in the elderly population. The consequences of these additional

Inflammatory responses

Interleukin - 6	Smaller increase (2-48h)
C-reactive protein	Smaller increase (24,48h)
Interleukin - 1ß	Smaller increase (0-6h)
TNF	Smaller increase (24,72h)

FIGURE 25.9. Physiologic response: laparoscopic versus open cholecystectomy.

Other Immune responses

Mono superoxide	Smaller increase
PMN superoxide	Smaller increase
PMN chemotaxis	Smaller increase
WBC counts	Smaller increase

FIGURE 25.10. Physiologic response: laparoscopic versus open cholecystectomy.

procedures must also be considered when comparing the laparoscopic with the open approach.

The prevalence of acute disease in the elderly population will clearly influence the outcome of any procedure, whether laparoscopic or open. In addition, the ability to complete procedures laparoscopically will be affected by the amount of inflammation and by the distortion of anatomy found in complicated cases. Again, using cholecystectomy as the example, Fried et al.[14] documented the causes for conversion from laparoscopic to open procedure, and identified five factors that could be used to predict the need for conversion. Age greater than 65 years, male sex, obese, thickened gallbladder wall, and acute disease were all noted as predictors of conversion. In univariate analysis, patients with acute cholecystitis were nearly nine times more likely to need conversion than were those in whom acute cholecystitis was not present.

The answer to the final question, "Can the laparoscopic route also help rapidly establish a diagnosis in cases where the signs and symptoms of abdominal disease are atypical," is most promising. Diagnostic/therapeutic laparoscopy has been suggested for several abdominal conditions, and the list continues to grow. In one series from Belgium,[15] 255 patients with nontraumatic acute abdomen were initially evaluated laparoscopically. The correct diagnosis was established in 93% of the cases, and preoperative errors in diagnosis were corrected by laparoscopy in 20% of the cases.

TABLE 25.5. Laparoscopic versus open cholecystectomy in patients <65 and >65 years old.

Complications	Laparoscopic age < 65	Laparoscopic age > 65	Open age > 65
Total	5.2	11.6	18–35
Pneumonia	0	0.9	6–13
MI	0	0.6	2–3
Wound	1	3	5–20
Urinary	0.4	3.6	
Confusion	0	0.3	19

Source: Fried et al., 1994.

Others confirm both the diagnostic and the therapeutic efficacy of laparoscopy in this setting, with as many as 96% of patients being successfully diagnosed and treated laparoscopically for intraabdominal sepsis in one series.[16] Cases reports of successful treatment of less common, but difficult-to-diagnose problems specific to the elderly, have appeared. Occult SBO from gallstone ileus[17] and incarcerated obturator hernia[18] are just two examples.

In summary, the laparoscopic approach to major intraabdominal disease in the elderly patient, although still a significant stress, appears to be less of an operative stress than are the open procedures. With careful preloading and close monitoring of $PaCO_2$, hemodynamic consequences of pneumoperitoneum are well tolerated. Most measures of hormonal, metabolic, and immune responses appear to be comparable or less significant in the laparoscopic than they are in the open operation. The outcome for cholecystectomy, which is the most widely studied procedure to date, is better in terms of postoperative complications and deaths, although the prevalence acute disease may have a negative impact on this improvement. For other procedures, such as colectomy, data are being accumulated that suggests there is also an improvement in outcome in these areas.[19,20]

It is likely that the applications of laparoscopy to the treatment of surgical disease in the elderly will continue to grow over the next decade. Caution must be exercised, however, when applying these techniques in acute or complicated settings where a complication of the laparoscopic procedure may present more of a stress than would an uncomplicated open operation.

References

1. Day JC. Population projections of the United States by age, sex, race and Hispanic origin: 1993–2050, Current population reports: U.S. Department of Commerce Bureau of the Census, 1993;25–1104.
2. U.S. Department of Health and Human Services. Health data on older Americans: United States, 1992, Vital and Health Statistics Series 3, No. 27.
3. Peebles RJ, Schneidman DS, eds. Socio-economic factbook for surgery 1996, The American College of Surgeons, Chicago, 1996.
4. Graves EJ. 1993 summary: national hospital discharge survey, CDC Advanced Data 1995; No. 246.
5. Boyd BJ, et al. Operative risk factors of colon resection in the elderly. Ann Surg 1980;192:743.
6. Escarce JJ, et al. Outcomes of open cholecystectomy in the elderly: a longitudinal analysis of 21,000 cases in the pre-laparoscopic era. Surgery 1995;117:156.
7. Harris SN, et al. Alterations of cardiovascular performance during laparoscopic colectomy: a combined hemodynamic and echocardiographic analysis. Anesth Analg 1996;83:482.
8. Schauer PB, et al. Pulmonary function after laparoscopic cholecystectomy. Surgery 1993;114:389.

9. Glaser F, et al. General stress response to conventional and laparoscopic cholecystectomy. Ann Surg 1995;221:372.
10. Jakeways MSR, et al. Metabolic and inflammatory responses after open vs. laparoscopic cholecystectomy. Br J Surg 1994;81:127.
11. Richmond HP, et al. Immune function in patients undergoing open vs. laparoscopic cholecystectomy. Arch Surg 1994;129:1240.
12. Fried GM, Clas D, Meakins JL. Minimally invasive surgery in the elderly patient. Surg Clin N A 1994;74:375.
13. Feldman MG, et al. Comparison of mortality rates for open and closed cholecystectomy in the Elderly: Connecticut statewide survey. J Laparo Endosc Surg 1994;4:165.
14. Fried GM, et al. Factors determining conversion to laparotomy in patients undergoing laparoscopic cholecystectomy. Am J Surg 1994;167:35.
15. Navez B, et al. Laparoscopy for the management of non-traumatic acute abdomen. World J Surg 1995;19:382.
16. Geis WP, Kim HC. Use of laparoscopy in the diagnosis and treatment of patients with surgical abdominal sepsis. Surgery 1995;9:178.
17. Franklin ME, Dorman JP, Schuessler WW. Laparoscopic treatment of gallstone ileus: a case report and review of the literature. J Laparo Endosc Surg 1994;4:265.
18. Bryant TL, Umstot RK, Jr. Laparoscopic repair of an incarcerated obturator hernia. Surg Endosc 1996;10:437.
19. Begos DG, Arsenault J, Ballantyne GH. Laparoscopic colon and rectal surgery at a VA hospital. Analysis of the first 50 cases. Surg Endosc 1996;10:1050.
20. Peters WR, Fleshman JW. Minimally invasive colectomy in elderly patients. Surg Laparosc Endosc 1995;5:477.

26
Minimally Invasive Surgery in Breast Pathology

E.A. Leandros, G.D. Kymionis, and M.M. Konstadoulakis

Carcinoma of the breast is one of the most common malignant neoplasms in women in the United States (Table 26.1). It is estimated that one out of every nine women will develop breast cancer in her lifetime. The incidence of breast cancer has been rising steadily over the past decade. It is exceeded only by lung cancer today as a cause of cancer death in women. In the 1990s, more than 1.5 million women will be diagnosed as having breast cancer, and nearly 30% of these women will finally die from this disease.

The increased number of breast cancer cases may be due to the widespread use of screening mammography. Many new patients are now diagnosed with breast tumors less than 2cm. In 1982, approximately 12,000 women were diagnosed as having tumors less than 2cm in diameter and negative axillary lymph nodes. This number had risen to 32,000 by 1986. In 1996, about 180,000 women were diagnosed with breast cancer in the United States (approximately one every 3 minutes). Twenty percent of breast cancers will be diagnosed between screenings,[1] and among those in which biopsy is performed, 34% will be cancer.[2] Benign lesions have some mammographic features that may mimic malignant lesions, and certain malignant lesions have mammographic features that mimic benign lesions.

Today, we are witnessing a revolution in minimally invasive surgical techniques. Laparoscopic cholecystectomy is now the preferred method for the removal of the gallbladder, whereas other abdominal and thoracic laparoscopic operations have also gained significant ground the last couple of years. For breast pathology, minimally invasive surgery has been used primarily in the diagnosis of nonpalpable breast lesions. Laparoscopic axillary dissection has been tried, and stereotactic removal of breast lesions less than 2cm is being done with increased frequency.[3-6]

Evaluation of Breast Lesions

Evaluation of breast lesions involves a lot of effort and has a high cost. Before the late 1980s, definitive tissue diagnosis for nonpalpable breast lesions required a mammographically guided localization procedure (with a

TABLE 26.1. Annual incidence of breast cancer by age.

Age range (years)	Mean no. of cases per 100,000 women
40–44	129.4
45–49	159.4
50–54	220.4
55–59	261.6
60–64	330.7
65–69	390.7
70–74	421.8
75–79	461.4
80–84	451.3

wire device or visible dye) followed by an open surgical biopsy. This method has many drawbacks. Surgical biopsies can be disfiguring and have an error rate from 0.2% to 22%.[7–10] Surgical biopsies also carry a small mortality risk (from anesthesia) and a moderate morbidity rate due to infection, wound healing problems, and fracture or migration of the localizing wire. In addition, considerable bleeding may occur during a surgical biopsy that obscures the operative field and precludes confident excision of deep lesions.[11] If the wire inadvertently dislodges, migrates, or is transected, then the surgeon can also become disorientated and excise the wrong tissue.[8,12] Furthermore, lack of communication between the radiologist, who has placed the localizing wire, and the surgeon can result in a surgical miss.[10] Postoperative hematoma, cellulitis, and poor cosmesis may also occur. Surgical biopsies are therefore generally time-consuming, potentially nerve racking, and require a great deal of resources.[13] The delays frequently encountered impose a psychological stress on the patient awaiting the procedure. Combining the time spent in radiology and then in the operating room, the needle localization and surgical excisional biopsy may require up to 3 hours. In terms of cost, this method is rather expensive considering the direct cost to the patient, and the indirect cost to society from the patient being away form work due to the surgical biopsy. In the United States alone it is estimated that open surgical breast biopsies are performed on 500,000 to 1 million women annually. Approximately 40–50% of these are for nonpalpable lesions. If one assumes 750,000 open surgical biopsies per year with a biopsy cost of $3,000 per biopsy, then the current cost of surgical breast biopsy only in the United States can be estimated close to $2.3 billion. Finally, it is important to remember that surgical excisional biopsy is not 100% accurate and that the reported lesion miss rate ranges from 0.2% to 20%.[14–20]

Stereotactic Core Needle Breast Biopsy

A different approach toward breast biopsy was born when Parker performed the first stereotactic core breast biopsy in 1988. This method introduced the minimally invasive surgical technique in breast pathology and

TABLE 26.2. Average costs of procedures.

Procedure	Average cost ($)
Mammography	84
Fine-needle aspiration biopsy	150
Needle core biopsy for nonpalpable lesion	850
Excitional biopsy	
nonpalpable lesion	2,800 (4, 22)
palpable lesion	2,400

promises to have a similar impact on the management of breast disease as laparoscopy has had on gallbladder disease.

The cancer miss rate of stereotactic core needle breast biopsies (SCNBB) is reported to be 1.2% (15 of 1,197 lesions) based on multiinstitutional series.[21] Stereotactic large-core breast biopsy also offers substantial advantages over surgical biopsy. The cost of SCNBB is 25–50% lower than surgical biopsy (Table 26.2).[4] The procedure can be scheduled promptly, even on the same day just after the mammogram, and lasts 20–30 minutes. The complication rate is negligible, and no disfiguring cosmetic results or pain have been reported. Core biopsy is well tolerated, and because it can be performed under local anesthesia the patient does not lose additional time by staying away from work. SCNBB obtains multiple needle localizations and may therefore be used to define the extent of malignancies, especially for patients with multicentiric or multifocal disease. Furthermore, a definitive diagnosis instead of equivocal mammographic findings eliminates the need for serial *46* month follow-up mammograms.[22,23] The anxiety among patients waiting for mammographically guided needle core biopsy is therefore reduced. In addition, when therapeutic breast surgery follows SCNBB, no cavity is present. On the other hand, when therapeutic breast surgery follows a diagnostic open surgical breast biopsy, the surgeon has to enter a recent surgical cavity containing hematoma and edema.

Technique of Sterotactic Core Needle Breast Biopsy (SCNBB)

An SCNBB begins with a two-view mammogram that demonstrates at least one lesion suspicious for malignancy.

The biopsy is performed using a dedicated prone biopsy table. The patient is placed in the prone position, and the lesion is identified using digital mammography. The breast is cleansed and prepared using povidone–iodine solution. The predetermined point of biopsy is marked on the stereo imaging using two small (5 cm × 5 cm) partial mammograms at −15-degree and at +15-degree angles. The two stereo images are exposed adjacent to each other on the same film. Computer-generated coordinates derived from the stereo images are dialed into the stereotactic unit. Local anesthetic is infiltrated into the skin and subcutaneous tissue. A small incision (2 mm) is made in the skin, and a 14-gauge needle in an automated longthrow biopsy gun is placed in the incision. The 14-gauge needles most consistently provide the highest quality intact cores because the breast frequently consists of extraordinarily friable and fatty tissue. Use of fine-needle aspiration or small cores (18-gauges) offers poor ability to make definitive benign diagnoses and distinguish between in situ and invasive carcinoma due to the insufficient tissue obtained. On the other hand, large cores (14-gauges) that allow one to obtain at least 70 mg of tissue are more accurate, permitting definitive diagnoses and complete characterization of malignant lesions. It is better to use a biopsy gun with a 14-gauge needle inside rather than the conventional 14-gauge needle because of the ease of the use of the gun. The use of the gun decreases patients' discomfort and increases specimen quality and integrity due to the split-second sampling and the ability of the gun to pierce both hard and mobile breast lesions before they have chance to move out of the path of the needle. The needle is positioned according to the coordinates, and prefire stereo pair images are obtained to document that the long axis of the needle is directed to the intended portion of the targeted breast lesion. The gun is fired and a final set of stereo views ensures that the needle has traversed the lesion. The needle is removed and the core tissue obtained is placed in formalin. Three to four passes are made through the lesion, to canvass it anteriorly to posteriorly in measured increments from the center of the lesion. All biopsy passes traverse the same skin entrance site. Digital stereo pair images are obtained after the first and last biopsy to confirm that the lesion has been traversed.

A typical procedure needs 35 to 45 minutes, although the actual biopsy procedure time is shorter. Hemostasis is achieved with manual compression. The pathology is reviewed the next day . If the lesion is probably benign (American College of Radiology, ACR: category 2) or benign (ACR: category 3), then the patient is placed into a computer-controlled mammographic follow-up program. If the lesion is premalignant or malignant, then the lesion is surgically removed. When the lesion contains microcalcification, a magnified radiograph of the core specimens is obtained to verify that calcifications proportional to the target calcifications have been obtained. The procedure is not complete until the core specimen contains calcifications that are proportional to the calcifications seen on the diagnostic mammogram (Fig. 26.1).

SCNBB is now performed on approximately 200,000–300,000 lesions per year in the United States. The theoretical accuracy of SCNBB is almost 1 mm. Its accuracy depends on many factors, such as breast or lesion movement and the experience of the surgeon who obtained the biopsy. An additional problem of SCNBB is that with standard mammography lesions close to the chest wall are not suitable for this method. These lesions can be pulled into the aperture of the compression plate and therefore

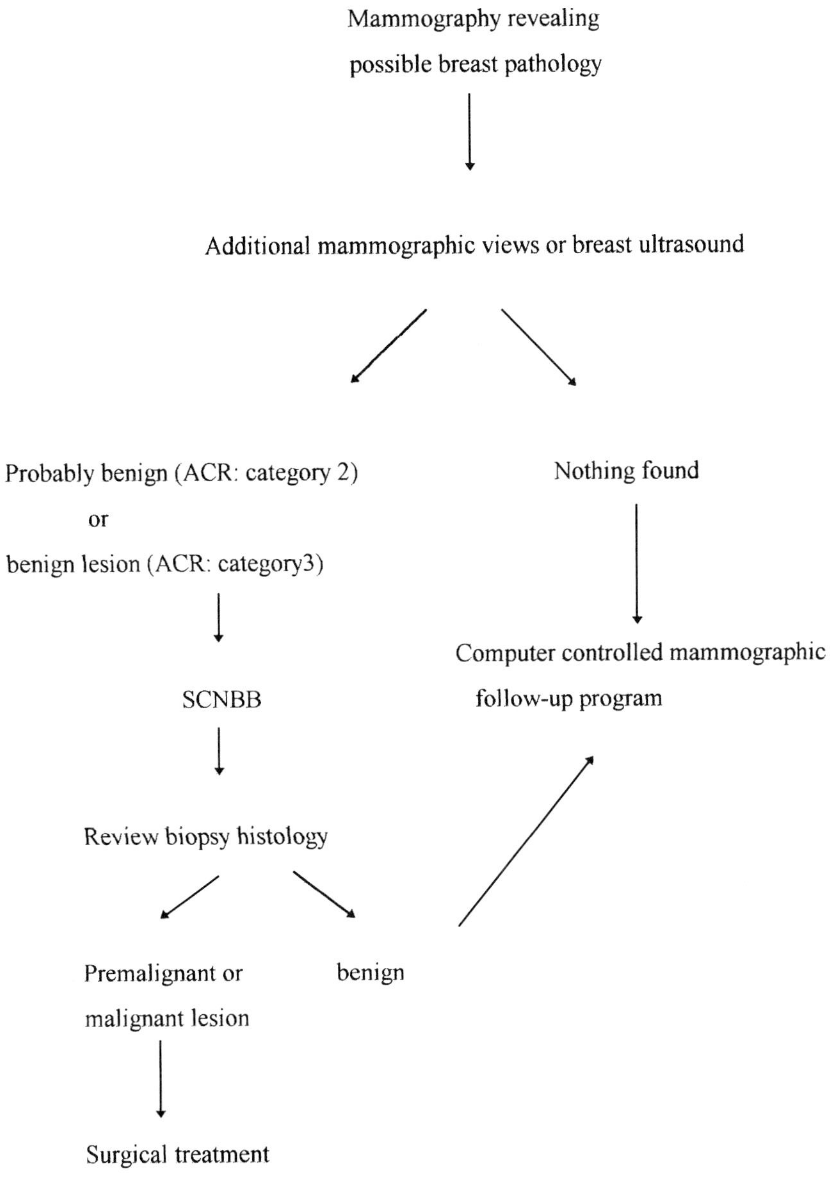

Mammography revealing

possible breast pathology

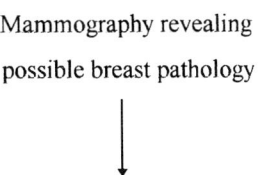

Additional mammographic views or breast ultrasound

Probably benign (ACR: category 2)

or

benign lesion (ACR: category3)

SCNBB

Nothing found

Computer controlled mammographic

follow-up program

Review biopsy histology

Premalignant or   benign

malignant lesion

Surgical treatment

FIGURE 26.1. Management of incomplete mammography finding using SCNBB.

appear to be accessible to biopsy. The tension created in the tracted breast, however, may cause the breast to retract slowly toward the chest wall, rendering the sterotactic calculations inaccurate. If the patient's arm and shoulder go through the aperture in the biopsy table, however, then the chest wall and breast can be placed directly on the image receptor of the stereostatic guidance system and the lesions will be included in the image.

Future Prospects

Due to the advent of efficient screening programs, more and more indeterminate lesions of the breast are found. A large number (40%) of breast cancers discovered today have a 20-mm or less median size range (minimally invasive breast cancers).[24] In parallel, an additional factor that contributes to the increase of the incidence of early breast cancer detection is the development of molecular biology, especially with BRCA 1 gene mutations analyses, which are found to be mutated in families with early-onset breast cancer.[25-30] The preceding data suggest that there is great need to extend the indications of minimally invasive surgical techniques in both the diagnosis of nonpalpable breast cancers and also in the treatment of small (20 mm or less) lesions.

During the last 100 years, the primary treatment of breast cancer has shifted from radical mastectomy to modified radical mastectomy to local excision (lumpectomy) with axillary lymphadenectomy. It seems logical, therefore, to extend the local treatment of breast cancer to minimally invasive surgery. Last year, new systems [e.g., Advanced Breast Biopsy Instrumentation (ABBI) system] which combine stereotactic X-ray imaging (a three-dimensional locating process that pinpoints a lesion to within 1 mm of accuracy) with a cannula containing a knife (2 cm) and a needle/wire marker assembly were produced. These techniques have the advantage that they combine larger biopsies with digitalized stereotactic mammography, thereby allowing the removal of the entire lesion, for smaller lesions, and permitting a significant margin around the specimen. If the specimen proves to be cancerous, but pathology reports that the entire margin is clear, then it is up to the clinical judgment of the surgeon whether additional tissue should be removed or if the procedure can be considered complete.

This is the first step for developing minimally invasive treatment procedures for small breast cancers. With large probes, a wider range of excisional biopsy with microscopically clear margins is possible. Initial pilot analyses show that continuous wave Nd:YAG laser hyperthermia, cryotherapy, and electrocautery appear to be promising methods for treating small, well-defined breast cancers with a minimally invasive surgical procedure.

With the progress of molecular biology, we will be able to detect a large number (today 6–10% of all breast cancers) of patients at high risk for developing breast cancer. These patients need to be enrolled in an intense life-long follow-up program. In this group of patients, the majority of the lesions discovered are going to be less than 1 cm, providing the need for a surgical system able to remove nonpalpable breast cancers with adequate margins, minimal deformation, good cosmetic effect, and maximum accuracy. The development of minimally invasive breast cancer equipment is crucial to meet the medical demands for breast surgery in the year 2000.

References

1. Baker LH. Breast cancer detection demonstration project: five-year summary report. CA Cancer J Clin 1982;32:194–225.
2. Bassett LW, Liut TH, Giuliano AE, et al. The prevalence of carcinoma in palpable vs impalpable, mammographically detected lesions. AJR 1991;157:21–24.
3. Lovin DJ, Parker SH, Leuthke JM, et al. Stereotactic percutaneous breast core biopsy technical adaptation and initial experience. Breast Dis 1990;3:135–143.
4. Parker SH, Lovin JD, Jobe WE, et al. Stereotactic breast biopsy with a gun. Radiology 1990;176:741–747.
5. Parker SH, Lovin JD, Jobe WE, et al. Nonpalpable breast lesions: stereotactic automated large-core biopsies. Radiology 1991;180:403–407.
6. Parker SH, Burbank F, Jackman R, et al. Percutaneous large core breast biopsy: a multiinstitutional study. Radiology 1994;193:359–364.
7. Kopans DB. Review of stereotaxic large-core needle biopsy results in nonpalpable breast lesions. Radiology 1993;189:665–666.
8. Landercasper J, Gundersen SB, Gundersen AL, et al. Needle localization and biopsy of nonpalpable lesions of the breast. Surg Gynecol Obstet 1987;164:399–403.
9. Norton LW, Pearlman NW. Needle localization breast biopsy: accuracy versus cost. Am J Surg 1988;156:13B–15B.
10. Yankaskas BC, Knelson MH, Abernethy ML, et al. Needle localization biopsy of occult lesions of the breast. Experience in 199 cases. Invest Radiol 1988;23:729–733.
11. Norton LW, Zeligman BE, Pearlman NW. Accuracy and cost of needle localization breast biopsy. Arch Surg 1988;123:947–950.
12. Davis PS, Wechsler RJ, Feig SA, et al. Migration of breast biopsy localization wire. AJR 1988;150:787–788.
13. Hall F. Screening mammography: potential problems on the horizon. N Engl J Med 1986;314:53–55.
14. Rissanen TJ, Makaranin HP, Matilla SI, et al. Wire localized biopsy of breast lesions: a review of 425 cases found in screening or clinical mammography. Clin Radiol 1993;47:14–22.
15. Hall FM, Storella JM, Silverstone DZ, et al. Nonpalpable breast lesions: recommendations for biopsy based on suspicion of carcinoma at mammography. Radiology 1988;167:353–358.
16. Homer MJ, Smith TJ, Safaii H. Prebiopsy needle localization: methods, problems and expected results. Radiol Clin North Am 1992;30:139–153.
17. Homer MJ. Nonpalpable breast microcalcifications: frequency, management and results of incisional biopsy. Radiology 1992;185:411–413.
18. Stein MA, Karlan M. Immediate postoperative mammogram for failed surgical excision of breast lesions. Radiology 1991;178:159–162.

19. Gallagher WJ, Cardenosa G, Rubens JR, et al. Minimal-volume excision of nonpalpable breast lesions. AJR 1989;153:957–961.
20. Hasselgren P, Hummel RP, Georgian-Smith O, et al. Breast biopsy with needle localization: accuracy of specimen x-ray and management of missed lesions. Surgery 1993;114:836–842.
21. Rosenblatt R, Fineberg SA, Sparano JA. Stereotactic core needle biopsy of multiple sites in the breast: efficacy and effect on patient care. Radiology 1996;201:67–70.
22. Schmidt R, Morrow M, Bibbo M, et al. Benefits of stereotactic aspiration cytology. Admin Rad, October 1990;35–42.
23. Jackson VP, Bassett LW. Stereotactic fine-needle aspiration biopsy for nonpalpable breast lesions. AJR 1990;154:1196–1197.
24. Curpen BN, Sickles EA, Solitto RA, et al. The comparative value of mammographic screening for women 40–49 years old versus women 50–59 years old. AJR 1995;164:1099–1103.
25. Hall JM, Friedman L, Guenther C, et al. Closing in on a breast cancer gene on chromosome 17q21. Science 1992;250:1684–1689.
26. Narod SA, Feunteum M, Lynch HT, et al. Familial breast-ovarian cancer locus on chromosome 17q12–23. Lancet 1991;338:82–83.
27. Narod SA, Ford D, the Breast Cancer Linkage Consortium. An evaluation of genetic heterogeneity in 145 breast-ovarian cancer families. Am J Hum Genet 1995;56:254–264.
28. Miki Y, Swensen J, Shattuck-Eidens D, et al. A strong candidate for the breast and ovarian cancer susceptibility gene BRCA1. Science 1994;266:66–71.
29. Smith SA, Easton DF, Evans DGR, et al. Allele losses in the region 17q12–21 in familial breast and ovarian cancer involve the wild-type chromosome. Nat Genet 1992;2:128–131.
30. Futreal PA, Liu Q, Shattuck-Eidens D, et al. BRCA1 mutations in primary breast and ovarian carcinomas. Science 1994,266:120–122.

27
Ethical Problems Posed by Laparoscopic Surgery

RONALD C. MERRELL

Ethics may be defined as a process for identifying, by consensus, the right course of action in a setting of uncertainty or ambivalence. When the right action is immediately obvious to almost anyone within a common value system, nothing is moot. Values guide us, and there is no need for ethical dialogue. The course of action indicated by a thoroughly ethical process may subsequently prove wrong. Error is not unethical. It is unethical to avoid dialogue when prevailing values fail to guide us.

Why would an ethical process be called for in laparoscopic surgery? Every new technology has critics who sincerely believe traditional values have been abandoned. Others disagree, and an ethical dialogue ensues. Laparoscopy is especially prone to ethical concerns because the technique is most often proposed as an alternative to established and effective therapy: cholecystectomy, herniorrhaphy, and so on. Laparoscopic techniques do not promise a cure for hopeless conditions. Departure from the tried and true to the untried and speculative requires an ethical dialogue. Laparoscopy per se does not challenge prevailing values of patients or physicians, as does technology associated with reproduction, or prolongation of life. There are enough features of concern in laparoscopy, however, to fuel debate until the technology is more thoroughly integrated into health care.

There are five areas of general or specific ethical concern that are apparent. First, laparoscopic surgery is a matter of research, which involves recruitment of subjects who agree to participate in unproven therapy. Research must be considered by a review panel that debates risk to the individual, likelihood the experiment will produce valid scientific results, societal good, and, indeed, bioethics. In other words, Is this experiment a proper action in the ethical context? A group consideration protects research subjects, scientific integrity, and the investigator. Vast profits have been made to provide the surgeon with laparoscopic products. Protecting the patient and investigator from conflict with commerce entails an ethical debate during research activities.

Second, the application of new technology to patient care assuring reasonable safeguards regarding the competence of the surgeon. This can be regulated through credentials and is not necessarily an ethical issue; however, full confidence in an individual or a system means some element of uncertainty at the outset. Bioethical dialogue must be part of that assurance to the public and among surgeons. Ethical debate during the monitoring of quality is also needed. For example, what does one do if there is a disastrous result in the tenth case of the experience for a given surgeon as opposed to the five-hundredth? Does a surgeon tell his or her precise quantitative and qualitative experience? What is an anecdote? What is a trend? What is acceptable? How does an institution justify an increased error rate for a new practitioner as opposed to one more experienced? Competence and quality, so obvious on the surface, are thoroughly ambivalent when technology is new.

Third, an institution or society must debate any departure from the standard of care. Innovation may be better, *res ipsa loquitur*, but that is rare and is subject to ethical debate even then. There are at least four steps to satisfy bioethics for an institution or individual surgeon to embrace an innovation. First, there must be a clear understanding of the standard of care, generally and locally. Second, the institution must be thoroughly conversant with the innovation as applied elsewhere. Third, the institution must be fully prepared to support the innovation with the equipment, training, and credentials. Finally, the institution must be prepared for a rigorous program of quality improvement to compare the innovation with the previous standard. These steps are *not* redundant to research; rather, they are necessary for any major new application within an institution.

Next, let us consider informal consent as a bioethical matter in laparoscopic surgery. At a minimum, a description of the old standard plus personal and general experience with the new approach should be added to the general terms of information. The areas of uncertainty include long-term outcome, ability of patients to comprehend complex clinical issues in order to render consent, enthusiasm of the surgeon for a new approach, or the unreasonable enthusiasm of the patient seeking a new therapy, which may be inappropriate. The latter issue has been especially troublesome in laparoscopic herniorrhaphy.

Finally, societal good is profoundly moot with regard to laparoscopic surgery. If medical expenditure is fixed in a hospital or a health system and a new, expensive technology is proposed, must some forms of care be abandoned? Can the budget expand for start up? Where in a priority rank does one put laparoscopy? What happens when a manufacturer or distributor offers inducements to the surgeon or hospital at the expense of patients? If a new technology is notably expensive, is access restricted to individuals with money or potential clout? Is the technology restricted to countries, communities or subjects on the basis of wealth? That hardly sounds comfortable. Laparoscopic surgery is actually a financial boon to the general society by rapidly returning patients to productive life. Laparoscopic surgery is advantageous for those who otherwise have acceptable surgical risks. Ethical debate is needed, however, in the ways actual education costs are compartmentalized and in the way economics are compartmentalized and in the way money is allocated.

Has laparoscopic surgery had any real problem with regard to bioethics? The answer is an emphatic, *yes*. Laparoscopic surgery in general surgery came about as an extension of laparoscopic gynecology. There was no clinical research phase of any serious dimensions. Surgery moved from case report to general application with great velocity and little reflection. On the matter of competence, surgeons were given credentials after a weekend course and began new procedures without appropriate backup. Institutions launched laparoscopic programs based on the aid of manufacturers' representatives rather than a committed infrastructure. Informal consent was eclipsed by market hyperbole and poor information on the part of patients and surgeons alike. Finally, laparoscopic surgery has come to define the difference between having and not having, privilege and its lack among nations and within many of them.

The reasons for this failure of bioethics in laparoscopic surgery are many, and some are not particularly palatable. The main problem, however, was time. For many patients and surgeons the benefits were so obvious that the plodding pace of a randomized control trial seemed itself unethical. Laparoscopic cholecystectomy was introduced at a time when length of stay was becoming the major focus of early managed care in the United States. Any tactic that could reduce hospital stay by many days *had* to be good. Competence problems could be excused by the sense of urgency to make laparoscopic surgery available generally, practiced by many surgeons, at the earliest date. On the other hand, competition among surgeons and hospitals almost certainly played a role. Many institutions were very poorly prepared for laparoscopic surgery, and some continue to have little depth for training, technical support, and quality programs. Informed consent was extremely different in the early series because of the enthusiasm of surgeons and patients, along with a dearth of data. The matter of societal good was rarely addressed in a coherent ethical dialogue at the outset. Treatment was initially restricted severely by finance because of startup costs.

Cholecystectomy electrified general surgery and inflamed the expectations of our patients. Have time and process caught up in the succeeding 10 years? Has laparoscopic surgery lost its special features, which set it apart from the bioethical concerns of more traditional general surgery? Perhaps standards for credentials and quality improvement are now in place in most institutions. There are many more scientific reports to support institutional and personal decisions of surgeons and patients. The initial costs have been paid and laparoscopic technology has been thoroughly incorporated into the infrastructure of most hospitals. There is still a great need for clinical research. There is a great need to regularize the education of new surgeons to include competence in laparoscopy. There is still a rapid growth of new applications and new instruments. Furthermore, there is a growing disparity in the availability of advanced laparoscopic procedures in centers of excellence as opposed to general hospitals.

Bioethical debate and process are adequately applied now to most areas of laparoscopic surgery. The debate now is more orderly, timely, and effective, and results in expansion of our medical value system to include laparoscopic surgery. It is not accurate to say, however, that our bioethical practices have completely caught up with the many issues of laparoscopic surgery. Progress in laparoscopic surgery has slowed to permit bioethical process to keep apace. The introduction of laparoscopic surgery to general surgery has been almost entirely salutary with benefit to patient, surgeon, institution, and society. New technology, however, cannot be assumed to be the perpetual friend of medicine, the ally of surgery, or the long-sought solace of patients. We must remember the first decade of laparoscopic general surgery as a time when technology slipped the bonds of even ethics and sailed a turbulent uncharted course. The basic values of surgeons and society were never lost completely. We should, however, take our lessons from this time. We should wish ardently and often for such a sweeping freshness in the wonder of technology; however, we are well advised to put in place a better bioethical map to accompany us on the voyage.

Index